RICHARD YOKLEY   ROZANE SUTHERLAND

EMERGENCY!
Behind the Scene

JONES AND BARTLETT PUBLISHERS
Sudbury, Massachusetts

BOSTON   TORONTO   LONDON   SINGAPORE

World Headquarters

Jones and Bartlett Publishers
40 Tall Pine Drive
Sudbury, MA 01776
978-443-5000
info@jbpub.com
www.jbpub.com

Jones and Bartlett Publishers
Canada
6339 Ormindale Way
Mississauga, Ontario L5V 1J2
Canada

Jones and Bartlett Publishers
International
Barb House, Barb Mews
London W6 7PA
United Kingdom

Jones and Bartlett's books and products are available through most bookstores and online booksellers. To contact Jones and Bartlett Publishers directly, call 800-832-0034, fax 978-443-8000, or visit our website www.jbpub.com.

Substantial discounts on bulk quantities of Jones and Bartlett's publications are available to corporations, professional associations, and other qualified organizations. For details and specific discount information, contact the special sales department at Jones and Bartlett via the above contact information or send an email to specialsales@jbpub.com.

Production Credits

Chief Executive Officer: Clayton Jones
Chief Operating Officer: Don W. Jones, Jr.
President, Higher Education and Professional Publishing: Robert W. Holland, Jr.
V.P., Sales and Marketing: William J. Kane
V.P., Design and Production: Anne Spencer
V.P., Manufacturing and Inventory Control: Therese Connell
Publisher—Public Safety Group: Kimberly Brophy
Acquisitions Editor—EMS: Christine Emerton
Associate Managing Editor: Robyn Schafer
Production Supervisor: Jenny L. Corriveau
Associate Production Editor: Jamie Chase
Director of Marketing: Alisha Weisman
Composition: PawPrint Media, Inc.
Cover Design: Anne Spencer
Interior Design: Anne Spencer
Associate Photo Researcher and Photographer: Christine McKeen
Cover Image: Courtesy of County of Los Angeles Fire Museum Association, Joe Woyjeck, photographer
Printing and Binding: Malloy, Inc.
Cover Printing: Malloy, Inc.

Copyright © 2008 by Jones and Bartlett Publishers,LLC

Library of Congress Cataloging-in-Publication Data

Yokley, Richard C.
  Emergency! : behind the scene / Richard Yokley and Rozane Sutherland.
    p. cm.
  Includes bibliographical references.
  ISBN-13: 978-0-7637-4896-8
  ISBN-10: 0-7637-4896-X
  1. *Emergency!* (Television program) I. Sutherland, Rozane. II. Title.
  PN1992.77.E44Y65 2008
  791.45'72—dc22
                          2007017416

6048

Printed in the United States of America
12 11 10 09 08 10 9 8 7 6 5 4 3

EMERGENCY! *Behind the Scene*

Contents

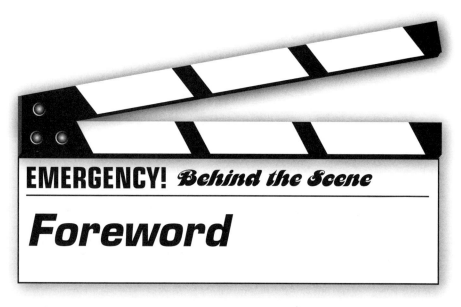

EMERGENCY! *Behind the Scene*

Foreword

You have just selected this book—but before you scan any further let me make a few judgments about you. I hope you won't mind. You probably either are or were:

- A firefighter or plan to be one, whether with a major metropolitan department or one of the thousands of smaller paid or volunteer companies that serve and protect our nation's communities.
- A member of a search and rescue team.
- A paramedic or EMT.
- A medical professional (for example, nurse, MD, pharmacist).
- One of the many "fire buffs" who support the activities of professional firefighters.

No matter which of these categories fits you, you probably learned the names of (and felt you personally knew) the cast of *Emergency!*: firefighter/paramedics Johnny Gage and Roy DeSoto; Drs. Kelly Brackett, Joe Early, and Mike Morton; nurse Dixie McCall; and the four-man crew of Los Angeles County Engine 51—Captain Hank Stanley, Engineer Mike Stoker, and firefighters Marco López, and Chet Kelly. You can probably hum the show's theme music in your sleep.

Was this show depicting something really occurring in Television Land? Or was it just showbiz? Was this when your career seed was planted?

Many paramedic programs or other emergency medical response programs were popping up throughout the United States starting in the mid 1960s, but it took this Saturday night TV show to educate the public that such activities were under way. *Emergency!* first aired on the NBC Television Network on January 15, 1972. For nearly an hour every week, millions of viewers watched this "reality" television program. Each episode was either taken from a real incident or simulation in which writers asked real fire-fighters to respond to incidents they created. A firefighter or paramedic served as a technical advisor for every show and at every filming location.

Emergency! ran for five and a half seasons, spawned six follow-up movies, and ran in syndication intermittently for several years. In many ways, *Emergency!* made history. The public demanded paramedics in their own cities and towns. Firefighters were cross-trained as emergency medical technicians (EMTs). The medical profession branched out, training true emergency room physicians and nurses for the first time. As a member of one of the categories listed earlier, you are a part of that history.

For its role in expanding the nation's EMS programs, *Emergency!* was ushered into the Smithsonian Institution's Museum of American History in Washington, D.C., on May 16, 2000. At a special ceremony in the museum's Presidential Suite, actor Randolph Mantooth signed over both his and Kevin Tighe's turn-out coats and helmets to be part of our nation's treasures. Much of the original paramedic equipment carried by Squad 51—including the first paramedic training manuals—were also deposited in the museum.

In his speech, Mantooth quipped that, "I am not so sure I like the word 'museum' used in close conjunction to my name, but what an honor for all of us who have participated in developing and building a concept that has saved countless lives. I am only a spokesman; it is those in the stations and in the field and hospitals that deserve the honors."

This book will bring back some memories and let you in on how *Emergency!* came about. As you read the words, put yourself in them. Take a moment to think back and ask yourself, "When was it that I was led into this career that I proudly follow today?"

— Richard A. Friend
Public Information Officer
Los Angeles County Fire Department (1967–1975 and 1979–1984)
Liaison to Universal Studios during the first four seasons of Emergency!

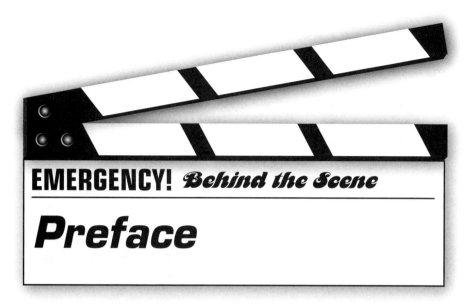

EMERGENCY! *Behind the Scene*

Preface

In 1928, NBC teamed up with RCA to operate the country's first television station—W2XBS in New York. A few years later, they produced the first on-air broadcast. Seven years later, the first mobile television vans (which were the size of buses) hit the streets of New York. On November 15, 1938, W2XBT (the mobile unit) broadcast the first on-scene, live disaster in the United States—a fire burning in a two-story building on Wards Island in New York. The NBC crew had been filming at a swimming pool in Queens when they spotted the fire and quickly turned their cameras to the fireboat and rescue.

The next year, the first regularly scheduled television operation began. W2XBS transformed into WNBT, which became WNBC-TV, now Channel 4. From these humble beginnings, television evolved as we know it today.

While this book is about the TV program *Emergency!*, it would not be complete without discussing the startup of the paramedic program within Los Angeles County, which includes the LA County Fire Department (LACoFD), the Los Angeles City Fire Department (LAFD), and several other fire departments and hospitals. It contains an extensive episode guide including title, filming date, air date, guest stars, writers, producers, directors, and a brief synopsis of each of *Emergency!*'s 124 episodes and six movies along with filming locations.

Although the word "city" has been officially eliminated from the LAFD, it will be used throughout the course of this book in order to make it clear when referencing the difference between LA County and the LA City Fire Departments. It is believed that the word "City" was added to the department's name more than 80 years ago with the formation of the LA County Fire Department. Brian Humphrey, LAFD public safety officer (PSO) states, "Fire buffs and journalists, including the Los Angeles Times, began referring to us in 1924 as the Los Angeles City Fire Department, so as to differentiate our agency from the newly founded Los Angeles County Fire Department." Humphrey added, "The addition of the word 'City' on LAFD apparatus graphics seems to appear first in the 1960s, especially on the ubiquitous Crown Firecoach fire apparatus."

On earlier apparatus, "city" was most likely applied when the vehicle went in for service, because archival photos of 1950s-era apparatus taken in the 1970s have the livery of "Los Angeles City Fire Department." "City" appears in both italicized and block lettering in the same font, sometimes slightly larger than the rest of the lettering on the engines. There are still several pieces of apparatus with "city" on the doors and ladder booms, including the helicopters, but the word was in the process of being elimi- nated from the new apparatus lettering orders as early as the year 2000. The department's turn-outs and work T-shirts still have the word "city" on them.

It is said that after Mayor James Hahn's successful campaign against the San Fernando Valley and Hollywood secession in 2002, the word "city" was removed at the request of the mayor to keep from alienating the Valley from the City of Los Angeles. However, Humphrey states that, "The endeavor to remove the word 'city' can actually be traced to a written order from Fire Chief Bill Bamattre mere days after he was named the 14th Chief Engineer of the Department on April 23, 1996. By his direction, we were no longer to refer to ourselves formally as anything but the Los Angeles Fire Depart- ment, and his title was simplified to that of Fire Chief."

> **Dr. Kelly Brackett:** "Squad 51, this is Rampart. Can you send us some EKG?"
>
> **John Gage:** "Ten-four, we're transmitting EKG. We're sending you a strip; vitals to follow. Pulse is 160; the victim is in extreme pain, Rampart. Patient is in V-fib. Rampart, we have lost the victim's pulse, beginning CPR. We're defibrillating victim, Rampart. Rampart, we have defibrillated victim, he has sinus rhythm."
>
> **Dr. Joe Early:** "Administer two-amp sodium bicarb, insert an airway. Start an IV, 51. Lactate Ringers."
>
> **Nurse Dixie McCall:** "Squad 51, continue to monitor patient and transport immediately."
>
> **John Gage:** "We're on our way, Rampart."

With this beginning, *Emergency!* took off. The audience was treated to an hour of entertainment unlike anything the nation had seen before. Before *Emergency!*, many of the viewers had never even heard of the word "paramedic."

This show dramatically changed the course of emergency medical response in the United States. Undoubtedly, it was the single most important factor in informing the public about the advancements being made in Emergency Medical Services (EMS) nationwide at that time. Five years before *Emergency!* aired, the first "fire department paramedics" hit the streets of Miami.

"The dramatic series *Emergency!* was responsible for spreading the word to the four corners of the United States, creating the almost instant demand for the services viewed on the family TV set," states Dr. Eugene Nagel, a noted cardiologist responsible for developing the paramedic program in Miami. He further states, "I can't think of anything that advanced emergency medicine in this country more than this program did." By February 1974, midway through *Emergency!*'s third season, Los Angeles County had 51 operational squads staffed by 406 certified paramedics, and more than 15 states had adopted the Los Angeles County paramedic training program.

No firefighter, EMS, or rescue program before or after has had the impact or sustained longevity of *Emergency!*. Like Jack Webb's earlier police drama, *Adam-12* (1968–1975), which changed the way America perceived its police officers, so *Emergency!* changed the course of firefighter/paramedic programs all across the United States. Although few television series at the time were syndicated while still scheduled as prime-time network shows, *Emergency!* went into syndication in various U.S. markets, even worldwide, as *Emergency One!* while it was in its sixth year on NBC. It was resurrected for a short time on cable's TV Land (1999–2001) and is still shown in some U.S., Canadian, and Australian markets, where a whole new generation can watch the exploits of LA County Station 51.

Yes, *Emergency!* had, and in some cases still has, its detractors, but they are few. Some felt that it glamorized rescue while demeaning ambulance companies to a back-seat role in EMS. Others say that many of the calls the fictional paramedics responded on were basic life support (BLS) that should have been handled by the ambulance companies. Of course, back in the early 1970s, there wasn't the distinction that we have today of BLS and ALS—it was all an emergency.

However, no matter how good *Emergency!* was (and still is), it would have never made it out of its first season without its fans, and it would not have had such a great impact on the community at large in its demand for paramedics across the country. Dr. Ron Stewart, Medical Advisor to the series, said, "I suspect that the most surprising thing that stands out in respect to the filming was by far the influence of the creation of this fantasy on the opinion of the public and their reaction to it. That has never left me—the power of that medium."

The ever-changing statistical information that included stations, apparatus (air and ground), and uniforms was most difficult to keep updated. The information was correct at the time of editing but could have changed by the time of publication. The authors regret any discrepancies.

The authors hope that this book is able to archive the history of an important aspect of EMS and of the health care system in general. This is the story of a series that has often been duplicated but never equaled, never given the honor it deserved, as there is no doubt, it changed EMS in this country.

"We're on our way Rampart!"

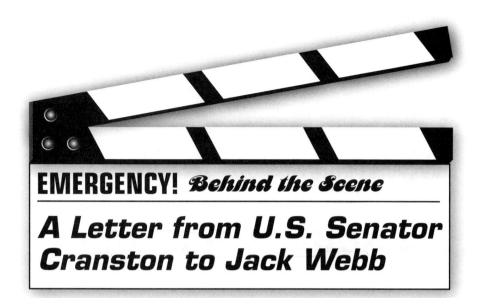

EMERGENCY! *Behind the Scene*

A Letter from U.S. Senator Cranston to Jack Webb

Emergency! was praised by U.S. Senator Alan Cranston (D–CA) for educating the public about the value of real-life paramedic programs. Taken from a 1974 NBC Press release: "Not only has *Emergency!* proven successful and popular television viewing, its graphic illustration of society's need for trained paramedics, has in the words of Senator Alan Cranston, '...alerted the public to the value of paramedic for better emergency care.'"

The release goes on to state, "In September 1972, the Senator wrote to Jack Webb to say, 'We unanimously passed a bill that, among other things would promote the training of paramedics to staff ambulances and emergency rooms in hospitals across the country. I introduced the provisions in the bill dealing with paramedics and emergency medical services in hopes that our nation will make greater use of the thousands of experienced, able young men who have returned from Vietnam with the medical skills America needs so desperately. They are to get top priority in the training programs. Jack, your *Emergency!* series fired the public imagination and was the harbinger for a medical idea whose time, I believe, has come. In the midst of a severe shortage of doctors, nurses, and trained emergency personnel, 175,000 die each year because they do not get adequate medical care in an emergency. Another 25,000 are left permanently disabled because of inept handling by untrained ambulance attendants. *Emergency!* has dramatized the potential of the paramedic. I hope the House of Representatives and the President will now follow the lead of 100 Senators—and Jack Webb! Thank you for the good work, Jack. And congratulations to you and all the people connected with *Emergency!*.'"

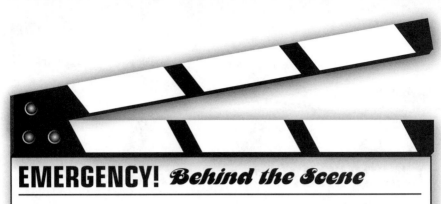

EMERGENCY! *Behind the Scene*

Acknowledgments

A special thanks to all these people for their valuable assistance in the research for this book, all of whom gladly (I think) shared their time, experience, and patience. Please forgive us if we have missed anyone. Without many of these contributors, this book could not have been written; more importantly, *Emergency!* would not have happened.

Cast of *Emergency!*: Michael Norell, Mike Stoker, Marco López, Tim Donnelly, Ron Pinkard, Betty Hammer (wife of Dick Hammer), and Robert Fuller

LACoFD Firefighter/Paramedic Technical Advisors: Joe Bartak, Jr., Bob Lee Hancock, Mark Hefley, Mike Lewis, Bob Belliveau, Rocky Doke, Bob McCullough, Gary Davis, and Bill Hoff

All LACoFD Personnel, current and retired, with special thanks to: P. Michael Freeman, Charles Gutierrez, Gary E. Lineberry, George Ashley, Ray Ribar, John R. Price, Cynthia Barbee, Joe Woyjeck, Alan Barbee, Veronie Steele, Jeff Brum, Lanny Cunningham, Kristina Hajjar, John De Leon, and Paul Schneider

Universal Studio personnel: Harold Frizzell, Johnny Miller, Barbara Michaels (wife of Mickey Michaels), Preston Wood, Dennis Donnelly, and Greg C. Jensen, Sr.

Harbor General staff: Ronald D. Stewart, Carol Bebout, and William Koenig

LAFD personnel: Blair Lamere, Brian Humphrey, Richard H. McClure, Jim Perry, and Bill Dahlquist

Museum staff: Paul Schneider and Joe Woyjeck, CLAFMA, the Historical Society of Long Beach, and Jane Rogers of the Smithsonian

Yosemite National Park staff: Ted Farmer, David Stone, Jack Morehead, and Butch Farabee

Sierra Madre Search-And-Rescue team: Dick Sale and Arnold Gaffrey

Crown Firecoach Enthusiasts: Mike Britt, Don Croucher, and Darrell Gilbert

Compton Fire Department: Scott B. Miller, Michael Shipman, and Charles Coleman

Lake Park, Florida, Fire Department: Mike Wells, Steve Waterman, and Bryan Fields

Thanks to "Nexxie" for reviewing countless hours of tape and for filling in a lot of the character gaps and identification.

A very special thanks to LACoFD Richard A. Friend for allowing access to his personal papers and for reading the draft manuscripts (several times), making sure we had it right. To Jim Page, for initial proofing and for always being there when we had a question. We deeply regret that both of these gentlemen passed away before the publication of this book, something they both were looking forward to. The information they provided to the authors was invaluable.

Additional thanks go to A.J. Heightman, Editor-In-Chief of *JEMS* Magazine; Nancy E. Barr, casting assistant and production coordinator; Carol Meyer, EMS director, County of Los Angeles; Stan Jackson, Long Beach fireboat operator, Boat 15; Sammy Fox, San Luis Obispo City Fire Department; Andrew Wakeford, Dinky Toys, England; Paul Keenleyside, *Emergency!* Equipment Manifest; Thom Dick, EMT-P, JEMS Communications; Stephanie A. Naoum, National Fire Protection Association; Sheila James-Kuehl, *Emergency!* guest star and California State Senator; Commander Jim Sommer, executive officer, District 11 USCG Los Angeles Air Station; Eric Ryan, Hollywood Fire Authority; Chin Thammasaengsri, CBS Television; Peter Gwilliam, Station Officer, London Fire Brigade (retired); Jack Kunstmann, Ward LaFrance Fire Engine; Laurence A. Spring, Dennis Specialist Vehicles; Ken Riddle, Deputy Fire Chief, Las Vegas Fire and Rescue; Bill Mensing, Sheetcraft Company; Carl C. Van Cott, former vice president, Biocom; Keith Campbell, Palm Beach County Fire-Rescue; David Epling, Portola Railroad Museum; Thomas Hibbard, former deputy to LA County 1st District Supervisor; Eric Green, Civil Defense Museum; J. Carl Lee, radiation safety officer; David Leonard, Pasadena Fire Department (retired); Raul Moreno, *Emergency!* extra; and Erika Bartlett, *Emergency!* convention program designer and emergencyfans.com coadministrator.

The County of Los Angeles Fire Museum and the television series *Emergency!* have enjoyed a long and lasting relationship. The late James O. Page—LACoFD Battalion Chief and technical advisor to the show, later hailed as the father of modern Emergency Medical Services—served as president of the museum board. Randolph Mantooth is the museum's Honorary Chairman and spokesperson. In 1999, the museum took ownership of and restored Squad 51, and helped sponsor the Project 51 tour to the Smithsonian. They also own the Crown engine used in the first two seasons, and hope to acquire the Ward LaFrance engine upon its retirement from service in Yosemite National Park.

The museum's goal to construct a new world-class fire and EMS event center to display these vehicles, along with their impressive collection of vintage apparatus and historical artifacts, for public education and appreciation, is moving toward realization as this book goes to press. The authors are pleased and proud that a portion of the proceeds from the sale of this book will be donated to the County of Los Angeles Fire Museum Association in support of their efforts to showcase the history of the American Fire Service and EMS professions, and preserve the rich and innovative legacy of the Los Angeles County Fire Department.

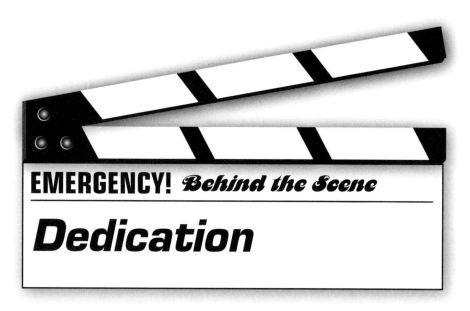

EMERGENCY! *Behind the Scene*

Dedication

To medical personnel and fans all over the globe.

Firefighters and EMS personnel, past and present and future, whose life direction this milestone program forever changed. Many became paramedics, joined the fire service, or dedicated their lives to the public good in so many other ways as a result of watching the exploits of Johnny and Roy, the Crew of Station 51, and the Doctors and Nurses at Rampart.

**Dedicated to those
who have made the ultimate sacrifice
in the performance of their duty.**

Los Angeles County Fire Department Firefighter Memorial

Patients Daughter: "What are they doing?"
Capt Stanley: "They're Paramedics!"
Patients Daughter: "What does that mean?"
Capt. Stanley: "They do this all the time."

—*From an unfilmed script written by Preston Wood
titled "The Reading Course"*

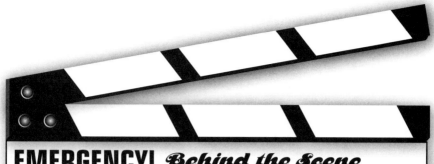

CHAPTER **1**

History of EMS in Los Angeles County

The Beginning of the Paramedic Program in Los Angeles

In its early years, the Los Angeles County Fire Department (LACoFD) responded to medical emergencies with conventional vehicles, usually Ford or GMC half-ton panel vans or trucks, which carried basic rescue gear, including:

- Porto-Powers
- Rope rescue equipment
- Fire extinguishers
- Cutting torch
- E&J oxygen equipment

The oxygen equipment included two steel oxygen tanks and was carried in a suitcase because it weighed more than 50 pounds. It had the capability for resuscitation and inhalation, and it could be used for aspiration.

1

Self-contained breathing apparatus carried on the vehicles would come later.

The job of the rescue squad firefighters was twofold: they would assist engine company crews at structure fires, and they would rescue people who were trapped in burning or collapsed buildings, wrecked cars, construction cave-ins, and other similar situations. They often responded out of their first-in district, or their main area of responsibility, when called upon for rescue situations.

This was an era when firefighters were not allowed to take a person's blood pressure, resuscitation was the "back pressure–arm lift" method, and cardiopulmonary resuscitation wasn't even a dream yet.

LA County had 27 of these rescue squad–type vehicles. They used one-man units in the beginning and upgraded to two-man units in 1968 to support the engine companies in fire suppression. The firefighters received no extra pay for being on the rescue squad, they were usually junior in seniority in the station, and promotions were limited. By 1974 all of the "rescue squads" would be converted to "paramedic squads."

LA County Firefighter Jim Page served on one of these rescue squads early in his career on Rescue 11 in Altadena, California. Some years later, in the early 1990s, he found and restored a 1947 Ford panel truck, his "hobby car," complete with working lights and equipment inside. It was just like the original he had driven, but instead of a flathead V8, the new rig ran with a 351-cubic-inch Ford "Cleveland" engine, a C-6 Ford automatic transmission, independent front suspension, power steering and power brakes, air conditioning, and stereo sound—a definite step up from the 6-volt system that couldn't handle lights and siren at the same time. This truck is now on display at the County of Los Angeles Fire Museum in South Gate.

The modern paramedic concept began in Belfast, Ireland, in the early 1960s, where Dr. J. Frank Pantridge created a program to increase the survivability of heart attack victims through treatment *before* they arrived at the hospital. A few years later, several doctors in cities across the United States were working on variations of Dr. Pantridge's approach. These included Dr. Eugene Nagel in Miami, Florida, where the first fire department paramedics hit the streets.

In the late 1960s, there were more than seventy separate incorporated cities within Los Angeles County, many with their own fire departments and others covered by the LACoFD. There was little, if any, coordination among the different fire agencies and the hospitals.

In 1969, Dr. J. Michael Criley and Dr. A. James Lewis were in the midst of developing a paramedic-training program in Los Angeles at Harbor General Hospital. The emphasis at this time was strictly on cardiac care and preventing unnecessary cardiac deaths with early treatment—not the expanded scope of the current program, which includes all phases of emergency care.

Bob Belliveau, one of the paramedics in the first Harbor General class, advises, "The Battalion 7 chiefs selected several people to go to paramedic training....It wasn't voluntary as much as a selection process where they wanted seasoned firemen with at least 3 years on the job and with rescue experience."

Extensive hands-on and classroom training began in August 1969 in emergency medical procedures, which included "following physician instructors on their rounds, checking vital signs, taking blood pressure readings, and interpreting electrocardiograms, basically performing as student medical assistants," according to an MCA/Universal press release. The firemen attended classes during the day and returned to their station if they were on duty that day.

Firefighter Gary Davis recalls that on the first day of class, Harbor General Hospital paramedic instructors Dr. Criley and Carol Bebout, RN, said, "We don't know what you all are capable of..." The firefighter/paramedics joined special cardiac care unit (CCU) nursing classes because initially they were going to be involved only in cardiac care in the field.

That all changed by the second class when the firefighter/paramedics related that they dealt with much more than just cardiac care. Each week in the course, the firefighters were involved in question-and-answer sessions with hospital interns. Dr. Criley would pose a series of questions to the interns, and if they could not answer, then he would ask the firefighters. More often than not, the firefighters would provide the correct answer, which did not make the interns very happy.

Through the leadership of Kenneth Hahn, Second District Supervisor for the County of Los Angeles, the paramedic program was implemented on December 8, 1969, when six LA County firefighters graduated. They staffed Squad 59 and earned the new title of fireman/paramedic.

Kenneth Hahn served as a county supervisor for a record 10 terms—more than 40 years. He was the force behind the implementation of the paramedic program. Additionally, it was through his leadership that the emergency phone system on freeways was established in 1962. Other highlights of Hahn's political career include helping to build a hospital in Willowbrook after the Watts riots and bringing the Brooklyn (now Los Angeles) Dodgers out west in 1958. Hahn was instrumental in the design and implementation of the original County seal in 1957. Coming full circle, he was still supervisor when LA County Fire Station 127 was dedicated to the executive producer of *Emergency!* as the Robert A. Cinader Memorial Fire Station.

Squad 59, "Los Angeles County Fire Department—Rescue Heart Unit," was assigned to County Fire Station 59 based at Harbor General Hospital, which housed an engine staffed only by a captain and a driver. Station 59 had previously been known among the firefighters as a "retirement station," due to the lack of activity. The station's sole purpose was for fire protection on the hospital grounds, and it was thus known as an "Institutional Fire Station." LA County had three such fire stations. The other two were Station 35 (located at Rancho Los Amigos Hospital in Downey) and Station 46 (located on the grounds of the Olive View Hospital, which was destroyed in the 1971 Sylmar earthquake). The activity at Station 59 soon changed with the assignment of a paramedic squad **(Photo 1-1)**.

That first squad, an old, green, Forestry Service Plymouth station wagon, was, according to paramedic instructor Carol Bebout, "old, dirty, and cruddy; it even had little seedlings growing in the tire well space in the back." However, after Supervisor Kenneth Hahn heard of the condition of the vehicle, he had the county shops deliver a new vehicle for use at RS59. Dick Friend commented that the paint was still "damp" at the dedication.

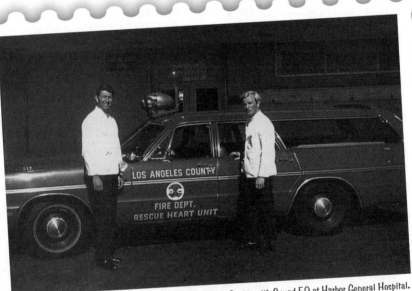

PHOTO 1-1   Firefighters/Paramedics Rocky Doke and Dale Cauble with Squad 59 at Harbor General Hospital.

Source: Courtesy of County of Los Angeles Fire Museum Association Collection.

The emergency lights on the roof were the old platter setup (see Chapter 10) that was on the rescue squads. Still, according to Bob Belliveau, one of the new paramedics who ran on RS59, "it was heavily overloaded with equipment." Bebout went on to state, "RS59 personnel hung out primarily in the cardiac care unit on '4 West' of the hospital, the actual location of the base station radio, where they could talk to patients, staff, start IVs, interpret EKGs, and gain additional experience. They also spent time in the emergency department honing their skills, getting to know hospital personnel and hospital practices."

Belliveau states, "Some of the hospital staff had problems with a bunch of us guys running around in uniforms with badges on, so it was decided we were to wear white smocks and coats." When a call came in for the paramedics during the day, the CCU Nurse, with drug box in hand, ran with them to the vehicle (as noted in the World Premier episode of *Emergency!*). If at night or otherwise in the fire station, the paramedics would have to call the CCU and notify them that a nurse was required for a call. The nurse would run down the corridor through the medical ward and down four flights of stairs to be picked up by the squad near the outside stairwell. The paramedics had to drive approximately 1500 feet from the station to the hospital. At least one nurse was always assigned to the squad. On those rare occasions that a nurse was not available, the squad then reverted to a first aid unit and did not function as a mobile intensive care unit.

Dr. Walter Graf, LA County Heart Association President and Chief of Cardiology at Daniel Freeman Hospital, approached McCormick Ambulance in late 1969 to participate in a different paramedic pilot program spearheaded by County Supervisor Kenneth Hahn. McCormick Ambulance, founded in 1962 as an outgrowth of McCormick Mortuaries, furnished a vehicle, which was then customized by the County Mechanical Department in cooperation with the County Heart Association. The HEART (Heart Emergency Ambulance Rescue Team) ambulance was staffed with an on-call coronary care nurse from Daniel Freeman Hospital to respond to heart attacks. Beginning in late 1969, it made pilot runs within a 5-mile radius of Daniel Freeman Hospital in Inglewood. Later, the ambulance would increase its response area. The HEART ambulance was in service, later staffed by paramedics, from August 1970 through June 30, 1972, at which time the County paramedic squads replaced it. McCormick is now part of Westmed Ambulance.

LA County firefighters from Station 18 attended the paramedic program at Daniel Freeman Hospital and became part of the Coronary Ambulance Rescue Team. In a cooperative effort between LA County and Daniel Freeman Hospital, the 4-week class (August–September 1970) had six

Inglewood firefighters, four LA County firefighters (RS18), and two fire-fighters from McCormick Ambulance. The second Daniel Freeman class (1971) had three LA County firemen, two from Inglewood FD, and one from McCormick Ambulance. These first classes launched the Daniel Free-man Hospital effort in the paramedic training world, and they still have an active paramedic program there today.

St. Francis Hospital in Lynwood was the third hospital to come online as a Base Station Hospital in November 1971. The recently graduated para-medics from Station 9 went into service as Squad 209 and contacted St. Francis for instruction and transportation to St. Francis. In some episodes of *Emergency!* on Squad 51's radio, broadcasts of Squad 209 responding to, or 10-7 at, St. Francis can be heard.

In contrast to the workings of the County unit, six LA City firefight-ers (Los Angeles Fire Department, LAFD) in the second paramedic class at Harbor General (along with six County firefighters) began in January 1970 and graduated July 1970. The City firemen were assigned to Rescue Ambu-lance 53. The City firefighter paramedics were housed at LA City Fire Sta-tion 53 at 483 North Mesa Street in San Pedro. Because of its distance from the hospital, nurses from Harbor General were assigned to the fire station on a rotating basis to ride with the crew until the Paramedic Act was passed and until the paramedics had completed their internship. Firefighter/para-medics on RA38 in Wilmington at 124 East I Street would soon follow.

Carol Bebout advised that, "Station 53 never had women assigned to it before, which caused the obvious problems. [LA City would not hire their first female firefighter until 1983.] To make it worse for the nurses that worked at night at the station, they were given the Battalion Chief's room and he had to sleep out in the dorm with the rest of the crew." And like Rescue Squad 59, if for some reason a nurse was unavailable to respond with RA53, it would revert back to a regular ambulance.

According to Captain Rick McClure, in LAFD's emergency medical ser-vices (EMS) Division:

> The initial training for the LAFD was completed utilizing firefighters as they were con-sidered first responders, trusted and trainable. The City of Los Angeles had two EMS systems prior to 1970. One, by the fire department in which firefighters handled the ambulance calls in the San Fernando Valley, South Los Angeles, and the Harbor. The rest of the City was provided service by the "Brown Bombers."

Brown Bombers were civilian ambulance drivers and attendants, dis-patched by the Los Angeles Police Department. They responded out of the receiving hospitals—Hollywood Receiving, Central Receiving (as com-monly seen on *Adam-12* and *Dragnet*), and Georgia Street Hospital.

In 1970, the Los Angeles City Fire Department was offered the opportunity to drop the ambulance service or acquire the civilian force; Fire Chief Raymond Hill accepted the ambulance service. "There was great heartache for the next few years," McClure says, "as these 'civilians' weren't used to a para-militaristic organization, someone there to tell them to get going when the bell went off and to explain that we are a public emergency service, there to provide care and compassion to the citizens of Los Angeles."

With an increased need for resources in 1972, the testing process for civilian ambulance drivers was established. The Fire Department sent senior ambulance attendants and drivers to paramedic schools, which formed a model for the civilian side of the show. RA3 and RA34 with civilian paramedics were the next staffed paramedic rigs. In 1980, the Fire Department reinstituted sending firefighters to paramedic school for workload relief. At that time, many ambulances were responding to twenty to twenty-five calls in a 24-hour period, on a consistent basis.

By putting three firefighter/paramedics on a shift, two could be on the rescue squad and one on the fire engine. Because fire suppression companies were not nearly as busy then, this allowed the firefighter/paramedics to switch off during the shift. "Most of the civilian paramedics were cross-trained as firefighters over the next few years," said McClure. "As for the firefighters that were first trained as paramedics staffing RA53 and RA38, they went back to tailboard working as firefighters, promoted, or retired when the civilians came on board. There are still single-role paramedics in the City, those former civilians that did not cross-train as firefighters, and are so identified by their distinctive blue helmets."

Currently in the City of Los Angeles, there is paramedic coverage in every station on assessment engines, and there are eighty-three paramedic advanced life support (ALS) rescue ambulances. According to LAFD Captain McClure, there will soon be an ALS or a Basic Life Support ambulance in every station.

The historical stations that first staffed paramedics for the City and County are no longer in service. LAFD Station 53 closed in the early 1990s pending the much-anticipated opening of new Fire Station 112 in 1995, which was built to combine the crews from nearby FS53 with the fireboats. LA County FS59 on the hospital grounds closed in 1970 after the passage of the Wedworth-Townsend Act, and the station number was reissued. The firehouse building, although not used as such, is still there, often with County ambulances parked nearby. Throughout the course of the TV series *Emergency!*, "Squad 59" can be heard several times from LA County dispatch as background voiceover in response to other calls.

Senate Bill 958/Assembly Bill 1711 was introduced to the California Senate and House in April 1970 by Senator James Q. Wedworth (D) and Assemblyman Larry Townsend. This bill made it legal for mobile care intensive care paramedics to save lives in emergency situations. It was not until the signing of the Wedworth-Townsend Paramedic Act by then California Governor Ronald Reagan that paramedics were allowed to run calls without the nurses in attendance. Townsend and Wedworth joined with Second District Supervisor Kenneth Hahn in watching Governor Reagan sign the historic bill into law on July 15, 1970 **(Photo 1-2)**.

Hahn recalls that Reagan asked if the program would cross city boundaries. Only after Hahn confirmed that it would did Reagan agree to sign the bill. Hahn always remembered that Governor Reagan told him after signing the bill, "My father died in Beverly Hills when a Los Angeles Police Department ambulance wouldn't cross the city line."

Squad 209 was placed into service at the end of 1971 and was unique to the LA County paramedic program. It would become the busiest squad in Los Angeles County. Squad 209 was not a Dodge with a utility body but a brand new Dodge Tradesman van originally destined for the Parks and

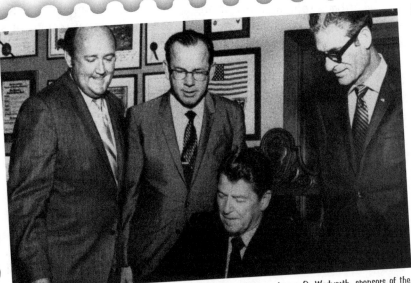

PHOTO 1-2   Assemblyman Larry Townsend (left) and State Senator James Q. Wedworth, sponsors of the Wedworth-Townsend Paramedic Act, join with Supervisor Kenneth Hahn to watch Governor Ronald Reagan sign the historic bill into law on July 15, 1970.
Source: Courtesy of Kenneth Hahn, LA County.

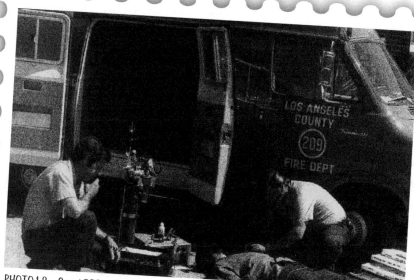

PHOTO 1-3   Squad 209 with Mike Lewis and Bob McCullough.
Source: Courtesy of Los Angeles County Fire Department, Photo Unit.

Recreation Department. The County mechanics raised the roof of the van and gave it a coat of red paint because it had already been painted green. Initially lettered "Mobile Intensive Care" with the County seal on the doors, it would later be lettered with the standard "Los Angeles County Fire Dept." with 209 within a circle, and a Twinsonic light bar replaced the Gumball rotator by the end of 1972 **(Photo 1-3)**.

Firefighter/paramedic Bob McCullough was asked why a van was used when the regular squads were already in service. "I believe the concept of the van was to test the waters as to whether it would be feasible to start doing critical patient transports," he replied. "We never did transport, although in theory it was what was considered when buying the van. The bubble top was added to give us head room if we ever did retrofit it to transport. It really got the private ambulance industry up in arms. LACoFD backed down to it, but LA City did not, hence their RA was born."

Firefighter/paramedic Mike Lewis recalls:

> When the program started, Squad 209 was County Supervisor Kenneth Hahn's baby. The supervisor came in to see it when we first received it; it was painted red but just had a driver seat and a passenger seat, it was an empty van—that is, no compartments or anything. The

morning he was to come in, I pulled it out on the ramp to wash it and the water pressure blew the
red paint off the right front hood and fender. When Hahn came in, he called me to the front and
with his group that was following him he said, "Mike, show me my squad," and when I opened
it and he saw all the equipment tied down with bungee cords on the floor in this empty van,
he said, "This is not my squad." He turned to his aid and said, "Take care of this." The squad
was sent up to the shops that afternoon. It was returned three days later complete with cabinets,
patient gurney, oxygen system, seating, and all set to go. The afternoon it was returned, I was
again called to the front and there was Supervisor Hahn with his group. Again he said, "Mike
show me my squad." When I opened the door all he said was, "That's my squad."

Was the supervisor thinking along the lines of eventual and possible
patient transport with the van? Lewis thinks he might have been, "We designed the interior using an LA City rescue ambulance, of course we never
did transport." Lewis said that the squad was still in service in 1974, and
it is unknown when the van was retired and replaced with a Dodge utility
truck. It is also unknown what the eventual disposition of the van was. This
was the only squad of this type placed into service. Station 9 was eventually
disbanded and equipment moved to Station 16 in Florence.

By 1971, LACoFD had several paramedic squads in service:

- Squad 36, Carson
- Squad 7, West Hollywood
- Squad 38, W. 54th Street, Los Angeles
- Squad 14, W. 108th Street, Los Angeles
- Squad 209, 7116 S. Makee Ave., Los Angeles
- Squad 18, Inglewood
- Squad 39, Bell Gardens
- Squad 3, East Los Angeles
- Squad 165, Huntington Park

As more and more firemen were being taught, numerous other cities
expressed interest in the program. By August 1971, Beverly Hills and Redondo Beach sent their firemen to Harbor General for paramedic training.
During this time Congress was working on legislation to standardize EMS
practices nationwide.

Politically, the paramedic program was not doing well at this time. The
paramedic program continued to be a "pilot" program, and LA County Fire
Chief Richard Houts, who supported the program, openly referred to it as
a "temporary experiment." Firefighter/paramedics were saving lives, but
criticism from the ambulance companies (who feared that the fire department was stealing their business) and physicians (who could not fathom
firemen "playing doctor") was playing in the press. Robert A. Cinader, the
executive producer of *Emergency!*, witnessed firsthand encounters with an-
tagonistic private ambulance companies during his ride-alongs.

According to Dick Friend:

> Chief Houts was a major supporter, and the program wouldn't have flown if not for him and one of the five LA County Supervisors, Kenneth Hahn, as well as Dr. Criley, who was also very prominent, working behind the scenes with many members of the medical profession that didn't want to see it happen. Chief Keith Klinger, who retired in June 1969, although highly [supportive of] firemen responding to medical emergencies, as it was he that introduced the use of resuscitators on all engines and trucks in the department, did not support the paramedic program.

Although there were several paramedic programs starting up across the nation, there was no coordinated effort to get together to combine thoughts, training, or funding. The general public in several of these cities was even unaware that such training was taking place. It wasn't until a television program debuted in January 1972 that the public really became aware of the paramedic program.

The First Los Angeles County Paramedics

The first six LACoFD firefighters, soon to be paramedics, began training in August 1969. They trained under the supervision of Dr. Michael Criley, Dr. A. James Lewis, and Carol Bebout, RN. It was initially the same training program that a CCU nurse received, but the curriculum was expanded after Dr. Criley and the LACoFD began to have a better idea of what a paramedic could/should be. They graduated December 9, 1969.

Bebout states, "The first class of six actually ended up with a great deal more practical experience and less didactic training." The program quickly developed into a training program, requiring 2 months of instruction, 1 month of clinical hospital experience, and a 2-month field internship. For the first 2 years of the program, nurses provided supervision in the field internship, but after that point, the newly certified paramedics supervised trainees in the field. The demand for training grew quickly, and the staff was soon teaching several classes at once, in overlapping phases of training. Eventually, they opened a second training facility at the University of Southern California, where Dr. Ron Stewart and Dr. Ron Crowell became involved.

Standing orders for the paramedics were nonexistent initially because all therapy required base station authorization—even starting IVs. Standing orders would take about 10 years to be introduced into the system.

Throughout the course of the television series *Emergency!*, technical advisors were always in uniform while on the set. On the set of *Emergency!*, the advisors and paramedics had to wear red "FOR REAL" nameplates above their name badges to signify who was an actor and who was a firefighter/paramedic.

At the time these first firefighters were being trained, neither the State nor the County had a system for certifying paramedics with formal licenses because this was a pilot program. It would take about 2 years after the first class graduated for certification to happen. Once the system developed out of the paramedic pilot program and became a full-fledged curriculum, paramedic certification numbers were issued retroactively, alphabetically by class.

The First Six LACoFD Fireman/Paramedics Taught at Harbor General Hospital (August–December 1969)

- Bob Belliveau, P0001 for LA County. TA (TA) on episodes 1.11, 2.6, and 3.19. Appeared in episode 6.6, "Rules of Order." One of the TAs for the movies, *Steel Inferno* and *Survival on Charter #220*. Retired as a Battalion Chief.
- Dale Cauble, PM0002. TA to the 2-hour *Emergency!* World Premier and episode 2.2. By 1975 he would hold the rank of Captain and become one of the department's chaplains.
- Gary Davis, PM0003. TA on episodes 1.10, 2.1, 4.7, 5.9, and 6.1.
- Gerald Nolls, PM0004. TA on episodes 1.6 and 2.8.
- David Phillips, PM0005.
- Robert Ramstead, PM0006. TA on episodes 1.4 and 2.12.

With the exception of Nolls, who was working in Lomita, all others came from Station 36 in Carson: Davis and Ramstead from A shift, Belliveau and Cauble from B shift, and Phillips from C shift.

The Second Class at Harbor General (January–July 1970)

- William "Roger" Crow, PM0007. TA on episodes 1.8 and 2.4.
- Roscoe "Rocky" Doke, PM0008. TA on episodes 1.9, 2.5, and 3.5.
- Richard Neal, PM0009. TA on episodes 1.7, 2.16, 3.16, 4.14, and 6.10.
- William Ridgeway, PM0010. TA on episode 2.19.
- Michael Stearns, PM0011. TA on episodes 1.2 and 2.14.[1]

---

[1] After being promoted to captain in July 1972, Stearns was required to relinquish his certification. At the time, fire department regulations did not allow promoted paramedics to practice. Captain Stearns was later appointed as one of two paramedic coordinators for the LACoFD. Stearns was a member of the team that went back to Elmira, New York, to pick up *Emergency!*'s Ward LaFrance and drive it back to Los Angeles (see Chapter 17).

These 11 medics, as well as future graduates, may have worked on additional episodes, but accurate records of all TAs were not kept. Paramedics would continue to be requested for TA duty from among later classes.

After the passage of the Wedworth-Townsend Act, a class photo was taken in August 1970 that included the 11 County graduates from the first two Harbor General classes and the six LAFD Paramedics who were also in the second class that would staff RA53.

The LAFD fireman/paramedics were:

- Ed Arnold, PM0012
- Ralph Brownell, PM0013
- Walter Hartsuyker, PM0014
- Claude Griggs, PM0014.5
- Dennis Grogan, PM0015
- James Nelson, PM0016

Also in the photo were Dr. A. James Lewis, Nurse Carol Bebout, and Dr. Criley. When the historic photo was taken, the first class at Daniel Freeman Hospital had just begun (August 1970). The third class at Harbor General Hospital (class 1970/71) did not begin until July 1971.

EMERGENCY! *Behind the Scene*

CHAPTER **2**

The Birth of Emergency!

It is said that the direct spark for the series began sometime in late 1969, when Sid Sheinberg, president of MCA/Universal, felt that a "variant of the action-packed realism" in *The Hellfighters* (a 1968 Universal Pictures film based on oil firefighters, starring John Wayne) would be just the thing for early evening television.

This may or may not be true, but one cannot discount the earlier production of *Rescue 8,* also airing on NBC. This widely popular program, airing 14 years earlier, starred Jim Davis, who later starred as Jock Ewing on *Dallas. Rescue 8* aired in worldwide syndication for many years and was dubbed into several languages including Chinese, German, and Swedish. This two-season (1958–1960), 73-episode series was also about two LA County firefighters on a (nonparamedic) rescue squad. Based out of the real LA County Station 8 in West Hollywood, the series chronicled the stories of the rescue squads in the early years of LA County. These squads provided an important rescue function but only the most basic of first aid.

Fire Station 8, built in 1953, would also feature prominently in the *Emergency!* World Premier (as Station 10) and as Station 8 in one other episode. Basically an island, the 2-square-mile district is surrounded by the Los Angeles Fire Department (LAFD) and the city of Beverly Hills.

However, even before there was *Emergency!* in the United States, there was *Emergency* in Australia. (Note the missing '!'.) Airing the same time as *Rescue 8*, this 1959 TV series on Melbourne's GTV-9 featured primarily the doctors and nurses in a hospital setting along with a nonparamedic ambulance crew. The episodes would open with a vehicle accident or other medical emergency with the ambulance crew responding, treating, carrying, and transporting injured patients to the hospital, where the balance of the treatment and remaining television program took place. The 30-minute live-on-film (kinescope) episodes were quite popular at the time. No firefighters were involved, but it is interesting to note the similarities to *ER*, and to Britain's popular *Casualty*, as well as *Emergency!*. Technical advice was provided by the Royal Melbourne Hospital, which loaned various items of medical equipment and provided coaching for the actors in its usage. The Victorian Civil Ambulance Service supplied an ambulance and an ambulance officer.

It is difficult, if not impossible, to verify the rumor that producer Jack Webb *(Dragnet)* outlined some sort of a fire and rescue series sometime before *Emergency!* and presented it to the networks that were, at the time, not interested. Unfortunately, all parties involved who could confirm or deny such a rumor are no longer with us.

However, sometime in late 1970 or early 1971, Jack Webb did meet with Sid Sheinberg in his Burbank office. Sheinberg asked Webb to consider developing a series with Universal about a firefighter rescue team. Jack Webb had Robert A. Cinader, creator of *Adam-12* and an executive producer for Webb's Mark VII Production Company, research the concept of a series about "rescue." Initially approaching the LAFD, Webb was turned down. The LAFD chief at the time wanted nothing to do with moving companies around to film a TV show. Webb initially wanted to use old LAFD Station 23 because it was only a training station at that time. Webb called County Supervisor Ken Hahn, who met with him and Cinader, and then later Dick Friend got involved—and that was the start of *Emergency!*.

Cinader and the Public Information Officer (PIO) for the Los Angeles Police Department, Lieutenant Dan Cook, had been friends since working as the Technical Advisor on *Dragnet* and *Adam-12*. Cinader asked Cook about the possibility of a new fire/rescue TV program. Lt. Cook knew

Dick Friend, his PIO counterpart for Los Angeles County Fire Department (LACoFD), and knew that they had a new paramedic program underway and advised Cinader to contact him. Cinader contacted Dick Friend, and after a lengthy phone conversation, Friend had Cinader meet with him and Captain Jim Page that same afternoon at Station 7 in West Hollywood, not far from Cinader's office. This historic meeting was on May 11, 1971.

Friend and Cinader met with Captain Page at Station 7, along with the rest of Station 7's C shift crew. They spent several hours going over station logs, discussing "interesting" runs (including the ten-story Playboy Club fire in 1970, the most challenging call of their careers), for a rescue-type television program, and eventually staying for dinner. Despite Page's efforts to interest Cinader in the new paramedic program, he seemed unenthused.

Page was later hired by Webb to research additional incidents for stories for a TV series about "physical rescue" and eventually submitted more than fifty story lines to Cinader, for which Page was paid $300.00. A couple of months after the first meeting, Jim Page was promoted to Battalion Chief, where he was assigned to Battalion 7B, headquartered at Station 36. He invited Bob Cinader to ride along with him and his driver Dale Cauble on medical emergencies involving the new paramedics. Typically, chiefs don't respond on routine medical calls, but Page wanted to make sure Cinader saw enough to make his TV series accurate and authentic. After Cinader saw the paramedics in action, he was convinced that a show featuring paramedics would make for good television.

About a month later, Friend and LA County Fire Chief Richard H. Houts went to Universal Studios for a meeting with Webb and Cinader. Several days later during a meeting with his other top LA County chief officers, Chief Houts gave his blessing to the show along with promising the full support of the Fire Department; he then told Friend, "Make it work." The rest, as they say, is history. It was hoped that if the TV program had some authenticity, the show could be a potent weapon if the viewing public suddenly "demanded" paramedics.

Dale Cauble, from LACoFD's first paramedic class at Harbor General, was appointed to the role of technical advisor for the World Premier. The studio paid for Cauble to be relieved from duty as a fireman/paramedic for about 2 months during the late summer and early fall of 1971. Cauble worked full-time in Webb's Mark VII office, reviewing the script and all its continuing changes. Whenever Page was on duty, Cauble would come by battalion headquarters at Station 36 to report on developments. Page recalls that from the start of his assignment, "Dale complained to me about how Webb and co-writer Harold Jack Bloom were trying to turn *Emergency!*

into a soap opera, with nurse Dixie [McCall] and Dr. [Kelly] Brackett engaged in a torrid love affair."

According to writer and producer Hannah Shearer, "After Bob Cinader's original script was done, Jack Webb hired Harold Jack Bloom to write hospital stuff for Dixie and Kelly's romance, which went nowhere. This was due to Webb thinking the paramedic stuff was not going to make the show work. Bloom had nothing to do with the show before, during, or after it, other than that one story line." Dr. Brackett and Dixie did date a few times that first season, most of which were interrupted.

As the script was developing, eventually reaching 113 pages and 398 scenes, the Fire Department and the paramedics were to play minor roles. Page conveyed Cauble's concerns to Bob Cinader. Cinader told Page to relax; the plan was to let Webb and Bloom just "do their thing," and Cinader would rewrite the script after they finished with it. Page went on to advise Cauble that he would not be blamed if the show turned into a turkey that embarrassed the department. Nonetheless, according to Page, "At one point, the tension of working with these high-powered, ego-driven personalities caused big chunks of Dale's thick hair to start falling out." Dick Friend commented that it looked like Cauble aged 20 years. On more than one occasion, Cauble asked to be replaced and to be given the opportunity to go back to his job as a firefighter/paramedic. Page pleaded with him to stick it out, which he did. After all this, Cauble would take over the reins as TA once again in season 2, for episode 2.2, "Kids."

Six months after that first meeting at Station 7, a script with all its revisions (dated November 19, 1971) was ready. Filming for the two-hour *Emergency!* World Premier began on November 22, 1971, and took 22 days to complete. It began, ironically, at LA County's Station 8—its fourth appearance in a firefighting TV series, but this time appearing as Station 10. It is here that firefighter Gage was assigned to a rescue squad. Roy DeSoto, one of six recently graduated paramedics from the first class at Harbor General, was holding interviews for prospective paramedics at Station 10 for the next class to be taught at Rampart. He was trying to convince Gage to become a paramedic, even though they were unable to practice at that time.

Historically, television and film production companies generally use fictitious fire station numbers when depicting an actual department so as not to confuse it with the real station and other legal issues. In this case, Station 10 (formerly in Downey) was an unused number in the department at the time of the movie. Later, in 1975, the number would be reassigned to a station in Carson. Likewise, station number 51 was also an unused number (see Chapter 9). During the series, real station numbers would occasionally be utilized.

The World Premier movie dramatized the vital need for paramedics. It started late in 1969 and concluded with paramedics who were able to respond from their stations directly to the scene without first having to pick up a nurse at the hospital.

There were two main fire/rescue plots in the movie. The first was a nighttime fire, a quasi night-drill put on by Page at the More-Glo Lighting Company (a warehouse in an unincorporated part of the county between Gardena and Carson, which had been recently gutted during a fire). It was located just east of the 110-Harbor Freeway and north of LA County Station 95. Filming involved many on- and off-duty LA County firefighters with equipment. The "drill" was coordinated by Chief Page. Ironically, firefighter Alan Barbee responded twice to this fire—for real the first time and then again on Engine 36 as a firefighter extra in the World Premier movie.

The second plot line was a rainy, nighttime rescue at a cave-in filmed in Bronson Canyon, an old rock quarry established in 1919 and in operation through 1930 in Hollywood's Griffith Park, again involving multiple pieces of equipment. This time, the rescue scene was coordinated by Dick Friend. Bronson Canyon has been the site of countless movie and TV locations such as *Whirlybirds* and the 1960s *Batman* series, *Star Trek, Gunsmoke, Bonanza, Rescue 8,* and the 1974 series *Firehouse*. The actual tunnel, with a faux concrete façade over the entrance, is, among other things, also known as the "Batman Cave" from the TV series. The tunnel interiors were filmed back at Universal. Friend recalls, "Webb wanted to see everything, so I dug out all kinds of tractors, funny-looking hose-laying devices, you name it; in all about 40 pieces of firefighting equipment that I could get my hands on surrounded the cave for the two-day shoot."

The executive producer and director for the January 15, 1972, World Premiere of *Emergency!* was Jack Webb. This was his only directorial role for the series, other than one proposed spin-off—*905-Wild*—at the end of season 4. The *Emergency!* World Premier was created and written by Robert A. 'Bob' Cinader and Harold Jack Bloom, with final revisions by Cinader, and would serve as the mold for the weekly series.

According to Friend, "Jack Webb directed us all as to what he wanted. Bob Cinader of course was behind the scenes 'directing' everything prior to the actual shooting." When it was announced that Webb would direct the World Premiere, Cinader grumbled about the decision. When Page asked why, Cinader said, "You'll find out." "The only reason I'm directing this," said Webb in an *LA Times* article (November 22, 1971), "is because we don't have time to fight with a director." "It's not my project," he went on to say, "it's Bob's." Page said years later, "Indeed, Jack's powerful presence and legendary impatience terrified most of the actors. I remember a scene at the tunnel site in Griffith Park where Randy (Johnny) was to speak a few simple lines of dialog. He blew the first take, and Jack Webb vented his anger. With each successive take, Jack got louder and more abusive. Eventually, it took twenty-three takes before Randy got it right."

Six 1-hour episodes were ordered up by NBC to start the mid-season schedule before the Premier had completed shooting. In the same *LA Times* article, Bob Cinader stated, "NBC bought it [the pilot] if we could deliver the movie by January 15 with the series to start the following Saturday. " Things were happening so quickly that the actors would be filming scenes for the 2-hour movie, then jump to filming scenes for one of the 60-minute episodes, and then back to filming movie scenes again. This meant that there were at least two complete film crews working at the same time in two different locations, along with all the additional fire equipment required. The 1-hour episodes were filmed in a 6-day shooting schedule. Eventually, a total of eleven 60-minute episodes were filmed and aired that first season in addition to the 2-hour premier. Later in the series, shooting for some of the episodes took longer because of the complexity of some of the fire and rescue scenes and filming locations.

Scripts for each of the programs were sent to Fire Chief Richard Houts, Battalion Chief Page, the LACoFD training section chief, the LACoFD firefighter/paramedic technical advisor assigned to that specific episode, as well as to Dick Friend. Their comments were sent back to Friend, who did the final review for the Fire Department. Scripts were also sent to Harbor General Hospital (soon to portray Rampart), where Dr. A. Jim Lewis (who was in the paramedic-training department run by Dr. Criley) and Dr. Ron Stewart (medical consultant for the series) and others reviewed them.

Friend, Page, and the technical advisors would meet with Cinader, the directors, unit manager, producers, writers, special effects personnel, and wardrobe staff every Wednesday at Universal for a final production meeting for the following week's episode. The purpose of this meeting was to review the script—page-by-page, scene-by-scene—and make any final changes or, as Friend said, "Forever hold your peace." Cinader once said, "Don't make Dick mad or he'll take his trucks and go home." Fortunately, that never happened.

Friend, Page, and the Fire Department technical advisor working on each episode often would review the dailies (the scenes shot that day) and make recommendations for editing, to ensure accuracy and protect the department's image. Along those lines, many of the LA County's departmental rules and regulations were adhered to throughout the making of the series to make it as accurate as possible.

One requirement that Friend and Page focused on early in the first season, as scripts were being submitted, was in regard to the banter, in the squad or engine, written in the scripts while the crews were responding to an incident. They advised that:

> Frivolous banter between the men while responding to an emergency situation is, in our opinion, inappropriate. The fact of a possible life-threatening situation, coupled with the serious business of traversing busy city streets with red light and siren precludes light-heartedness, to indicate a possible unsafe response. In reality, the men would be entirely concerned with transporting themselves and their equipment to the scene as quickly as possible. We are very concerned that this [banter] conveys an undesirable impression of our priorities.

Many later firefighting and paramedic TV series do not seem to share these priorities, but maintaining this degree of professionalism was important to the producers of *Emergency!*. For example, when the squad is responding to an incident, they will always have their helmets on, as per Fire Department policy at that time. The helmet policy is now no longer in effect, and today, the only position that must still wear a helmet at all times, while driving, is the tillerman on the open-cab tillers.

Just like *Rescue 8,* which featured two LA County firefighters on a rescue squad, the principal characters in *Emergency!* would also be two firefighters, but in this case newly trained paramedics. As stated in the 1974 book *TV Doctors* by Louis Solomon, "The paramedics go to where the action is, make the rescues, give first aid; the doctors make the repairs, give second aid." Randolph Mantooth and Kevin Tighe, relatively unknown actors, who earned only $250.00 per episode in the beginning, would forever become known as "Johnny" and "Roy." By the spring of 1974—the middle of the third season—they were reportedly earning $1250.00 a week and both asked for $7500.00 an episode in July of that year.

Sometime during the negotiations, Randy was hospitalized in Santa Barbara with an intestinal infection, which shut down the filming. Some thought it coincidental to happen during the negotiation period, but the infection was, in fact, real. Coincidentally, neither Randy nor Kevin received extra pay for doing the voiceovers for the Saturday morning cartoon series *Emergency + 4.* Webb offered a $40,000 bonus if Mantooth and Tighe would see out their seven-year contract at their current salary. They turned that offer down, but with Webb and the studio rumored to be looking for replacements (a typical negotiation ploy), they settled a few weeks later for $4500.00 per episode.

Robert Cinader said that *Emergency!* had a budget of $225,000 per episode in 1972, with approximately 100 cast and crew members. Squad 51 responded throughout LA County, even across the ocean to Catalina Island. Many of the fires and rescues in the show were composites of incidents from all over the county—ones that Cinader responded to and wrote into the story lines and ones from the actual station logs of rescues and fires from the LACoFD.

One week after the premier, the series began on 205 NBC affiliate TV stations nationwide. *Emergency!* was produced with the full cooperation of the LACoFD and Fire Chief Houts. Houts said in a 1973 interview for *Fire Engineering* magazine, "We believe that *Emergency!* has been good for the image of the fire service in general. That is why we have been willing to extend our full cooperation to the producers." The producers also had the assistance and cooperation of the County Department of Hospitals, the LA County Board of Supervisors, and the Department of Health Services.

The popular program would eventually air five and a half seasons through September 1977, with 122 original 1-hour episodes. It continuously maintained high viewer ratings, even though it aired against tough competition such as *All in the Family* and *M*A*S*H*. To date, *Emergency!* has been the only firefighting show that remained in this range of popularity during the entire course of the series. Others have "peaked," but none have maintained like *Emergency!*.

By 1976 *Emergency!* was being seen in 41 countries worldwide, and in the United States it was named one of TV's "Top Ten Shows." By contrast, the drama *Third Watch* (1999–2005) aired in only 20 countries worldwide. In a 1999 fan-oriented poll conducted by UltimateTV, *Emergency!* was among the "Top 100 TV Shows of All Time." *Emergency!* continues to air in several countries around the world; in Germany it is called *Notruf California*, literally translated, "*Emergency call, California*," and in Mexico it is called *Emergencia*.

Emergencia began airing in Argentina on Channel 13 shortly after the series was cancelled in the United States and continued until 1982. *Emergencia* climbed very rapidly to second place among the most watched series in the country, only exceeded by *Bonanza*. It aired again in Argentina briefly in 1997 on the Uniseries channel.

After the Series

By series end, the LACoFD had thirty-one paramedic squads and four paramedic engines in service. In 2005, the department served a population of 4,102,163, covering just a bit more than 2300 square miles.

LA County Fire Department 2005 Statistical Summary
• 91 paramedic squads
• 21 rescue/fire boats
• 3 paramedic air squads
• 18 paramedic assessment engines
• 6 paramedic engines
• 2 EMT-D lifeguard rescue units with an engine and a patrol (stationed on Catalina Island, 20 miles off the California coast)
• 165 fire stations* (includes 4 CFF stations)
• 239 engine companies
• 20 truck companies
• 20 quints
• 8 hazardous materials (HazMat) squads
• 13 USAR vehicles
• 7 emergency support teams
• 4547 total personnel
• 635 certified paramedics
* At the time of the survey, five additional stations were under construction.

The Air Ambulance Program

About the same time the paramedic squads began service, the LACoFD's air ambulance service began as a 6-month pilot program under a federal grant in 1970. It graduated from a Bell 206 with a pilot and an LA County firefighter crewmember (later an EMT-1) to the current staffing of four Bell 412s, three Sikorsky H-7015 FireHawks, and one Bell 206 JetRanger air squad—each staffed with a pilot and two firefighter/paramedics.

The paramedic air ambulance program currently stands at three 24-hour units. They use the 412s and the FireHawks for this mission. According to Gary E. Lineberry (LACoFD Helicopter Pilot, 1974–2000), "The air squads carry essentially the same complement of medical equipment and drugs as the ground rescue squads, but don't carry any extrication equipment as a part of their standard inventory."

On January 1, 2006, a 10-hour air squad was converted to a 24-hour air squad. The West County was the 10-hour airship, based at Camp 8 during the day, shut down at Barton at night. Also, the deployment of the East County 24-hour air squad, which is based out of a temporary heliport at

Configuration for the Deployment of the Three 24-Hour Air Squads

North County Air Squad—Based out of Fire Station 129, primarily serving the Antelope Valley.

East County Air Squad—Based out of Fire Station 64 (temporarily), primarily serving the San Gabriel Valley. Daylight hours are spent at Eastern Air Operations (EAO), which will revert back to Helispot 17-A when FS064 (temp) will be designated at EAO. Nighttime hours are spent at Camp 2 or Barton Heliport in Pacoima.

West County Air Squad—Based out of Camp 8 during the daylight hours and Barton for the remainder of its 24-hour shift, primarily serving Catalina Island and the south and west portions of the County, and serving as a backup to both the North and East County Air Squads.

Fire Station 64 in the City of San Dimas, is the result of a collaborative effort between LACoFD and the County of Los Angeles Board of Supervisors, San Gabriel Council of Governments, and the Department of Health Services.

Firefighter/paramedic personnel are assigned to the section through the Department's bid assignment system. These air operations crewmember positions are very desirable and generally require at least 8 years seniority to obtain a successful bid. Once assigned, they are required to complete an extensive 80-hour course in flight operations, flight safety, specialized equipment such as hoist operations and urban search-and-rescue techniques, flight physiology, and other subjects pertaining to the care and transport of the sick and injured in helicopters.

Lineberry stated, "Our first pilot, Roland J. Barton (seen in episodes of *Emergency!*) and pilot mechanic, Sewell Griggers, comprised the entire unit. Barton was not only a pilot, but also a leader in the development of helicopter firefighting. Through his efforts, the Jeb Aircraft Company constructed the first aluminum drop tank, which could carry 105 gallons of liquid and could be attached to the helicopter in two minutes. This was a vast improvement over the helicopter's initial method of carrying 50 gallons of water in a canvas bag! The new aluminum drop tank was piloted in the 1961 fire season with great success."

This year marks the 50th anniversary of helicopter operations in the LACoFD. On September 22, 1957, the first Bell 47G-2 two-place helicopter was purchased at a cost of $40,000 for the Department, after a year and a half of aggressive campaigning for a helicopter fleet by then-Fire Chief Keith Klinger.

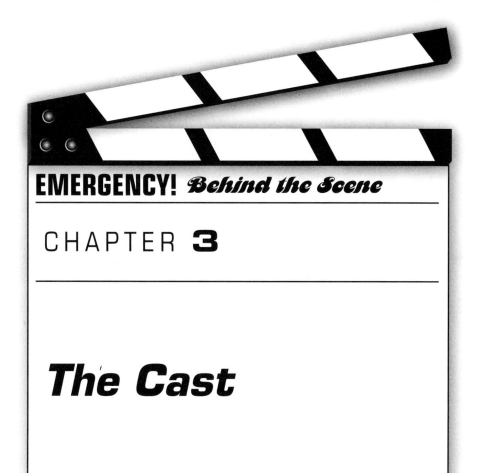

EMERGENCY! *Behind the Scene*

CHAPTER **3**

The Cast

Squad 51

The crew of Squad 51 consisted of two LA County firefighter/paramedics. Randolph Mantooth ("Johnny") and Kevin Tighe ("Roy") both made themselves available for several ride-alongs with Squads 36 in Carson and 59 at Harbor General in preparation for their roles. Tighe rode along with firefighter/paramedics Dale Cauble and Rocky Doke on Squad 36. The on-duty paramedics went over the equipment that Tighe and Mantooth could expect to use on the new show. Both actors also spent time in Harbor General's mobile intensive care unit to learn the hospital routine.

Randolph Mantooth

Mantooth was born in Sacramento, California, on September 19, 1945, and attended Santa Barbara City College. It was during this time that he felt that acting was his true calling. He left school and enrolled in the American

Academy of Dramatic Arts in New York. After graduating, he was spotted by a Universal Studios talent agent in a play and was offered a contract. Mantooth's first role on television was in Dennis Weaver's *McCloud* (1970–1977) series. In the first episode of this series, "The Man from Taos," airing September 16, 1970, Mantooth appeared as a hospital intern.

Mantooth appeared in several small roles when a part on *The Bold Ones* changed his life. Robert A. Cinader spotted him and wanted him for the role of a firefighter/paramedic in *Emergency!*.

Mantooth was advised to change his name for television, meaning his last name, but not realizing that, he simply changed his first name from Randy to Randolph. Even so, he quickly gained popularity. During the airing of *Emergency!*, both Randy and Kevin Tighe reportedly received more than 90,000 fan letters a week. On the show, there is no mention of Mantooth's character, Johnny Gage, ever taking the Engineer's exam as Roy did in "The Promotion" (episode 3.7).

Before *Emergency!*, Mantooth appeared in an episode of *Adam-12* that aired on April 1, 1971. In this episode ("Log 88–Reason to Run") directed by Chris Nyby, Sr., Mantooth portrayed a drifter suspected of theft.

After *Emergency!* Mantooth starred in *Operation Petticoat* and *Detective School*. He also appeared on several other TV series and mini-series including *Vega$, Diagnosis Murder,* and *The Fall Guy.* He later moved back to New York where he became a regular on ABC's *Loving, General Hospital, The City,* and *As the World Turns.*

Some biographies have suggested that Mantooth served as a firefighter before his acting career began, but this is incorrect. Jim Page recalls, "I was with Randy on the day in 1971 when he was dispatched by Bob Cinader to Fire Station 36 to see what firemen do, what they look like, how they talk, etc. At that time, he didn't know a spanner wrench from a nozzle. He was already under contract to Universal as an actor." LA County Firefighter Alan Barbee (now a retired Captain) was working at Station 36 at the time and confirms that Mantooth knew nothing about firefighter gear or the uniforms before the show and even put the helmet on backwards.

It was during this orientation tour at Station 36 that Mantooth was told to cut his hair in compliance with LA County Fire Department (LACoFD) standards. Mantooth was not happy with the order but reluctantly complied. After the World Premier was completed, Page asked the cast to autograph his copy of the script. Mantooth did so but added the phrase "Make room for a long-haired fireman" to his signature. As the show progressed through the seasons, so did Mantooth's hair.

More recently, Mantooth has been hard at work for several years on his project *USAR-1* based on the work of the LACoFD's Urban Search and Rescue teams. Randy Mantooth has spoken in several cities around the country about paramedic and EMT preparedness in the United States. In October 2004, he was the keynote speaker at the New Jersey First Aid Council's convention in celebration of its 75th anniversary. In March 2005, Mantooth spoke at the EMS Today Conference in Philadelphia, where he participated in a tribute to Jim Page.

Kevin Tighe (John Kevin Fishburn)

Kevin was born in Los Angeles on August 13, 1944, and was already trying out for acting parts by the age of 10. This was not surprising because his father was also an actor. He was working with the Royal Shakespeare Theater in London when he was selected for the role of Roy DeSoto with Universal. He was hired after reading only four lines of script, 1 week before shooting was to begin for the *Emergency!* World Premier movie.

During the series, Roy DeSoto, on at least three occasions, thought about quitting the paramedic program or changing careers: (1) in the "Problem" (episode 2.1); (2) in "The Promotion" (3.7), when he actually passed the Engineer's test and was promoted to engineer, which would have forced him to leave the paramedic program (which he knew about before taking the exam), but he eventually turned the promotion down; and (3) in the crossover *Sierra* episode titled "The Urban Ranger," when he considered becoming a Park Ranger.

"The wonderful thing about our show," Tighe said in 1974, "is that lives have been saved because of it. Paramedic programs have been set up all around the country as a result of [*Emergency!*]. They are not all necessarily associated with fire departments; some are voluntary. Los Angeles County gets requests from all over the [United States] asking how to set up paramedic programs. It's just great."

Tighe has kept busy appearing in dozens of movies, stage plays, and TV programs, including *What's Eating Gilbert Grape, Roadhouse, City of Hope, Another 48 Hours, Rose Red, Law and Order,* and most recently appearing in *LOST*. He appeared as a Los Angeles city battalion chief in an unaired pilot about firefighters filmed in 1997 titled *The 119*. Tighe is currently deeply involved in providing hospice care for terminally ill patients and their families.

Engine 51 Captains

There were three main Captains serving on A shift at Station 51. There actually was a fourth, presented in Chapter 4.

Richard "Dick" Hammer

Prior to joining the fire department, Dick Hammer was a basketball player for the University of Southern California (USC) Trojans. His team made it to the NCAA Final Four in 1954, where Hammer was named the Most Inspirational Player.

Hammer joined the LACoFD in 1959, graduating the academy January 25, 1960. He later earned a spot on the fifteen-man U.S. Olympic volleyball team that went to Tokyo in 1964. The guys in the station covered for him during practice and during the Olympics. After the Olympics, Hammer continued playing and coached volleyball teams at Loyola and USC, where he met Tom Selleck. They later became good friends, often auditioning for the same commercials. Later, Dick and his wife visited Selleck in Hawaii while he was filming *Magnum P.I.*

Hammer was later stationed at Fire Station 60 at Universal. While there, he earned his Screen Actors Guild (SAG) card and began appearing in commercials. Ironically, his first would be as a firefighter in an Aunt Jemima pancake commercial. The casting director, inquiring if Hammer was a real firefighter, stated that they needed someone who knew what he was doing because the scene required him to slide down a firehouse pole. Hammer went on to appear in more than 100 commercials. During the 1970s Hammer portrayed the Marlboro man, even though he did not smoke and, unlike the other Marlboro actors, was the only one not a real cowboy. Although Hammer was paid for his time during the shoot, he never received any residuals for his television or print advertisement appearances.

According to Hammer's wife Betty, Cinader knew him from working together at Universal. Hammer's crew from Station 60 was often on the set during fire scenes or other hazardous filming for safety. Cinader asked Hammer to try out for the role of the Captain in *Emergency!* because Jack Webb insisted that a "real" firefighter be involved in the show.

Hammer used his real name and appeared as Captain Hammer in Episodes 1.1 through 1.9. Hammer left the series prior to the end of the first season because he had too many irons in the fire, so to speak. According to his wife, "Learning the lines was difficult for him on top of all the other work he had to do as head Fire Captain of the Studio." The series took up just too much of the rest of his time off that he wanted to spend with his family. Dick Friend recalls while on a break from filming, Hammer and he discussed that he was not sure about continuing with the series and Friend stated, "Dick, you're a Captain, so just be yourself." Hammer left the series prior to season's end.

In 1973 Hammer graced the cover of Jim Page's book *Effective Company Command*. It was a photo of Hammer standing up in the open-cab Crown,

Engine 60, on the lot at Universal. Subsequent reprints, the latest in 1996, in paperback (original was hardcover with dust jacket) would have only a red cover with the title and author's name.

Dick Hammer was also a popular substitute teacher for the Long Beach School District. In 1983, after 24 years in the department, he retired. His wife Betty says that Hammer kept the magnetic "51" disk from his engine as a memento of the show; she still has it on her refrigerator and is saving it for their grandchildren.

John Smith (Robert Earl "Dutch" Van Orden)

Smith was hired to finish the rest of season 1 as the Captain at Station 51. He was credited as Captain Hammer in end credits in Episodes 1.10 and Episode 1.11. Smith's real name "Van Orden" is on his turn-out coat, not "Hammer." Smith and Robert Fuller (Dr. Brackett) appeared together in an earlier television program, *Laramie,* as Slim Sherman and Jess Harper, respectively. They starred together in the western, which aired from 1959–1963. And like Dick Hammer, Smith also appeared in print advertisements, including ones for Del Monte Foods. He was also listed as one of TV's Top Stars in 1959. Smith was unavailable to commit to continuing the series during the show's hiatus.

Michael Alden Norell

The third Captain in the series, who would remain until the series ended, was Mike Norell. He joined the cast in season 2 as Captain Hank Stanley. Norell had been in California for several months without getting an acting job, and, in the summer of 1972, his agent sent him to an audition with Cinader for the part of a deputy sheriff. There were only about ten actors at the casting call, and Norell recalls:

> As we waited outside the producer's office, the first guy, then the second guy, came stomping out saying, "I'm calling the Guild." We all wondered what the hell was going on in there. I was third. I went into the office. Robert Cinader sat behind his chair wearing red glasses. Behind him was a police radio. We talked for a minute, and then another guy in the room began asking me questions. He was obviously a cop—crew cut, cheap suit, white socks. He asked me, "Mr. Norell, when was the last time you were arrested?"
>
> I was pretty startled, but I managed to try for a joke. "Well, you caught a pretty big criminal," I said. "My last arrest was in 1959 by the Virginia State Police. They nailed me for speeding."
>
> The cop said, "How did you feel about your treatment at the hands of the law at that time?" I sort of laughed and said, "Hey, I was guilty...."
>
> "Mr. Norell," [the cop] said, and he had sort of a high-pitched cop voice, "In your depiction of a law enforcement officer on television, would you wish in any way to take revenge on

the law enforcement establishment for your treatment at the hands of the law at the time of your last arrest?"

"For Christ sake," I said, "my father was a general in the Army. I was a captain in the Army. I don't hate cops. You want me to play a cop, I'll happily cut my hair and take your money and do my best. Now if that's out of the way, would anybody like to hear me read anything?"

They all stared at me.

I went home and called my agent and said we could forget *that* job.

That evening, Norell recalls, his agent called and told him that they wanted him for the part of the fire captain and were offering him a role in twenty-two episodes. Dick Hammer and John Smith were no longer available, and Cinader thought that Norell would be good for the part. "I purely lucked into the job!" Norell insisted.

In preparation for his role, Norell did a ride-along with LA County Fire Captain Morgan Peterson at Station 95. He also talked with LACoFD staff associated with the program, including Public Information Officer Dick Friend, because he wanted to "do it right," a sentiment shared by many of the cast and crew of *Emergency!*. For the most part, Norell advises, "We just all did what the TAs (and Mike Stoker) told us to do."

Norell recalls that when he first took over the role of Captain, some of the LACoFD chiefs and captains complained that his part didn't have enough action or authority. "That was, of course," Norell explains, "because Randy and Kevin were the stars and I wasn't." However, he insists that these complaints resulted in greater dialogue for his character and, hence, a more realistic depiction.

"About halfway through my first season," Norell shares, "some visiting Fire Chief came up to me on the set and said, 'You know, you seem to get a little too excited when you pull up on a response. What you have to remember is that the Captain has been to a thousand house fires. It's routine.' I thought this was a terrific note and I immediately started trying to be as cool as possible."

Norell enjoyed being a part of the show and seeing its impact on the field of emergency medicine. "It became evident as the show went on," he relates, "that it was having a huge impact, which made all of us feel really good. LA was really one of the first cities to have firemen/paramedics and it was working great. I can't tell you how many people have told me personally or written to me over the years that they had been inspired to become firefighters or EMTs from watching *Emergency!*. It's nice to feel that we were part of something a little more important than just entertainment."

Norell sought out the "day players," actors who were hired for just one day on the set, to make friends and help them with their parts. "I always offered to rehearse as much as the guy wanted, and told him not to worry if he dried up or got it confused, because I'd bail him out and either ask the right questions or ad lib something myself," he relates. These actors were often very nervous, Norell recalls, because large special effects like fires or explosions often meant only one take per scene, so they had to get it right the first time.

Norell enjoyed his job on *Emergency!*, but he also remembers the downside—lots of waiting around, often outside in the heat. But, he says, "When I was actually working, I enjoyed it. Of course, I enjoyed it a lot more on those fairly rare occasions when I had a really nice part in the episode."

To show you Mike's humor, we had what may be the best of the 'dog ate my homework' stories ever. During our correspondence with Mike, while working on this book, Mike 'sent' the bulk of the information to co-author Rozane. Unfortunately he hit the 'delete' key and lost all his work, including, the questions. Mike said in his defense, "By the way, the best one [excuse for not turning in work] I came up with was in seventh grade with my art notebook, which I hadn't completed. I told the teacher that my grandmother had just passed away and her last dying wish was that my art notebook be buried with her. The teacher said that was pretty damn good, so if I turned it in the next day, I would only lose one grade." So, Mike stated, "I have copied the questions into a document in Windows, so if I lose them again, it will be because my grandmother has died and requested that my entire hard drive be buried with her."

Fortunately, it did not get lost the second time.

Engineer—Charles Michael "Mike" Stoker

The Fire Department insisted that only a real firefighter drive LA County engines, both on and off camera. Notices went out to all the stations looking for a driver with a SAG card. Stoker, who had a SAG card, saw the notice on the bulletin board at Station 65 (where he worked most of the time while filming the show) but did not think much of appearing on camera. It was not until after the insistence of Jim Page and Dick Friend that Stoker applied for the job as the engineer on *Emergency!*.

He had worked with Page earlier when both were at Station 69 in Topanga Canyon, and, like Dick Hammer, had been doing some commercials and print ads for several years. Stoker was also one of four members of the group to bring the Ward LaFrance engine, which replaced Engine 60 and Engine 127, at the beginning of season 2 (see Chapter 17).

Stoker relates that he received the script about 1 week in advance so he could arrange his work schedule to appear on the set when needed. He traded shifts with several other firefighters so that he wouldn't miss important shoots and would work longer hours to make up for the favors. "As I was under contract, the pay was the same, whether I appeared in an episode or not," Stoker said, but he never had to miss an episode due to conflicting obligations. There were, he admits, a few times he asked to be excused if he had only one or two lines, and on those rare occasions, the Transportation Captain would move the rig for the scene.

Stoker met his future wife Peggy on the set toward the end of the series. She was a paramedic instructor at Harbor General who occasionally read over the scripts and was invited to a shooting. Stoker said he invited her to an end-of-season wrap party, and they were married 6 weeks later and had three children together.

Stoker said that people on calls that he responded to often recognized him, and he recognized that the attention given to *Emergency!* was making an impact on a larger scale. "Fire Chiefs from all over the country frequently visited the set to report of the impact the show had on their budget etc. in their respective cities," he said.

While his role on *Emergency!* was as an Engineer, this term changed in the late 1970s to Firefighter Specialist, because the job entailed being an inspector, truck engineer, and camp foreman among other duties. The position of apparatus driver is still called engineer in most other departments, although it may be called driver, chauffeur, or motor pump operator in other communities.

Stoker served on the LACoFD for more than 30 years. He was actually promoted to Engineer about midway through the series. He was promoted to Captain after the series ended and was assigned to Station 106 for a time before retiring in 1996. When asked about taking the promotional exam for Battalion Chief (BC), he said, "It was obvious after awhile that trying for BC would be futile. I was not willing to do the necessary things to build a background for the job...no training, fire prevention, or central city experience. I chose to work close to home and be a family man." He currently divides his time between Montana and his rental in Buenos Aires, Argentina, and his beach home in Punta del Este in Uruguay.

The Jump Seats

Rounding out the rest of Engine 51's crew is Marco López (who used his real name for his character), considered the best cook at the station, and Tim Donnelly as Firefighter Chet Kelly, the station jokester. Because of the skill and ease with which they portrayed their characters, many people thought Tim and Marco were real LA County firefighters. Marco López said, "People always thought that I was a real fireman, probably because I

used my real name in the show like Mike Stoker did. That has been a com-
pliment all my life." Both Tim and Marco were in several early episodes
of *Dragnet* and *Adam-12,* but they never appeared together in the same
episode.

Marco Antonio López

Marco López had worked for Jack Webb since 1966 at the Mark VII studios. He appeared in seven episodes of *Dragnet* as a police officer, but he
was primarily Webb's stand-in and double during the series. López also
worked at Paramount Studios (in two episodes of *Mission Impossible*) and at
20th Century Fox (where he worked on Irwin Allen's *Voyage to the Bottom
of the Sea*).

López recalls, "I was told that I would be on a new show called *Emergency!* and that I would be a permanent cast member. This was in 1971 and
I worked on the show through 1977. My salary was at the bottom of the list
along with Mike Stoker."

López underwent a rigorous 2-week training session before starting
the pilot and also went on several ride-alongs. His character was written
to mirror his own real-life enjoyment of cooking. López says that none of
the recipes used on the show (such as the infamous "Roy's Beef Whatever,"
"Capt's Clam Chowder," "Butterscotch Bean Dip," and "Johnny's Green
Stew") were real; they were simply a figment of the writer's imagination.
López's real recipes, however, were enjoyed by cast and crew behind the
scenes and during cast parties so much that he eventually opened his own
catering business as well as published a cookbook of his favorites.

Timothy "Tim" David Donnelly

While Tim Donnelly's father was working as Unit Manager for Jack Webb
on *Dragnet 1967,* Webb discovered that Tim was an actor, and Webb was
quick to offer him a job. Webb got a script, handed it to Donnelly, and said,
"We shoot next week." Donnelly went on to work in five more *Dragnet*
episodes, and Webb soon became his mentor.

Several years later, after returning home from a trip to Europe, Donnelly's mother told him to go immediately to Universal Studios, where his
father and Cinader were waiting. They were working on casting for *Emergency!* All Donnelly had to do to get the part was cut his hair and shave his
beard. Although he admits he felt a bit naked, it was worth it to play the
part of Firefighter Chester "Chet" B. Kelly.

To train for his new role, Donnelly ran with the paramedics in Carson
for about 2 weeks. The "jokester" character emerged in the fourth or fifth
episode, and the producers just went with it. "I guess I sort of followed the

character," he recalls. Chet studied for the Engineer's exam in at least three episodes, although apparently he never took the test.

Donnelly realized early on what a large impact the show was making, and he appreciated the real firefighter/paramedics and the difference they were making. He recalls, "We had lots of town heroes, young ones that visited our set. We all embraced them for what they did."

Donnelly now helps run a soup kitchen in his hometown, and he says it's the best experience he's ever had. "The first day," he relates, "they had me cooking for 250 people for lunch. I now cook Mondays and Tuesdays and help wash dishes or anything else that is needed." He insists that "working for the homeless and needy is a great teaching tool for all involved."

The "Voice" of *Emergency!*

Sam Lanier

Sam Lanier was a real dispatcher for LA County from 1958 to 1977. He was heard in every episode and occasionally seen in the communications center. After retiring from the Fire Department, he became a fire safety advi-

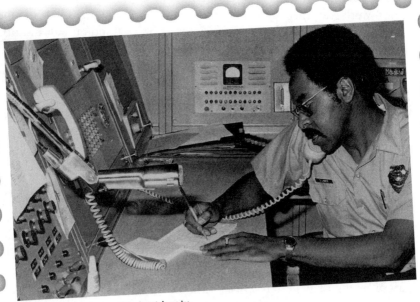

PHOTO 3-1   Sam Lanier at the dispatch center.
Source: Courtesy of Los Angeles County Fire Department, Photo Unit.

sor to film and TV production companies throughout the Los Angeles area (**Photo 3-1**).

Rampart Hospital Staff

A December 1971 press release from Universal Studios and NBC gave top billing to Robert Fuller, Julie London, and Bobby Troup, the hospital staff actors. They all spent time at Harbor General in preparation for their roles.

Robert Fuller
Fuller played the role of Dr. Kelly Brackett, head of the hospital's Emergency Department, modeled after Harbor General's Dr. J. Michael Criley.

Fuller recalls, "When we started *Emergency!* everything went so fast. From the day I walked into Jack Webb's office and walked out with twelve pages of the World Premier, we were to start shooting in ten days. I had just taken my cowboy boots off, put a white coat on, and Jack handed me a 12-pound Dolan medical dictionary…" Just a few days before filming began, Fuller spent one day at Harbor General Hospital and one at the Fire Department in preparation.

He felt very close to the rest of the crew and says that he "dearly loved Julie and Bobby and got along great with the boys." Long after *Emergency!* Fuller teamed up in 1997 with Randy Mantooth and Kevin Tighe's daughter Jennifer for an episode of *Diagnosis Murder*, which was directed by Chris Nyby II. When asked what it was like working together again, Fuller stated, "It was like old home week."

Fuller relates, "As the show progressed I saw the statistics rise across the country about the work the paramedics were doing and was very proud to be a part of *Emergency!*. I'm not surprised the show is still popular after 30 years, it was a great show for children and adults…"

Robert Fuller received his Hollywood Walk of Fame star in 1975. He was driven to the ceremony in Squad 51. When asked about his current plans, he replied, "The only work I plan to do is catching a big fish."

Julie London (Julie Peck)
London played the part of Nurse Dixie McCall, the Emergency Department's head nurse, which was modeled after Nurse Carol Bebout at Harbor General. London was nominated for a Golden Globe Award in 1974 for "Best TV actress in a Drama Series" for her work in *Emergency!*. She has a Hollywood Walk of Fame Star for her music work. Her last acting role was Dixie in the *Emergency!* TV Movie, *Survival on Charter 220*. London was married to Jack Webb from 1947 through 1953 and to Bobby Troup from

1959 until his death in 1999. Julie also appeared in an episode of *Laramie* with Robert Fuller and John Smith, "Queen of Diamonds" (episode 2.1), which aired September 20, 1960.

Robert "Bobby" Wesley Troup, Jr.

Emmy award winner Bobby Troup, as Dr. Joe Early, portrayed a wealthy Beverly Hills neurosurgeon in private practice who frequently volunteered his services. On the first day of shooting for the World Premier, Webb told Troup, who was sporting a ponytail, to get a haircut.

Ronald Fredrick Pinkard

Pinkard played the role of the third physician at Rampart, Dr. Mike Morton, joining the cast in the fifth episode. Pinkard made his first appearance as Dr. Tom Gray in the *Emergency!* World Premier. Pinkard was hired for what was supposed to be a one-scene, one-day shoot. "I was supposed to help Robert Fuller in an operating room scene," says Pinkard. "They didn't realize how much I knew. After my Navy training, twirling instruments around and using bloody sponges was natural. So when they said 'Action,' I just went into it like I was treating a patient in crisis, and that one-day job turned into eight years as Dr. Mike Morton." Pinkard appeared in the pilot, under the name of Dr. Gray, but he did not like the name and it was changed it to Dr. Mike Morton for the remainder of the series.

Like Tim Donnelly and Marco López, Pinkard had been appearing in other Jack Webb productions (such as *Adam-12*) prior to being cast in *Emergency!* and, like Randy Mantooth and Marco López, he also spent time on ABC's *General Hospital* later in his career. Pinkard worked as a Naval consultant on Tom Clancy's blockbuster hit *The Hunt for Red October*. Since *Emergency!* Ron Pinkard served with the Mayor's Office in Denver, Colorado, as the Deputy Director of Art, Culture, and Film from 1991 until his retirement in 2002.

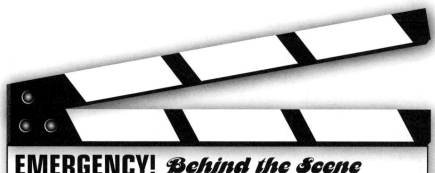

EMERGENCY! *Behind the Scene*

CHAPTER 4

Supporting Cast and Guest Stars

The following are just a few of the recurring supporting cast members and guest stars that Universal Studios relied on over the course of *Emergency!*'s run.

Firefighters

Colby Chester
Colby Chester appeared in the pilot episode and *Emergency!* movie as Fireman Tony Freeman—as Gage's partner on Rescue 10—and in "Transition" (episode 4.15) as firefighter/paramedic Gil Robinson. He later appeared as Ranger Matt Harper in *The Rangers,* the pilot for the 1974 NBC short-lived series *Sierra* (see Chapter 15).

James Gilbert Richardson III
Richardson played Craig Brice, a highly respected paramedic whose perfectionist attitude and by-the-book philosophy made him a very difficult

person to work with. He was paired briefly with Roy while Johnny was in the hospital, and even easy-going Roy had problems dealing with him. Craig served on the paramedic advisory committee and competed in the Fireman's Olympics. He was promoted to Captain at the same time as Johnny and Roy. Richardson appeared in three episodes, two of which he wrote.

He also starred in *Sierra* in 1974 (another Webb and Cinader project) in the role of a paramedic Park Ranger named Tim Cassidy (see Chapter 15).

Art Balinger

Balinger portrayed Battalion Chief Conrad in fourteen episodes, including the pilot. He also appeared in several episodes of *Dragnet* and *Adam-12*. He also appeared in *Towering Inferno* as a TV announcer.

Art Gilmore

Gilmore appeared in two episodes as a Battalion Chief. An accomplished radio and television announcer, he portrayed himself or a narrator in more than 100 movies and TV series. He also appeared in several episodes of *Dragnet* and *Adam-12*.

William Boyett

Boyett appeared in season 6 as a Captain at Station 39 and in six episodes and two post-series movies as Battalion Chief McConnike.[1] He also appeared in *Rescue 8* and several episodes of *Dragnet*. In *Adam-12,* he appeared as Sergeant MacDonald. In his many roles on TV and film, he often portrayed a police officer, including two *Star Trek: TNG* episodes. Boyett was among many of *Emergency!*'s supporting role characters who appeared in the western *Laramie* with Robert Fuller and John Smith.

William Bryant

Bryant appeared as an Engine Captain in twelve episodes and both post-series movies filmed in Los Angeles, all from different stations. Ironically he was the Fire Leader in the original *Battlestar Galactica* series episode, "Fire in Space." Prior to *Emergency!,* he appeared in three *Laramie* episodes.

Dick Bakalyan

Bakalyan appeared in three episodes of *Emergency!* in two different roles. He played Charlie (or Charley), the department mechanic on Repair 14, the department repair vehicle, in episodes 6.15, "Breakdown," and 6.19, "The Boat." This character was profiled as a grouchy station mechanic who was very pro-

---

[1] Before Stanley was promoted to Captain, he was an Engineer under then Captain McConnike, and they had quite a past. There was an incident of the burning of McConnike's hat by then Engineer Stanley and we never discovered why.

tective of the fire department's vehicles and had a short temper. Bakalyan portrayed a different character in episode 5.6, "The Indirect Method."

Bakalyan also played a a retired LA County firefighter and tavern owner named Charlie in *Pine Canyon Is Burning* with Kent McCord, and he appeared in an episode of *Laramie* with Robert Fuller and John Smith.

Dick Friend
LA County Fire Department's Public Information Officer appeared as himself in "Inferno" (episode 3.21) and "The Screenwriter" (episode 4.1). He also did several voiceovers.

Scott Arthur Allen
Allen reprised his role as Firefighter/Paramedic Kirk in three episodes: "Nurses Wild" (episode 1.6), "Weird Wednesday" (episode 1.8), and "Not Available" (episode 6.2).

John Anderson
Although he appeared only once, Anderson is included here because he was the fourth Captain serving at Station 51. This well-known actor appeared in "The Smoke Eater" in season 4, taking over for the vacationing Captain Stanley. He also appeared in several *Laramie* episodes with John Smith and Robert Fuller.

Gary Crosby
Son of legendary crooner Bing Crosby and the uncle of Denise Crosby (Lt. Tasha Yar and Sela on *Star Trek: TNG*), Crosby appeared in four episodes of *Emergency!*. In two, he played Fireman Tom Wheeler from Station 110, and he also appeared in the spin-off *905-Wild* as an animal control officer. He had a reoccurring role as Officer Ed Wells in *Adam-12*.

Donald Mantooth
Randy Mantooth's brother, Donald, appeared in two episodes of *Emergency!*: "Green Thumb" (episode 3.17) as a paramedic and "Foreign Trade" (episode 4.9). He also appeared in *Sierra*. He and Randy worked together in an episode of *Battlestar Galactica* ("Greetings from Earth," episode 1.19), which aired February 25, 1979. He is a freelance photographer who worked with Robert Pratt (*Emergency!* guest star) in Pratt Tooth Productions and once photographed President Ronald Reagan.

Bryan Cutler and Larry Manetti
These two men both portrayed the same character, Fireman/Paramedic Bert Dwyer. Cutler appeared in season 4's "Daisy's Pick" and "Fugitive"; Manetti appeared in "Rules of Order" in season 6.

Other Guest Actors

Ronne Troup

Bobby Troup's daughter, Ronne, appeared in three episodes of *Emergency!*, including one with her sister Kelly. She also appeared in four episodes of *Adam-12*. Her latest work was in *Cold Case* in 2003, episode 1.23.

Randall Carver

Carver appeared in three episodes (2.9, 4.2, and 5.8) and the post-series movie *Survival on Charter 220*—all as different characters. He said that he really admired the technical advisors, who "made sure all the situations were handled accurately, even at the risk of redundancy."

Kenneth Tobey

Tobey appeared in several episodes and as the Ferry Boat Captain in the *Emergency!* movie *Most Deadly Passage*. He was also one of the stars of an earlier rescue drama, *Whirlybirds*, which aired from 1957 to 1960.

Katherine Kelly-Wiget

Wiget played Roy's wife Joanne DeSoto in the *Emergency!* pilot and in "The Wedworth-Townsend Act," episodes 5.15 and 5.16 (the pilot rerun in flashback format). She is referred to (over the phone) as Ann in "Hang-Up" (episode 1.10). Her only other appearance in the series was that of Betty Snyder in "Musical Mania" (episode 2.11).

Tom Williams

Williams is probably remembered most on *Emergency!* as the heart attack victim in the "Stewardess" (episode 5.1). He was in episode 6.22 "Upward and Onward" as the TV director and appeared as a conventioneer in the *Emergency!* movie *The Convention*. Williams also had roles in episodes of *Adam-12* and in *Code R*, produced by Ed Self.

Kip Niven

Niven appeared in four episodes (1.7, 2.5, 2.14, and 3.11), all portraying different characters. He appeared in *Sierra* and portrayed Reverend Marshal on *The Waltons*.

Ann Morgan Guilbert

Probably better known as Millie Helper on the *Dick Van Dyke Show*, Guilbert appeared in the World Premier movie as well as in various episodes in seasons 2 and 4.

Ted Gehring

Gehring appeared in several episodes in every season of *Emergency!* as various characters and in the *Emergency!* movie, *Most Deadly Passage.*

Sheila James-Kuehl

James-Kuehl appeared in only one episode, "The Tycoons" (episode 5.23). She is probably most remembered on TV as Zelda Gilroy on *The Many Loves of Dobie Gillis.* She graduated from Harvard Law School in 1978 and served as a California Senator for Los Angeles Senate District 23. After her election in 1994, she served for 6 years in the State Assembly serving the 41st district and was elected to the State Senate in 2000 and 2004. She was the first woman named President pro Tempore of the California State Assembly.

Boot and Henry

There were two canine mascots throughout the series. In seasons 2 through 5, Boot, a Benji-looking dog, inhabited the station. Boot's original name was Duke in the first script draft.

In season 6, a Bassett Hound named Henry (as Captain Hank Stanley insisted, "Don't you call it Hank!") became Chet's (played by Tim Donnelly) pride and joy. When asked about Henry during an interview, Tim recalls, "Henry was a very slobbery, smelly, and shedding dog and was going to be fired from the show until I offered to do scenes with him." Tim recalls that the dog's trainer said that if Henry couldn't work on the show, he would be put to sleep, so Tim agreed to work with him. "Actually," Tim said, "I knew that if I worked with the dog I'd get a lot more scenes!"

Both of the dogs were given mysterious traits. Boot had ESP, knowing when a call was coming in, and Henry made his food and dish magically disappear without moving from the couch.

Police Officers

Many actors worked on the show as police officers, mostly uncredited. Those who stand out are listed here.

Vince Howard (Vince House)

Howard appeared in 29 episodes of *Emergency!* and the two Los Angeles–filmed movies as Motorcycle Officer Vince Howard. He was often the policeman on the scene when the engine or squad arrived. He was always ready to lend a hand when the firefighters needed extra help. In almost ninety guest appearances on series television, he would most often portray a police officer. Vince was a member of the quartet singing group, The Rhythm Aces, in 1950s and later was part of the group, The 4 Jays and The Magic Notes.

James McEachin

McEachin appeared in four episodes as several different characters, including Police Lieutenant Ron Crockett. He later had a recurring role in the Perry Mason movies as Lieutenant Brocklin. McEachin is a Korean War veteran and the recipient of the Silver Star, Bronze Star, and Purple Heart. In September 2005, McEachin was appointed as Army Reserve Ambassador.

William Bryant

Bryant was previously mentioned as an Engine Captain, but his first appearance in *Emergency!* was that of Police Sergeant Pierce in "Kids" (episode 2.2).

Scott Smith (Francis Smith)

Smith is one of the few Los Angeles County Fire Department employees credited as appearing in an episode of *Emergency!*. He appears not as a firefighter, but as a Sheriff in "Cook's Tour" (episode 1.3).

Colby Chester

As well as appearing as a fireman in two episodes, Chester appeared in "Nurses Wild" (episode 1.6) as a Deputy Sheriff.

Scott Gourlay

Gourlay appeared as Officer Scotty in several episodes. Throughout the series, he also played many other characters and worked as a stuntman (see Chapter 11).

Jim B. Smith

Smith appeared as a police sergeant in three episodes and as a different character in the *Emergency!* movie *Survival on Charter 220*. He portrayed a police officer in several episodes of *Dragnet* and *Adam-12*. Ironically, he portrayed a fireman operating an LA County foam truck in an episode of *CHiPs*, "Green Thumb Burglar" (1.8), directed by Chris Nyby II. He also appeared as Park Ranger Jack Moore in Cinader's *The Rangers*, the pilot for *Sierra*.

Rand Brooks

Rand Brooks appeared as a police officer in the World Premier *Emergency!* movie. Brooks gained a small niche in film history with his performance as Charles Hamilton, the ill-fated first husband of Scarlett O'Hara (Vivien Leigh), in the 1939 movie *Gone With the Wind*. He spent the next several years in Westerns, most frequently appearing as Lucky Jenkins in the Hopalong Cassidy series. On television, Brooks was seen as Corporal Boone on *The Adventures of Rin Tin Tin* (1956–1958). Rand Brooks was at one time married to comedian Stan Laurel's daughter, Lois, with whom he owned and operated the largest private emergency ambulance service in Los Angeles County (Professional Ambulance Service) until selling it to the AMR ambulance company. Brooks appeared in *Rescue 8* as a Rescue Firefighter on Squad 3.

Ambulance Attendants

Some of the attendants on *Emergency!* were off-duty LA City paramedics or EMTs from Snyder or Goodhew ambulance companies. Many times, the stuntmen on contract to Universal would perform the duty (see Chapter 11).

Raul Moreno

Moreno was not a credited member of the cast or even paid when he appeared because he was only in background scenes as a teenager. He grew up in Wilmington, California, not that far from Station 127, and he often hung around to watch the crew filming. He appeared as an extra or stand-in in about ten episodes, including the warehouse fire scene in "Zero" (episode 3.10) and stock footage of Squad 51 driving around. "The assistant director told us to sit on [our] bikes and look natural, which we did," Moreno recalls. "During breaks and after filming, most everyone would come over to sign autographs....Marco and Tim were the best. They would let kids sit on the truck and put the helmets on."

Nurses

Deidre Hall

Hall appeared in six episodes in season 2 as Nurse Sally Lewis at Rampart. She was also a nurse at Rampart in the *Adam-12* crossover, "Lost and Found." Hall went on in 1976 to portray Marlena Evans in the daytime soap *Days of Our Lives*.

Patricia Mickey

Mickey appeared in five episodes in season 1 and one episode in season 2, as Student Nurse Sharon Walter, who was chided by Dixie for running in the hallway. Before appearing on *Emergency!*, Mickey appeared as one of Dean Martin's Golddiggers in 1971 and was once married to Phil Everly of the musical group The Everly Brothers.

Anne Schedeen

Schedeen appeared in five episodes, two as a Rampart Nurse.

Virginia Gregg

Gregg portrayed Wilma Jacobs, RN, in several episodes of *Emergency!* in seasons 1 and 3.

Molli Benson

Benson played Rampart Nurse Gail in four episodes.

Chris Forbes

Forbes appeared as Student Nurse Ellen Bart in five episodes.

Lillian Lehman

Lehman portrayed Nurse Carol Williams in seven aired episodes and one unaired, but on the cast list.

Karen Philipp

Philipp appeared in episodes 2.21 and 3.1 as a Nurse. She is more well known as one of the singers in *Brazil 66* and as Lieutenant Dish in the television series *M*A*S*H*.

Michele Noval (Michele Noirae)

Noval played Nurse Mary in "Details" (episode 4.12) and "The Boat" (episode 6.19).

Dena Dietrich

Dietrich appeared in "Surprise" in season 4 as Nurse Betty. This famous actress is best recognized in her white gown, adorned with a crown of daisies, as Mother Nature in the Chiffon Margarine commercials that ran from 1971 through 1979. Her utterance, "It's not *nice* to fool Mother Nature!" gave her worldwide recognition.

Brit Lund (Britt Lind)

Lund appeared as Nurse Daisy in "Daisy's Pick" (episode 4.7), the object of Johnny's attention. She also appeared in the TV movie, *Pine Canyon Is Burning*, as a school teacher.

Gretchen Corbett

Corbett played Johnny's physical therapist in "The Nuisance" (episode 5.24), as well as the Stewardess in "The Stewardess" (episode 5.1).

Carole Cooke

Cooke portrayed Nurse Beauxchet in "The Nuisance" (episode 5.24).

Famous Guest Stars

For some of these guests, it was one of their first TV appearances, and they would go on to star in television programs, feature films, and other endeavors. Other actors were already established celebrities in their own right.

Famous Guest Stars	
Name	**Episode**
Kareem Abdul-Jabbar	"Foreign Trade," 4.9
Robert Alda	"Syndrome," 2.16
John Anderson	"The Smoke Eater," 4.16
Elizabeth Baur	"Saddled," 2.6
Shelley Berman	"The Screenwriter," 4.1
X. Brands	"Alley Cat," 3.3
Dick Butkus	"The Hard Hours," 3.18
Ruth Buzzi	"Grateful," 5.21
Patti Cohoon	"The Girl on the Balance Beam," 5.18
Jackie Coogan	"Trainee," 2.8
Cathy Lee Crosby	"Virus," 2.4
Gary Crosby	"Brushfire," 1.4; "Publicity Hound," 1.7; "Crash," 1.11; "905-Wild," 4.22
Larry Csonka	"The Screenwriter," 4.1
Tony Dow	"Brushfire," 1.4
Dick Enberg	"Zero," 3.10
Erik Estrada	"Details," 4.12
Jamie Farr	"Boot," 2.19 (not credited)
Melissa Gilbert	"Dinner Date," 2.10
Sharon Gless	"Fuzz Lady," 2.7; "Election," 5.3
Linda Gray	"That Time of Year," 6.4; *Steel Inferno,* movie
Mark Harmon	"905-Wild," 4.22
Mariette Hartley	"Zero," 3.10
Harold "Happy" Harriston	"The Firehouse Five, Plus One," 6.18

(continues)

Famous Guest Stars (continued)

Name	Episode
Wolfman Jack	"The Inspection," 5.5
Sheila James	"The Tycoons," 5.23
William Katt	"Weird Wednesday," 1.8
Audrey Landers	"Computer Error," 3.14
Anne Lockhart	*Steel Inferno*," movie
Kent McCord	*Emergency!*, pilot; "The Wedworth-Townsend Act," 5.15 and 5.16
Patty McCormack	"Dinner Date," 2.10; *What's a Nice Girl Like You doing...*, and *The Convention*, movies
Jock Mahoney	"The Mascot," 1.1; "Boot," 2.19
Martin Milner	*Emergency!*, pilot; "The Wedworth-Townsend Act," 5.15 and 5.16
Donny Most	"Computer Error," 3.14
Nick Nolte	"The Hard Hours," 3.18
Marion Ross	"Inheritance Tax," 3.9
Mike Roy (TV chef)	"Pressure 165," 5.7
Neil 'Bing' Russell	"Computer Error," 3.14; "I'll Fix It," 4.2; and "Pressure 165," 5.7
Mort Sahl	"Hang-Up," 1.10
Pamela Susan Shoop	"That Time of Year," 6.4
Bobby Sherman	"Fools," 3.16
Laurette Spang	"Dinner Date," 2.10; "The Old Engine," 3.2
Mark Spitz	"Quicker Than the Eye," 4.8
Larry Storch	"Saddled," 2.6; "Computer Error," 3.14
Vic Tayback	"Boot," 2.19
Kenneth Tobey	"Body Language," 3.12; "Surprise," 4.6; *Most Deadly Passage*, movie
John Travolta	"Kids," 2.2
Cicely Tyson	"Crash," 1.11
Dick Van Patten	"Women!," 2.9; "Grateful," 5.21
Adam West	"The Bash," 4.14
Joanne Worley	"Zero," 3.10

EMERGENCY! *Behind the Scene*

CHAPTER **5**

Production Staff

Producers

Jack Webb

Webb took on many roles including actor, producer, writer, and director. He began his radio career as a private detective in 1949 in *Pat Novak for Hire*. Later that same year Webb produced and starred in *Dragnet* for the NBC Radio Network. In 1951 *Dragnet* began its move to television. It became the highest rated police show in television history, and it was the first to be produced, directed, written, and starred-in by the same person.

In 1968 Webb's Mark VII productions produced *Adam-12,* which ran through 1975. During this time Webb produced two other series, but it would be *Emergency!* that would match the success of *Dragnet* and *Adam-12.*

Although only involved in the incipient stages of *Emergency!*, and as the World Premier director, Webb's presence was felt throughout the series. Many wonder why Webb was not given more credit for the creation of the program because without Webb there would not have been *Emergency!*. This may be true in part, but it would be his producer, Robert A. Cinader, who brought *Emergency!* to life in the form in which it was eventually seen on television.

According to Jim Page, "Jack Webb was a powerful influence on the show. Without his contacts at NBC, it would have never been created, but without the brilliance of Bob Cinader, following Jack Webb and his cronies, picking up the pieces, and turning them into a realistic action-adventure series, *Emergency!* would have had a short life." Jack Webb has two stars on the Hollywood Walk of Fame, one for Radio and the other for Television.

Robert A. Cinader

Prior to getting his start in television, Cinader worked at the United Nations in the publications division. Shortly after leaving the United Nations he joined CNP (California National Productions), a subsidiary of NBC in New York, where he eventually attained the post of vice president of programming and became involved in the distribution of *Badge 714,* the syndicated version of the original 1950s *Dragnet* series. He later transferred to Los Angeles, where he developed his first television program for CNP, *The Silent Service,* in 1957.

By 1962 Cinader became vice president and general manager of the Red Skelton Studios (formerly the Charlie Chaplin Studios), until the studio was sold to CBS and he moved to Warner Brothers. The studio is now owned by Jim Henson Productions. Cinader joined the staff of Jack Webb's Mark VII Ltd. at Universal as the associate producer of *Dragnet 1967.* During this time he became deeply involved with the Los Angeles Police Department (LAPD) in obtaining story ideas for the series. In doing so, Cinader conceived the story idea behind *Adam-12,* airing 1968–1975, although Jack Webb is credited as its creator. After leaving *Adam-12* in 1969, Cinader began to work on story lines about the Los Angeles County paramedic program in 1971. And as stated before, the rest is history.

Like he did with *Adam-12,* riding with police officers, Cinader would often ride along with the Fire Department and even respond to incidents on his own to garner ideas for fire and rescue scenes for the show. It is said that Cinader made more than 500 trips with the squads in his search for authenticity and ideas.

Cinader stated during an interview published in the August 1973 issue of *Fire Engineering* magazine, "*Emergency!* is not designed to be a documentary report of the fire service or emergency medicine, but a dramatic hour with human entertainment values." Once the scripts have gone through all their reviews by the appropriate people, Cinader said that he "locks himself up" to revise the scripts into their final form.

Besides working on *Dragnet, Adam-12,* and *Emergency!,* Cinader would work on two more of Webb's Mark VII fire- and paramedic-related features, *Pine Canyon Is Burning* and *Sierra.* Cinader was working up until his death in 1982 on *Knight Rider* as the series co-executive producer along with many other former *Emergency!* writers, producers, and directors.

Robert Cinader received several awards and citations for his contribution to emergency health services including those from the International Association of Firefighters; the LACoFD; the American Medical Association; the California Fire Rescue and Paramedic Association; the American Trauma Society; the California Fire Chief's Association, Southern Division; the California State Fireman's Association (now the California State Firefighters Association); and the County of Los Angeles. In May of 1972, Cinader and *Emergency!'s* cast and crew were commended by the Joint Rules Committee of the California State Legislature with Senator Wedworth and Assemblyman Townsend presenting the commendation to Cinader.

He was appointed to the LA County EMS Commission in 1975 and served until his death in 1982. In his honor, LA County Fire Station Station 127 in Carson, the home of TV's Station 51, was dedicated in 1985 as the Robert A. Cinader Memorial Fire Station. This is the only fire station in LA County that bears someone's name. Cinader also played a crucial role in the establishment of trauma centers nationwide.

Cinader had a slogan, "Educate through Entertainment." His theory was, you can teach through entertainment, without the audience realizing it. That most certainly was the case in this television program—like none before, or since.

Harold Jack Bloom

Although credited as being a co-creator, Bloom did not have much to do with the program other than writing a love story between Dr. Kelly Brackett and Nurse Dixie McCall for the World Premier (see Chapter 2).

Edwin "Ed" Self

Not only a writer for *Emergency!,* Self was also its producer during seasons 3, 4, and 5. He first worked on *Emergency!* during the second season while working at NBC as manager of current programming. He also produced *The Rangers* (*Sierra* pilot), and *Code R.* Self also wrote for the original *Batman* series. Ed's father, William Self, was at one time head of television programming at 20th Century Fox.

Directors

Dennis Donnelly, 1st Assistant Director

Donnelly directed eighteen episodes of *Emergency!* and one episode of Cinedar's *Sierra*. He also directed the *Adam-12* crossover ("Lost and Found") with several members of the *Emergency!* cast. Donnelly directed many other episodic television programs, including *Adam-12, Hawaii Five-O, Charlie's Angels, Dallas, The A-Team, Simon and Simon,* and many others. Previously, Dennis Donnelly had worked with his brother Tim on several *Dragnet* episodes. The brothers come from a long line of performers in the entertainment business, starting with their great-grandfather, a San Francisco and New York stage actor who has the name of another but infamous stage actor, John Wilkes (Booth). Their grandfather, Pat O'Malley, starred in silent movies, and their aunt, Kathleen O'Malley, appeared in more than fifty television programs and movies, including the *Tool Box Murders,* directed by Dennis and in which Tim also appeared.

Donnelly directed the aerial unit in *Terminal Velocity.*

Christian Nyby and Christian I. Nyby II

This father and son were often confused with each other, because both were often credited as "Chris Nyby." Both would direct several *Emergency!* episodes. Nyby, Sr., directed early western television series such as *Gunsmoke, Rawhide,* and *Wagon Train* and several episodes of *Bonanza.* Christian I. Nyby II got his start directing episodes of *Ironside* and several of Jack Webb's Mark VII projects such as *Adam-12, The Rangers, Sierra,* and *Pine Canyon Is Burning.* He would go on to direct many episodes of the *Perry Mason* series and would again direct Randy Mantooth and Robert Fuller in a *Diagnosis Murder* episode, "Malibu Fire."

Kevin Tighe

Tighe directed four episodes: 3.22, 4.3, 5.4, and 6.5.

Randy Mantooth

Mantooth directed two episodes: 5.24 and 6.14.

Cinematographers

Ellis "Bud" Thackery

The Nybys weren't the only father-and-son team working on the show. Bud and his son Frank, both cinematographers, worked on *Emergency!*. Bud sat with his camera in an unused wheelchair being pushed down a New York street as he filmed chase scenes. That was in 1964, when he was director of photography for a Kraft Theater sequence entitled "Once Upon a Savage Night." Bud Thackery began his career in 1923 at the old Warner Brothers/Sunset Boulevard Studios and was nominated for an Emmy.

Frank Thackery

Bud's son Frank worked on several of Cinader's projects, including *Sierra, Pine Canyon Is Burning,* and *Emergency!* For mobility and taking a cue from his dad, and long before the invention of the Steadicam®, he would often use an extra wheelchair as a platform in the scenes shot at Rampart with a handheld camera on his shoulder. Frank Thackery worked on many of Universal's projects, including the original *Battlestar Galactica.*

Additional Production Staff

Paul Donnelly, Executive Unit Manager

Father of Tim (*Emergency!*'s Chet Kelly) and Dennis (*Emergency!* director), Paul Donnelley had worked with Jack Webb and Robert A. Cinader on other projects, namely *Dragnet 1967.* Donnelly was the head of production for Universal Pictures and TV in the 1950s and 1960s when Lew Wasserman, president of MCA, set out to make television programs. Paul Donnelly was the first assistant director for the 1953 movie *The Wild One,* starring Marlon Brando. Although Donnelly retired in 1968, Robert A. Cinader hired Donnelly to help him put together *Emergency!.*

Mickey S. Michaels, Set Designer and Decorator

Michaels was hired to be *Emergency!*'s set decorator and would remain so for at least the first three seasons. He was very meticulous in his designs and recreations. Michaels took many photos of Fire Station 127 and Harbor General ER and measured almost every square inch to recreate them on Universal's sound stages.

Michaels matched everything from the "real" hospital interior and emergency entrance to recreate the standing sets on Universal's Sound Stage 41, which is where the interior scenes for Rampart were filmed. He included details the average viewer would not even notice (or care about), such as the correct color-coding of electrical outlets to signify which outlets are powered by the hospital's emergency generators in the event of a power failure. Sound Stage 41 was also the area where many apartment rooms and offices were constructed and used throughout the series.

The standing set on Sound Stage 33 replicated Station 127 and was virtually exact, even down to the turn-out lockers and name brands of appliances and fixtures in the kitchen and elsewhere throughout the station. According to LA County Firefighter Ray Ribar, the firefighters and technical advisors who were on the set were very impressed and could not believe they were on a sound stage—except instead of a ceiling there was a multitude of lights. LA County Firefighter Bob Hoff worked at FS127 at the time and recalled the conversations Michaels and his crew would have over getting the "correct" color of brick that would be reproduced back at Universal. (Hoff would later become a paramedic and TA for the show.)

The buildings that house Soundstages 33 (building 3265) and 41 (building 3225) are literally across the street from each other on Conopy Street at Universal. This made it quite convenient if actors had to go from one building to another to do scenes. Ironically, they are across the street, to the west, from Soundstage 30, where the *Backdraft* attraction is currently located.

Michaels was obviously just the man Webb was looking for to recreate the sets. Years earlier when Webb's *Dragnet* on NBC (1951–1959) was just getting started, Webb's meticulous eye for detail and accuracy, set him apart from the rest. According to an interview with *Time* magazine in 1954, Webb purchased the same calendars that were hanging on the walls in the real police station. There were many other details that the viewer would not notice: the telephones on the set had the same extension numbers "from downtown" when called to get to various departments such as R & I (Records and Identification), and Webb had castings of the doorknobs at City Hall made and copied to be used on the *Dragnet* set.

Michaels was honored by the Set Decorators of America and received two Academy Award nominations and two Emmy nominations. Dick Friend says of Michaels, "He would occasionally stop by at an LA County station for a ride-along. Everyone loved and admired him." LA County firefighter/paramedic Rocky Doke, a technical advisor on the show, said that both Cinader and Mickey Michaels spent many months at Station 36 during the course of the show.

Ralph Winters and Joe Reich, Casting Directors
Both Winters and Reich are credited as casting directors on many of the episodes. Reich was Universal Television's staff casting director from 1960 through 1981.

Cinnie Troup, Script Supervisor
Cinnie was Bobby Troup's daughter from his first marriage. She would work on two seasons of *Emergency!* as script supervisor and is still in the business. Her latest was a 2003 *Murder She Wrote*. She is usually credited as Cynnie Troup.

Gina Casey, Universal Studios Seamstress
Casey's role in *Emergency!* is discussed in detail in Chapter 18.

Technical Advisors
LA County Sheriff's Office (LASO)
The Sheriff's Office for the County was deeply involved in the first season of the show. They assigned deputies from the Public Information Office to act as technical advisors. During this season, all the actors portraying sheriffs and their vehicles sported the official LASO logo. However, Cinader never did develop good rapport with the LASO and decided to develop his own police force early in 1972 after repeated confrontations with the LASO technical advisors.

Location Manager and Scouts
To make the fires look realistic, the scouts kept track of the fires that made the news, examined the buildings, and checked with the owners to determine the status of repairs. If a building was usable and available for filming, it was worked into a current or future script. With the help of the set decorators, the studio would restore the burned building somewhat, to be usable for filming, and then burn it down again.

Writers
There are several writers who, for some reason, don't list *Emergency!* among their writing credits such as Carey Wilbur, who also wrote for *Lost in Space and Hawaii Five-O* and who wrote the *Star Trek* episode "The Space Seed," which inspired the movie *The Wrath of Khan.*

Many who worked for Jack Webb also wrote for other projects of his such as Preston Wood and Michael Donovan, who not only wrote for *Emergency!* but also wrote for *Dragnet, Adam-12, The Rangers,* and *Sierra.*

Another *Emergency!* writer, the writer of "Nurses Wild" in season 1, Fred Frieberger, would become executive producer of the original *Star Trek, Space 1999, The Wild Wild West,* and others as well as write for many of the popular series of the 1950s, 1960s, and 1970s.

Michael Norell (Captain Stanley)
An accomplished stage actor and writer, Norell wrote four *Emergency!* episodes (4.12, 5.6, 5.21, and 6.22). He recalls:

> I only wrote those four that aired. And let me tell you how it worked. I never wrote and submitted a script. I would be invited by Bob Cinader to pitch ideas. You'd spend an hour or so throwing out ideas for rescues and hospital stories and firehouse stories and eventually there were enough that he liked and he'd tell you to go to work. A couple of weeks later, you'd turn in a first draft. On that show, there were no rewrites by the actual credited writer. There would

be a set of pink pages that would reflect Ed Self's rewrite, then a set of blue pages that reflected Cinader's rewrite…there was no arguing. If Cinader killed your babies (as writers like to say), too bad.

Norell relates the following story about controversial episode 5.6, "The Indirect Method," about a female paramedic before LA County had any women in the department:

> It was just a story that came into my head. I wanted to deal with it much more deeply, and I wanted to deal with that, but they wouldn't let me. I tried to sell them on the idea of a female firefighter, but they wouldn't touch that either. Fact is, firefighters' wives are really the ones who hate the idea, not so much that they think there'll be hanky-panky in the firehouse, but because they are comforted to believe that whoever is beside or behind their husband is strong enough to save his life, to carry him out of danger, and most women just aren't.

Norell also tried to pitch an episode dealing with firefighters' job satisfaction, as related to property loss and trauma, but, he says, "they wouldn't touch that one either":

> I was probably not alone among writers trying to dig a little more deeply, but *Emergency!* was a "sweetheart" show, hand-in-glove with the LACoFD, and was not about to say anything remotely negative about firefighting or life-saving. Some nameless Fire Chief once told me, "The difference between a fireman and a firebug is that the firebug has his ejaculation setting and watching the fire, and the fireman has his talking about the fire the next day, and if you tell anybody I told you that, I'll have you killed."
>
> It was certainly an eye-opener when I rode about with 95's, and they pulled around the corner to a burning trash can. My reaction as a civilian was "Whew!, an easy one." Their reaction was disgust and disappointment. They wanted a big fire—all of San Pedro ablaze or a building fully-involved. That was job satisfaction. That was fun. It was what they'd been trained for, and who can blame them. It was just a bit of a shock to me. But, as I say, Bob Cinader would not touch that subject with tongs.

After the series ended, Norell penned scripts for *The Love Boat, Magnificent Seven, I Spy Returns,* and *Nash Bridges,* as well as more than forty-five movies and TV series and pilots to date.

Kevin Tighe
Tighe wrote episode 6.21.

Jim Page
Three of Page's scripts were accepted and filmed. Page also wrote a teleplay titled "Hardwood County Rescue Squad" based on his experiences with North Carolina's volunteer paramedic program, but it was rejected by NBC.

Steve Downing

Downing was an LAPD officer (and later, Commander), who wrote several scripts for Webb's *Dragnet* and *Adam-12,* and eleven scripts for *Emergency!* under the pseudonym Michael Donovan. Downing was the co-executive producer of *MacGyver* and wrote and produced the TV movie, *Without Warning: Terror in the Towers*, about the 1993 World Trade Center explosion, featuring George Clooney as a firefighter.

Preston Wood (W. Preston Wood II)

Wood wrote twenty-two episodes of *Emergency!*, more than any other writer. He also wrote for several other Mark VII projects, including *Dragnet, Adam-12, Sierra,* and *The Rangers.* Yet, among all the television writing that Wood has done over the years, he says he considers *Emergency!* his favorite.

Wood went on a few ride-alongs. He says, "They were not 'absolutely' required but were a fixture of all Jack Webb's Mark VII shows going back to the original *Dragnet* two decades earlier….I did a couple but they quickly became unproductive, as I found on writing for *Adam-12.* Sitting in the stations, trading war stories over a cup of coffee with the guys was much more efficient. I also spent a great deal of time in ERs with doctors since 40 percent to 50 percent of each episode was set in the ER with doctors who were in basic control of medical procedures in the field."

Wood worked as a program development executive for NBC from 1958 to 1961. He contributed to scripts for all three major networks and many Top 10 shows of that period, including *Bonanza, Gunsmoke, Hawaii 5-0, The Addams Family, The Wild Wild West, The Man from U.N.C.L.E, Quincy M.E.,* and many others.

Wood remarked that he was "very much aware of the impact the series [*Emergency!*] was having across the land and how radically EMS was changing the role of fire departments."

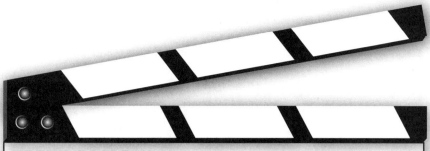

EMERGENCY! *Behind the Scene*

CHAPTER **6**

Los Angeles County Fire Department Staff

Fire Chiefs

Chief Engineer Keith Klinger, Fire Chief Emeritus

Klinger joined the LA County Fire Department (LACoFD) in 1934, became Chief Engineer in 1953, and retired in 1969.

The next year, after becoming Chief, he co-hosted the very first television program about firefighters—a 30-minute program titled *ALARM*. It starred Richard Arlen as Fire Captain London, Chick Chandler and J. Pat O'Malley as firemen, and Dick Simmons (Sgt. Preston of the Yukon) as Police Lt. Larry Jones. This show was produced with the full cooperation and assistance of the LACoFD by Roland Reed Productions. The fire station and rescue squad in the show were from LA County Fire Station 8 in West Hollywood. However, the series never developed beyond a single episode, and it was another 4 years before the debut of *Rescue 8* and 18 years before *Emergency!*.

Klinger was the first Fire Chief to introduce helicopters for firefighting. It was also Chief Klinger's innovative decision to put a resuscitator on every fire apparatus. After Klinger's retirement, the Los Angeles County Board of Supervisors named the present Fire Department Headquarters after him.

Chief Engineer Richard Houts (1969–1977)

Chief Houts's picture hung above Captain Stanley's desk at Station 51, and he appeared in episode 5.20, "Above and Beyond...Nearly," to award Johnny and Roy Act of Bravery medals.

Houts's determination to implement the paramedic program provoked a great deal of controversy among many other Fire Chiefs at the time. He retired from the LACoFD in 1977, after 8 years as its Fire Chief and 35 years of service in the department.

Fire Chief Clyde A. Bragdon, Jr. (1977–1984)

Beginning his career in 1956, Bragdon served as county Forester, Fire Warden, and Fire Chief for the County of Los Angeles from 1977 to his retirement in 1984, when he was appointed to be Administrator of the United States Fire Administration, Federal Emergency Management Agency, by President Ronald Reagan. Bragdon also served as administrator of the U.S. Fire Academy.

In this role, he testified before the Occupational Safety and Health Administration regarding occupational exposure to bloodborne pathogens as to the duties of firefighters that place them at risk. He stated: "Today's firefighter is not just a firefighter. He is also an emergency health care worker, often the first to arrive at the scene of an accident. In fact, 80 percent of all field emergency medical care is provided by the fire service. The occupational exposures inherent to their jobs necessitates that the Rule cover all firefighters, emergency medical technicians, and paramedics."

Fire Chief John England (1984–1988)

England donated the 14-year-old Ward LaFrance pumper that was used on *Emergency!*, and was then inservice as a reserve rig at Station 60, to the fire department in Yosemite National Park. In exchange, the park donated its 1937 Seagrave to the Los Angeles County Fire Museum (see Chapter 21).

Fire Chief P. Michael Freeman (1988–)

Chief Freeman took over the reigns in 1988 and continues to lead one of the largest fire departments in the country. At the 1998 *Emergency!* Convention, he honored the cast and crew of *Emergency!* with honorary firefighter

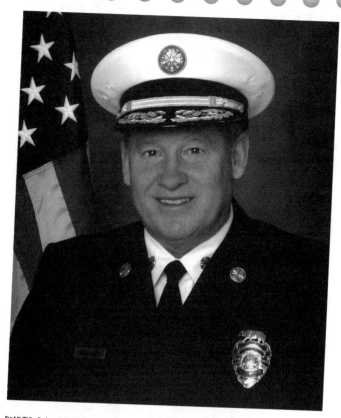

PHOTO 6-1   LA County Fire Department Fire Chief P. Michael Freeman.
Source: Courtesy of John DeLeon, Head Photographer, Los Angeles County Fire Department, Photo Unit.

plaques for their realistic portrayal of the Fire Department and the show's influence on the startup of paramedic programs all across the country **(Photo 6-1)**.

Chief Freeman also spoke at the Smithsonian on May 16, 2000, when authentic LACoFD equipment, uniforms, and artifacts from the TV program were inducted into the museum's archives at the culmination of the Project 51 tour.

Chief Freeman recognized that "*Emergency!* sparked public recognition and appreciation for the new paramedic profession. Watching Johnny and Roy in action was a reflection of how early LACoFD paramedics really worked. Decades later, the show's influence is evidenced by the number of paramedics worldwide and how it redefined the scope of the fire service. It was truly one of America's first reality shows."

Public Information Officer

Richard "Dick" A. Friend

Friend began his fire service career at the age of 14 as a volunteer auxiliary fireman in the Rolling Hills area of Palos Verdes **(Photo 6-2)**. With a short-

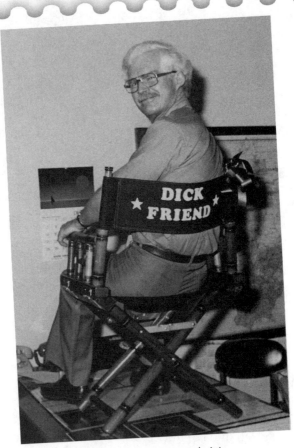

PHOTO 6-2   Dick Friend sitting in his director's chair.
Source: Courtesy of Rozane Sutherland, author.

age of manpower because of World War II, he was one of a dozen teenagers to be trained on the County's Engine 6—a 1924 American LaFrance engine. In the same year, he took a summer position with the LACoFD weed abatement crew to assist the County with burning off brush in the residential area. In July 1948, Friend was assigned a paid position as one of two callmen attending fires, performing drills, and working overtime at the station. He worked 24-hour shifts and lived in a trailer next to the shed that housed Engine 56, a surplus pumper. Fireman Dick Houts eventually replaced him, and the two would meet up again some years later for a very important project. Friend continued to attend fires during his work as a reporter for the *Los Angeles Mirror* and later as an editor at the *Long Beach Press-Telegram*. In 1967, he joined the LACoFD as its Public Information Officer (PIO).

As the PIO, Friend often assisted local TV stations and film studios in providing fire footage, granting interviews, or providing technical assistance. Fire Chief Richard Houts named Friend the production coordinator for *Emergency!,* and in this role, he oversaw script preparation and final review, ordered necessary fire equipment, arranged off-duty personnel, assigned TAs, and helped coordinate the major incidents filmed on location.

Even though it was good publicity, Friend advised that the production company should not get the services of the LACoFD for free. All equipment used on the program (with the exception of Universal Studios Engine 60) was rented for a fee. Off-duty firefighters were hired to drive the apparatus and perform on camera as required.

Friend did several voiceovers and appeared in two episodes, "Inferno" (episode 3.21) and "The Screenwriter" (episode 4.1) as himself. In three additional episodes, his character is played by an uncredited actor. Friend left the department after season 4 (1975) to publish the *Western Fire Journal* (later to become the *American Fire Journal* in 1978). Even though no longer "on the job," he would continue to have lunch about every other month with Cinader and Chief Houts. He would return to the fire service, once again as LA County PIO, in 1979 and serve in that capacity until 1984.

Battalion Chiefs

James "Jim" O. Page

In August 1957, after working as a $1.00/hour ambulance attendant, Page joined the City of Monterey Park Fire Department on his twenty-first birthday. He joined the LACoFD 2 years later in November 1959 **(Photo 6-3)**.

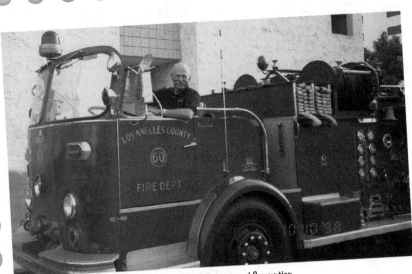

PHOTO 6-3   Jim Page in Engine 60 at the 1998 *Emergency!* Convention.
Source: Courtesy of Rozane Sutherland, author.

In 1971 Page was directed to coordinate the implementation of the Department's paramedic rescue services. He also served as technical consultant to *Emergency!* in its first two seasons. Prior to Page's retirement from the Fire Department in September 1973, he penned two scripts under the pseudonym "Jim Owens." He penned one script that aired in season 3 under yet another name (see "Snake Bite," episode 3.6). He did submit other scripts, but they were not used. Page's scripts tried to show the problems that actually were occurring within the Fire Department such as in his "Drivers" and "Trainee" scripts (episodes 2.13 and 2.8, respectively), which aired in season 2. The writers for the series were paid approximately $4000 for each script, and Jim received residuals of $12.00 every time one of the episodes he wrote aired.

About the time the primary casting decisions were being made, Dale Cauble informed Page that Webb had decided to name the paramedic (to be played by Mantooth) "Jim Page." Webb had often used the real names of some Los Angeles Police Department personnel in *Dragnet*. Page met with Webb the next day, expressed his appreciation for the honor of having a TV character share his name, but explained that his boss already thought he was too visible with the paramedic program. Page was later advised that the character was to be named the similar sounding "John Gage."

In 1973, after serving 14 years with Los Angeles County, Page took an early retirement and accepted the position of Chief of Emergency Medical Services (EMS) for the State of North Carolina and spent the next 10 years based on the East Coast. In 1976, he was selected as executive director of the nonprofit Advanced Coronary Treatment Foundation in New York.

In 1979, he founded JEMS Communications, publishers of the *Journal of Emergency Medical Services* (*JEMS*) (previously *Paramedics International*) and *FireRescue Magazine*. In 1984, Jim returned to the California fire service at Carlsbad Fire Department while maintaining a leadership role in *JEMS*. In 1986 he became the Fire Chief for the City of Monterey Park, where he had first stared his firefighting career some 40 years earlier, retiring in 1989. He then returned to full-time service as Chairman and Chief Executive Officer of JEMS Communications and held the post of Publisher Emeritus.

In 1995 the International Association of Fire Chiefs honored him when they created the annual James O. Page Award of Excellence. He also established and funded an EMS educational foundation in 1996 at Palomar College in San Marcos, California (north of San Diego), near his home. In 2000, he was featured by *Fire Chief Magazine* as one of the twenty most influential Fire Chiefs of the 20th century. In 2002, JEMS Communications created the annual James O. Page/JEMS Award, presented annually to an organization or individual who excels in EMS leadership in the face of extreme political or organizational pressures.

Page has been associated with the County of Los Angeles Fire Museum Association since 1996 and served as its president until his death. A fitness enthusiast, Page died September 4, 2004, of cardiac arrest while swimming in a pool in Carlsbad, California.

George Harms

Harms headed the Fire Department's Training Division and took over the role as consultant to *Emergency!* after Page's retirement in 1973. Both Harms and Friend worked together in scouting filming locations (off the Universal lot) for fire and rescue scenarios.

Bob Hanson

Hanson filled in for Dick Friend as department liaison to the series when Friend went on vacation and eventually replaced Friend when he took leave to publish *Western Fire Journal*.

LACoFD Dispatchers

Around 1973 the Department began to phase out the civilian dispatchers and convert to an all safety service crew. As the civilians retired, they were replaced with firefighters. They worked a 24-hour schedule just like the stations and operated with a staff of four to five, usually with a fire captain as the supervisor. Over the next few years, the Department also began to phase out satellite dispatch centers such as Malibu and the Valley dispatching center in El Monte; some firefighter personnel retired, returned to the floor, or were reassigned to the LA dispatching center.

In 1992, the County replaced the old dispatching center with a new state-of-the-art center and once again went back to civilian dispatching. They do not work a 24-hour shift but work 10- or 12-hour shifts.

Samuel G. Lanier, Jr., A Shift Civilian Dispatcher

Lanier was a Korean War army veteran and was an LA County dispatcher from 1958 to 1977. He was the voice of *Emergency!* Although his face is seen on several occasions, a lot of stock footage of Lanier was utilized throughout the series. Sometimes just his back is shown, or he is handed a piece of paper by another dispatcher before flipping a toggle switch and leaning into the mike. Although not always seen, he is heard in virtually every episode. As a civilian dispatcher, and like all the others, he wore a uniform and a dispatcher badge.

After his retirement he became a fire safety advisor to TV and film production companies. He also was a badge-carrying fireman for the Hollywood Park Fire Department, which was responsible for the Hollywood Park horse racing track in Inglewood.

Lanier died as he lived, trying to save others. He heard a traffic collision in front of his home in Culver City, reported it, and went out to assist. Lanier suffered a heart attack at the scene and, in art-imitating-life, LA County paramedics responded on the call to assist Culver City.

Duane Lewis, A Shift Firefighter Dispatcher

Lewis was one of many dispatchers who often appeared in the background, handing Sam Lanier the alarm information. In the sixth season, Lewis was the first of these firefighter/dispatchers to be identified. Lewis retired in 2003 as a fire captain working at Station 144.

Lanny Cunningham, B Shift Firefighter Dispatcher

Cunningham would often pull an overtime shift and work with Sam Lanier and Duane Lewis. Although he was not directly involved with the show, he commented:

I asked Sam once, how do you come up with the addresses on *Emergency!*? He told me
he would look up a street in the Thomas Brothers Map book and looked at the addresses for that
street. He made sure he made up an address that DID NOT exist. EXAMPLE: Let's say there is
a street called Tristen Lane. In the map book it shows Tristen Lane goes from 4500 to 6299.
He would pick an address like 7122 Tristen Lane, knowing that address does not exist.

In other words, the street names, including cross streets, are real streets; the hundred block numbers are bogus. The cross streets are somewhere else altogether and don't intersect with the incident location. And neither has anything to do with the filming location.

Repairman

George Ashley

Ashley worked as a fire apparatus repairman for the LACoFD as "Repair 10," and among several other stations on his route was Universal Studios FS60. Before joining the Fire Department, he worked at Ward LaFrance for 15 years, where he oversaw the delivery and service of all new Ward LaFrance fire apparatus sold in California, Oregon, and Washington. In this capacity, he serviced the Ward that was used on *Emergency!* (see Chapter 8).

"Mickey Michaels was at my shop all the time," Ashley relates. As the set director, he was in charge of all the props, including the Ward E-51. "He would always be inspecting some repair work I had been doing to the rig," says Ashley:

Mickey could be a real pain at times as I had other work at the shop that had to get done
for other departments and he would have E-51 sent down for a lot minor repairs that could have
been handled at the Universal shops. One time one of the rear compartment doors came open
underway and got badly bent so I had to order a replacement from the plant and when it arrived
I had to paint it with the right color and install it. I got along good with him but I had a very
small crew (3 men) in handling the LACoFD delivery plus other deliveries on the West Coast,
and Mickey always expected me to drop everything to take care of E-51.

There were fourteen Repair vehicles that covered the County. My service truck, which I
took home with me, as all the repair units were virtually on call 24/7, looked very similar
to the rescue squads but were a bit smaller. Mine was a 1975 3/4 ton GMC cab and chassis
with a service truck body. I carried most everything I would need to do minor overhauls on the
apparatus including tools such as an electric welder, cutting torch, hydraulic jacks and a porto-
power unit. Tire replacement was done in the field, and I also carried replacement parts for
Crown and Ward engines, Dodge squads, and the Plymouth and AMC staff cars."

Ashley was a civilian employee but as a member of LACoFD, he wore an LACoFD uniform and carried a badge. "Where the firefighters had their station number," he said, "mine said 'R 10.'"

Helicopter Pilots and Crew

Chief Pilot Roland Barton and Senior Pilots Alan MacLeod, Joe Kelly, Ted Hellmers, and Frank Pino flew all LACoFD aircraft that appear in the series, most of the time uncredited. In all the scenes where helicopters are utilized, rarely are the pilots' faces clearly seen, if at all; usually only the exterior of the helicopter is in view.

In the episode "Above and Beyond...Nearly" (episode 5.20), LA County Firefighter Dave Bowers is sitting in the left seat as a crewman. Firefighter Larry Younkers is the crewman in "Right at Home" (episode 5.17). They both later became paramedics, as did many of the crewmen, and continued work at Air Ops.

An interesting note: Pilot Roland Barton appears in the first season wearing a ball cap with a patch from Fire Camp 9 in one episode. Gary Lineberry, former pilot for LA County, states that they did not start wearing the helmets until 1973, which you will see in later episodes.

All pilots and crewmen are identified in the episodes in which they appeared.

Technical Advisors

The studio paid the firefighters' salaries for the 6 to 8 days (or more) that it took them to confer and film. They usually got the script 2 weeks before filming, attended Wednesday production meetings, and were always at the director's side during filming. On occasion a second technical advisor (TA) was required to replace the credited/assigned TA for an episode during shooting because of a prior commitment, an illness, or something similar.

Universal was not consistent as to what they called the TAs. Various examples on the scripts are "L.A.C.F.D. T/A," "F.D./TA," and "FIREMAN T.A." The advisor's name will follow, sometimes after "FM" (fireman).

Kevin Tighe had this to say about the TAs on the program:

> When we first started the show, Dale Cauble and Rocky Doke were the two paramedics I went out with as we went out and rode with the paramedics before the pilot. That helped me draw the character and that's how I found who I was going to be. I mean, we depended upon them for who we were on the show. They also served such an extraordinary function on the show day after day. They had to see every single scene and if it wasn't right, it was shot again. We wanted as much technical expertise and wanted to make it as honest as we could and yet still make it entertaining and it looks to me like we succeeded.

To give you an example of where we were when we first started, I remember a scene where I was reading a blood pressure. I had the stethoscope and I'm getting it. I loosen the cuff and give it to the radio and they yell, "Cut!"; I thought everything went perfectly. Then I see the advisor come over to the director. Then I went over to them and the advisor kind of timidly says, "Well, it was a good scene, but it's just that if you're going to do a reading, it's better to have the stethoscope in your ears."

The issue of technical accuracy is always a problem no matter what the subject. Recreating the life of a firefighter isn't a simple task, especially when dozens of pages of the script with many scenes must be shot in a single day and often out of order. Be it a program about police officers, lawyers, firefighters, or a hospital setting, the writers and producers take liberties, theorizing that the average viewer would not pick up the inaccuracies. The same complaints are always aired regarding "fire" programs: "No smoke in the building," or "That's not the way it's done." *Towering Inferno's* million gallons of water on the roof and other similar issues are a TA's nightmare. *Emergency!* even had its problems where occasionally drama overwrote the scene being portrayed correctly.

Pete Gwilliam, retired from the London Fire Brigade and often an extra on several British programs including the long-running fire program *London's Burning* (fourteen seasons), said, "The underlying concept with all TV film producers is that a documentary is just that. A drama series, however, must give the viewing public what they want: action, disaster, sex, romance, and that 'hero' figure. When working on *London's Burning* I remember the director saying to me after I wanted to reshoot my accidental fall on a line, 'It's Drama, Luvie,' the director said."

Yes, some procedural mistakes were made on the program, as they continue to be made in current programming. Loading victims into the ambulance feet first was done on occasion on *Emergency!*. Many of the ambulance crew were actual off-duty members of an ambulance company, but most were "extras" who did not know which end of the stethoscope to stick into their ears. Defibrillator placement was mostly correct, but there were times where correct placement gave in to camera angle. This was, however, corrected by the Harbor General staff (see Chapter 7).

Additional information and comments from the TAs listed here are also found in the episode guide (see Chapter 12).

Bob Belliveau
Belliveau was in the first class of six paramedics LA County trained at Harbor General and was issued paramedic license number PM0001 as a result of numbers being issued alphabetically by class.

Bob says, "It must be remembered that the medical community had some reluctance to the program as well as many of the top staff of the Fire Department." While training began in September 1969, and would continue for almost 1 year, the first unit was already in service in December. Because there wasn't any enabling legislation at that time, all rescue calls responded with two firemen and one nurse from the CCU. The nurse had to run down four stories of stairs to meet RS59," Bob relates. "The nurses were a very good asset on the rescue calls due to their bedside manner and empathy for the patients."

"At the start of the show," he recalls, "Randy Mantooth had problems demonstrating starting IVs. It looked like he was sewing. So I showed him how to do it correctly and let him start an IV on me, and he never had a problem after that."

Belliveau became the TA on three episodes, "Crash" (episode 1.11), "Saddled" (episode 2.6), and "The Floor Brigade" (episode 3.19), and appeared as himself in "Rules of Order" (episode 6.6) but was not the TA for that show. He was also one of three TAs for the *Emergency!* movie, *Survival on Charter 220*.

Belliveau went to San Francisco and Seattle to study the feasibility of doing full-length *Emergency!* episodes with their fire departments and emergency medical systems. He recalls. "I spent about 5 days at each city and studied the locations for incidents, types of equipment, and possible script material. I also spent time with the writers. The Technical Advisors for these movies came from the local fire departments."

Belliveau retired after 34 years on the job with the rank of Battalion Chief.

Dale Cauble

Prior to joining the LACoFD in 1966, Cauble was the Fire Chief for the Palos Verdes Fire Department and was also among the first class of six paramedics LA County trained at Harbor General (PM0002). He was TA to *Emergency!*, the 2-hour World Premier movie; he was also Chief Jim Page's driver for a time while stationed at 36. He eventually became the department chaplain.

Gary Davis

After joining the Department in 1966, Davis went through the initial training along with Dale Cauble. After becoming a paramedic (PM0003), Davis worked the rest of his career as a firefighter/paramedic. Before he retired in 1997, he was the longest continuously certified paramedic in the United States. He was working on the air squad when he retired. Davis is currently an "on-call" fire marshal for the film studios, taking care of safety, fire safety, and special effects procedures.

Recalling how he was advised of the new paramedic program starting up, "I don't know what the station captains on the other shifts said but ours said, 'There is a new program starting up at Harbor General, anyone interested in sticking needles in people's hearts?'"

While working as a TA, he would recall that whenever Robert Cinader would come on the set everybody would get real nervous. However, "he 'loved' us firefighters," states Davis. "Cinader had an open-door policy at the studio. Whenever one of us needed to talk with him, we would show up at the gate, say we needed to see Cinader, and the guards would let us by."

Rocky Doke

Doke was PM0008. He relates that the nurses at Harbor General had a big impact on the show: "Carol, Peggy, and so many others who made it all come together for us." According to Doke, Dr. Ronald Stewart helped the firefighters learn and understand all the new medical terminology. "Looking back," says Doke, "the impact the show had on EMS worldwide is incredible."

Mike Lewis

Lewis was in the third class of paramedics trained at Harbor General, becoming #37 in the state. At one point Lewis said, "Initially, the first class of graduates set a lot of firefighters against the paramedics and the paramedic program in general. They felt because they wore the white coat they no longer had to get dirty."

Lewis was a paramedic for 9 years when he took the test for engineer in 1980; he passed and had to give up the paramedic program. During his tenure as a paramedic, he was a TA for three of the *Emergency!* Programs: "Frequency" (episode 3.1), "Computer Error" (episode 3.14), and "The Smoke Eater" (episode 4.16). Lewis retired in 1997. Currently he is involved as "Sparky, the Fire Prevention Clown" and travels all over, attending fairs, parades, and schools to teach fire safety. He is a recipient of *Firehouse Magazine*'s Heroism and Community Service Award.

Bob McCullough

McCullough started his fire service career in 1967, and his first captain was Jim Page. He became interested in the paramedic program while working at Station 36, where he saw the crew in action. McCullough was in the same class as Mike Lewis and graduated #38 in the state. After their practical training at Stations 59 and 36, they would be assigned together putting Squad 209 in service at Station 9, at 7116 South Makee Avenue in Los Angeles.

The station still had the old standard rescue squad as Rescue Squad 9 (similar to the TV program *Rescue 8*) and kept that in service to respond as manpower to fires. McCullough's partner, Mike Lewis, stated that Squad 9 was later manned by EMTs with Paramedic Squad 209 being placed into service. Instead of a Dodge truck with the utility body, the department obtained a Dodge van as its squad and it was numbered *Squad 209* (see Chapter 8).

McCullough was the TA on "Inheritance Tax" (episode 3.9), "Nagging Suspicion" (episode 4.4), "Equipment" (episode 5.4), "The Nuisance" (episode 5.24), and "Computer Terror" (episode 6.9). The TAs were rarely seen in the series, but McCullough made it into one of the last movies; he was TA on *Survival on Charter 220*. He is the driver of the apparatus in the opening scene responding to the tower rescue. McCullough retired in November 1993 as a result of an on-the-job injury.

McCullough said, "[I] took my work too seriously at the time as I felt that I did not want any of my shows to embarrass the men and women of the LACoFD. I loved my job both as a firefighter/paramedic and as a technical advisor."

Kirk Kington

Kington (PM0063) placed Squad 20 into service upon graduation. He was a TA on "It's How You Play the Game" (episode 4.19), "Right at Home" (episode 5.17), and "Not Available" (episode 6.2).

Bob Hoff

Hoff (PM0071) was in a class of about thirty firefighters going through paramedic instruction at Harbor General. His first assignment was Squad 18 in Lennox and then Squad 36 in Carson with Chief Page. "Working on the episodes was fun," Hoff recalls, "I think what we as firefighters brought into the series was the camaraderie and practical jokes we play on each other. The regular actors got so good at what they were doing I just stood back and watched most of the time." Hoff worked on "It's How You Play the Game" (episode 4.19), "Back-Up (4.21), "The Indirect Method" (episode 5.6), and "Fair Fight" (episode 6.5). He also appeared in the movie, *Survival on Charter 220*.

Hoff states that much of the stock footage seen in the series from the cab of the squad, looking out the front windshield, was filmed using Squad 18: "The cinematographer, using a small handheld, sat between us for about two shifts as we drove the area so they could get different responding scenes."

Hoff appeared in a *Quincy M.E.* episode and on *CHiPs* as a paramedic at accident scenes, credited in "The Sheik" (episode 2.09) and uncredited in several others including "E.M.T." (episode 3.17). He also appeared on the syndicated Dinah Shore program *Dinah* with Kevin Tighe and Randy Mantooth discussing the paramedic program and the TV show.

Joe Bartak, Jr.
Bartak (PM0073) was TA for "Above and Beyond…Nearly" (episode 5.20).

Mark Hefley
Hefley (PM0079) was the TA on "Magic" (episode 4.18), "Pressure 165" (episode 5.7), and "Paperwork" (episode 6.11). He recalls that, in the days of *Emergency!*, being a paramedic was not readily accepted. "We were labeled prima donnas," he recalls. "As with any new program we had to sell ourselves to our peers, hospital personnel, and the public as well. *Emergency!* helped a lot with the public….Many of us spent a lot of time with the writers coming up with different situations and how to resolve them. Before too long, other firemen in the station would sit down with us and retell some of the incidents they had been on or had heard about."

Bob Lee Hancock
Hancock (PM0177) was TA on "That Time of Year" (episode 6.4) and "All Night Long" (episode 6.21). Hancock advised the actors, including Randy Mantooth, that firefighter/paramedics talked about their actions while they were doing them, for example, "I have the IV going," or "Did you get the BP?" Hancock says, "I remember telling Randy that we talked up things while we were doing them, like, 'I have the IV going; did you get the BP?'—things like that and I know that they did ad lib a lot of that."

Alan Barbee
Barbee worked at Station 36 when the paramedic actors showed up for their first walk-through familiarization tour. He would later work at Station 127 and, along with other firefighters, would often be utilized as a firefighter extra. Barbee would often assist Paramedic Bob Ramstead (PM006) when he was assigned as a TA and even served as TA for one episode himself. Barbee retired in 2003 as a Fire Captain. He remembers that being an extra on the set at Universal and on location was a lot of fun, initially, but, he says, "There was a lot of sitting around and waiting that made the day long."

LACoFD and *Emergency!*

The Los Angeles County Fire Department capitalized on the popularity of *Emergency!* and their close association with the program by using a photo of Johnny and Roy in a fire prevention flyer (**Photo 6-4**).

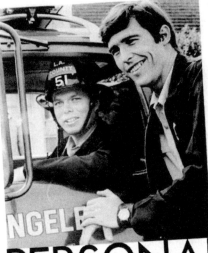

A Message to You from
John Gage and Roy DeSoto:

"OUR FIREMEN ARE DEDICATED
TO SAVING LIVES AND PROPERTY.
IT TAKES THE EFFORT OF ALL
OF US TO HELP SAVE OUR HOMES,
FAMILIES, AND SCHOOLS FROM
DESTRUCTION BY FIRE. PLEASE,
BE CAREFUL WITH ALL FIRE!"

Kevin Tighe • Randolph Mantooth

Fire safety is everyone's **PERSONAL RESPONSIBILITY**

Uncontrolled fires destroy our natural resources, our homes, factories and schools.

Fire's annual toll in the United States:
- 12,600 people killed, including 3,800 young people, under 15 years of age
- 91,000 apartments lost • 537,000 homes burned • 15,000 schools burned

Find the emergency phone number for your community in the telephone directory under "FIRE."

The telephone number from my home to report a fire or request the fire department paramedic rescue squad is:

"WE'RE HERE TO HELP!"— The Los Angeles County Fire Department

PHOTO 6-4   Los Angeles County Fire Department fire safety flyer.
Source: Courtesy of Los Angeles County Fire Department, Photo Unit.

EMERGENCY! *Behind the Scene*

CHAPTER **7**

Harbor General Hospital Staff

During the 1960s and 1970s, Harbor General Hospital's affiliation with the University of California at Los Angeles (UCLA) School of Medicine continued to grow **(Photo 7-1)**. To make this association more evident to the public, the Los Angeles County Board of Supervisors changed the name of Harbor General Hospital in 1978 to the Los Angeles County Harbor–UCLA Medical Center. Paramedics and mobile care intensive nurses (MICNs) still continue their training at this hospital. Several of the staff doctors and nurses at Harbor General became directly involved during the production of *Emergency!* with overseeing the scripts and technical aspects of the program's emergency room scenes.

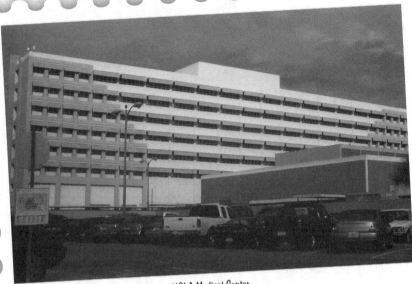

PHOTO 7-1   Los Angeles County Harbor–UCLA Medical Center.
Source: Courtesy of Harbor/UCLA Medical Center; Rozane Sutherland, photographer.

Doctors

John Michael Criley, MD

Dr. Criley was the head of the Cardiology Division at Harbor General Hospital and approached the La County Fire Department (LACoFD) because they provided rescue services to the largest area of the county. Dr. Criley and the first class of LA County paramedics officially began service in December 1969 with a station wagon obtained from the LACoFD Forestry Division, lettered "Rescue Heart Unit." A nurse was required to ride along with the new paramedics to administer drugs and start IVs. It was not until July 1970 that the Wedworth-Townsend Act authorized paramedics to operate in the field on their own. Paramedics still received medical supervision through the BioPhones, which the medics carried aboard their squads.

Dr. Criley, and Dr. Walter Graf from Daniel Freeman Hospital, invited Dr. J. Frank Pantridge, from Royal Victoria Hospital in Belfast, Ireland, to view the LA paramedic program. In the early 1960s, Dr. Pantridge discovered that treating patients in the field saved lives. The Belfast system had coronary care nurses and physicians staffing their cardiac care unit (CCU). According to Dr. Koenig (see later discussion in this chapter), Dr. Pantridge was not very impressed with the "nonphysician" concept being developed in Los Angeles and other communities.

Dr. Criley advocated the use of defibrillators in office buildings before this was common practice, claiming that, "Defibrillators have saved more lives than fire extinguishers," and insisting that, "If you could train people in factories, office buildings, in virtually every public place how to use a defibrillator, we could save countless lives."

In 2001 the American College of Physicians–American Society of Internal Medicine (ACP–ASIM) bestowed its highest classification of membership upon Dr. Criley, awarding him Mastership status. Among his accomplishments as Chief of Cardiology at Harbor–UCLA Medical Center, he founded the first Los Angeles County paramedic program and was on the team that performed the first successful heart transplantation in southern California. He has been a Fellow of ACP–ASIM since 1973 and is currently emeritus professor of medicine and radiological sciences at UCLA. Dr. Criley continues to serve on the faculty of the Division of Cardiology at Harbor–UCLA Medical Center and maintains an active role to support fund raising for UCLA's Research and Education Institute as a board member on the Harbor–UCLA Collegiums.

Many years later during the "Project 51" tour, at a reception in Washington, D.C. sponsored by the IAFF in honor of the *Emergency!* team, Doctor Criley recounted the problems that he and Dr. Nagle of Miami, Florida, encountered in those early years. They remarked that they were almost physically attacked when they made presentations to the medical community and to their peers on the training of firefighters to provide advanced medical procedures in the field. *Emergency!* was, in his eyes, "a major force in not only legitimizing the paramedics but also for exporting the idea across the country. It put the spotlight on LA County and its Fire Department."

Ronald D. Stewart, OC, BA, BSc, MD, FRCPC, FACEP, DSc

Dr. Stewart was the Medical Director for paramedic training in the County of Los Angeles and was one of the main architects of the paramedic program in California. He wrote the first paramedic and mobile intensive care unit (MICU) nurses training manuals and was one of the medical consultants at Harbor General for *Emergency!*.

He recalls his years with *Emergency!* with great fondness:

> I particularly remember Bob Cinader, the power behind the whole initiative. He was a great bagpipe lover, and I, being a piper, was fair game to participate in his excursions to every

pipe band that blew through LA. Unfortunately for them, a reluctant duo of Kevin Tighe and Randy Mantooth was usually "invited" (aka coerced) into accompanying Bob and me to these usually second-rate performances. But Bob thoroughly enjoyed them.

There are lots of great memories I have, how much I learned about the portrayal of life and its problems, and the close teamwork that developed among the people on the show, plus Randy's allergy to bee stings that frequently caused panic in on-location shooting...

Like many of those involved, Dr. Stewart recognized the influence the show was having on the entire field of emergency medicine:

I fully credit this TV series as an important element in increasing the public awareness about EMS in the United States, if not the world, at the time. We were struggling to get the attention of the academics, politicians, administrators, and the public to explain the importance of this new medical specialty. I believe that this program, with all its warts, helped do that. Granted it was a soap opera, but there is no rule that says soap operas can't influence public opinion, in fact the opposite is true...

For me personally and professionally, I came to realize the immense power of the medium of television. How it could influence public perceptions and opinions, and how persuasive it was in the life of the United States and its people. I viewed it since as a great instrument, much like a very sharp scalpel, ready and able to cut and heal, but equally sharp to do damage.

Dr. Stewart said that he was appointed the medical consultant to the series by default because he was recently appointed head of the paramedic program in the County. As a medical consultant to the show, Dr. Stewart was responsible for the accuracy of in-hospital procedures and surgical techniques. He says that this required him to be on the set quite often, but, "only if I could squeeze it in to a bruising schedule. I was still on the streets with the paramedics most of the time and in the emergency department humping charts almost every day."

Dr. Stewart recognized the important role that *Emergency!* played in developing a national paramedic program. "I became aware of the power of the program late in the first year [of the show], when we began receiving fan letters saying things like, 'I saved my Granny by doing what I saw on Emergency!'.....I never thought for a minute when I started that so many people would be exposed to the ideas..."

When asked about the manuals that he had to write, he said, "Part of our problem when I started to direct paramedic education in the County was that there were no texts written that reflected either the background of the paramedic trainee (firefighters) or the environment in which they would practice (the streets). So I was forced to write the texts that built on their previous experience and training. So I headed off to the 'tower' of LA County Fire and sat in on the classes given to recruits. I realized that they were talking about pumps, pressures, electrical stuff, energy (fire), gases, etc. All readily translated to medical principles and I used these as a base for anatomy and physiology and clinical teaching." Firefighter Rocky Doke, a member of the second paramedic class, recalled Stewart's tireless work: "Translating all that medical jargon into layman's terminology, firefighters speak if you will."

Dr. Stewart said that he spent "every spare minute" in the streets, learning from the firefighters and watching what they did with the new knowledge they were acquiring. He said that he wrote the manuals early in the morning, after his shifts at LA County/University of Southern California (USC) Medical Center ended, because this was the only free time he had. "I remember it as an exciting and productive time," he said.

The manuals were used in the County Training Institute and later at Daniel Freeman Hospital; they also became the basis for training programs in Canada and Australia. "I never dreamed that these rough drafts, with stick figures that revealed my very un-artistic bent, would become so well appreciated and well recognized—to the point that I was asked to donate the originals, which I never could find, to the Smithsonian."

In 1978 Dr. Stewart left Los Angeles for Pittsburgh to serve as medical director of the Pittsburgh EMS system, where he established the Department of Emergency Medicine and the Center for Emergency Medicine. In 1987, he returned to his home in Canada, where he continued his work in emergency medicine. In 1993, he ran for political office and was elected to the provincial parliament and later appointed minister of health, a post he held until 1997. In 2000, he attended the Project 51 ceremony at the Smithsonian, where he donated copies of his original manuals to the Smithsonian Museum.

The Ronald D. Stewart Medical Humanities Bursary Award was established in his name, in recognition of his significant contribution to medical education and student life at Dalhousie University, particularly in the field of the medical humanities. Dr. Stewart is director of medical humanities, professor of anesthesia, professor of emergency medicine at Dalhousie University in Halifax, Nova Scotia, Canada.

William J. Koenig, MD, FACEP

Dr. Koenig's career in emergency medicine began when the specialty was just in its formation. He graduated from UCLA School of Medicine and completed his emergency medicine residency at Los Angeles County/USC Medical Center in 1976. After starting practice, he immediately became involved in the training of paramedics in Los Angeles and later served as the director of the J. Michael Criley Paramedic Training Institute. He also assisted Dr.

Stewart with the development of the paramedic training manual, which was being requested from all over the country.

Dr. Koenig states, "The public awareness of the television program *Emergency!* was, at best, a weekly advertisement for the paramedic program. Paramedics and their work would have eventually happened, but it was a TV program that caused the public to 'demand' this kind of service in their communities all across the nation. The initial expectations of training were solely on cardiac care, but it was quickly discovered that the role of the paramedics could be expanded to cover all facets of emergency care."

Dr. Koenig recalls that the demand for paramedics was great, and Harbor General had difficulty keeping up with the demand from fire departments and private sectors. Even so, paramedics often considered themselves firemen, not doctors, he says.

Dr. Koenig was the chairman of the State EMS Commission and president of the Emergency Medical Services Directors Association of California. He served as the medical editor of the *Journal of Emergency Medical Services* and the medical director of the Emergency Department at Long Beach Memorial/Miller Children Hospitals. He is currently on the boards of EMS Best Practices and The Prehospital Care Research Forum and is a member of the Emergency Medical Directors Association of California, where he chairs the legislative committee. He currently serves as the EMS medical director of Los Angeles County EMS.

Mobile Intensive Care Nurses

The position of MICNs began with the passage of the Wedworth-Townsend Paramedic Act. Previously, state-licensed registered nurses (RNs) rode with the newly trained group of firefighter/paramedics to provide medical and legal coverage for what they were doing in the field. MICNs are the link between the paramedics in the field and the physicians in the hospital. They do periodic ride-alongs as part of their continuing educational requirement.

The first nurses certified as MICNs worked in the CCU at Daniel Freeman Hospital or the CCU at Harbor General Hospital. Because paramedics were based out of both of these hospitals, nurses needed to be certified as MICNs to give orders over the base station hospital radio.

MICNs at Harbor General Hospital were CCU nurses who underwent additional training in medical control and direction of paramedic field care. With the help of verbal reports from the paramedics in the field, they identified patients' needs and chose the appropriate treatment. Teamwork between the field paramedic and the MICN to give the appropriate care helped save lives.

The Daniel Freeman Hospital concept was a Mobile Coronary Care Unit on wheels, driven by a McCormick Ambulance driver and staffed with a CCU nurse from the hospital. Only after the state law passed and after the first MICUs out of Harbor General Hospital were so successful did Dr. Walter Graf switch the emphasis to mobile intensive care with a broader scope of care.

The first MICN, Carol Bebout, was certified in 1969. Two more RNs, Judith Anderson and Delia Daylo, were issued their MICN certification in November 1970, and Mary Jane Wilcox followed in December. The next year, five more RNs became MICN-certified. As of 2003, there were approximately 640 active MICNs working in 23 base station hospitals in Los Angeles County.

Carol Bebout, RN

Carol Bebout was the first of the MICNs trained to accompany the new paramedics, and she graduated along with the first paramedics in December 1969. Bebout was the head nurse in the CCU at Harbor General Hospital at the time. She had previously worked for the County of Los Angeles Department of Health Services (1962–1968) and later became a paramedic instructor at Harbor General Hospital.

"I was truly in the right place at the right time and was fortunate enough to be working for Dr. Criley, a physician ahead of his time," says Bebout. "He was intrigued by other paramedic programs working in Ireland and elsewhere and thought that something was similarly workable in LA County."

Dr. A. James Lewis, Dr. Criley, and a few other physicians taught most of the classes, and Bebout was the principal nonphysician instructor. The doctors taught subjects including pharmacology, electrophysiology, electrocardiograms, and cardiac function; Bebout and the other CCU nurses taught the more fundamental subjects like anatomy, physiology, vital signs, and drug administration. Bebout taught, prepared exams, supervised training, and provided clinical experience in the hospital for the paramedics while she was running the CCU. She says that, "After the program was so imminently successful and after it captured the attention of the County Board of Supervisors, a full-time paramedic training program facility was established, and funds made available to hire personnel." This included Gaylord Ailshie, a retired Army Lieutenant Colonel, who had trained paramedical military personnel at Fort Sam Houston. At that time, Bebout transferred out of the CCU to become the first full-time paramedic instructor.

The CCU nurses at Harbor General took turns riding along with RS59 and RA53 before the passage of the Wedworth-Townsend Paramedic Act to provide medical and legal coverage for the paramedics. Bebout says that she "scheduled nurses to ride from all three shifts. All of the nurses…rotated riding with whichever units required ride-alongs at the time. Keep in mind though that the County's Rescue Squad 59 personnel were trained and ready to be cut loose prior to the City RA 53 people being trained, so things happened in a staggered fashion **(Photo 7-2)**.

Bebout didn't work with the actors. Mostly, she contributed to the show by checking scripts for accuracy (along with Dr. Lewis and Dr. Criley) and sometimes meeting with Bob Cinader and suggesting story lines. The technical advisors were responsible for the accuracy of what was filmed on the set. Bebout recalls, "They really tried to keep things straight, accurate, and honest, but the need for drama really was the overriding concern. Fortunately, the really big blunders (like defibrillating on the wrong side of the chest) did get fixed."

Bebout admits that Dixie McCall's role was loosely based on her own real-life role, although the character worked in the Emergency Department and not a CCU. "Actually," she shares, "unrealistic though it was, Cinader had her working everywhere in the hospital—even the operating room!"

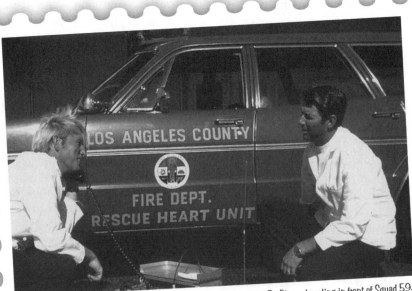

PHOTO 7-2   Firefighter/paramedic Rocky Doke and Dale Cauble with BioPhone, kneeling in front of Squad 59.
Source: Courtesy of County of Los Angeles Fire Museum Association Collection.

Bebout shares that the show was "excellent publicity for what we were doing in real life," although she admits that it may have been too dramatic at times. "I was tickled to death that it was so popular with kids," she said, "The program made firefighters true heroes to children, which was great! I was constantly amused at the letters that came in from adults...the ones that said, 'This program is such a good idea—why doesn't someone do it?' We were, of course, doing it in real life every day, but [the average person] didn't know that! The fan mail that came into the show was priceless."

Bebout says that she learned a great deal about firefighting and felt that her ride-alongs were very rewarding, even though she remained in the squad or engine while they went off to fight fires. She recalls:

> It was a very big adjustment for me as a nurse...working in a hospital was a very big adjustment for the firefighters and working in the field was also a big adjustment for all of us nurses....We learned a great deal about mutual respect, team effort, sharing education, etc. Of course, I also learned about playing cards for the dishes, etc.!

New to this aspect of firefighting culture in which card games determine dishwashing duty, Bebout says that she ended up doing more than her fair share of dishes, due to her poor card-playing abilities. "I didn't understand the whole business of playing cards for several hours for 15 minutes worth of dishes," she shares, and at first, "I said, naively, that I would just wash the dishes if it was my turn, but I was told...that wasn't the point. We all live and learn about the cultures that exist in every profession. Firefighters had to learn about the cultures that existed in the hospital setting, too, so turnabout was fair play." (See "Dealer's Wild," episode 1.5.)

> I'm sure that I speak for all of the CCU nurses when I say that we really enjoyed riding with RS59, not just initially, but for the whole duration of the experience. For us, it was fun and challenging and very different from our in-hospital experience. We quickly found that starting IVs in the dark, defibrillating patients in a 4-foot-by-6-foot bathroom, and trying to do fluid replacement while the patient was being extricated from a car was very challenging.
>
> There's no way that I could ever convey to you how important my experiences were as a young nurse involved in the paramedic program! I was very fortunate to have been in the right place at the right time....It was fun to be a pioneer and, in many ways, make up the rules as we went along. The program was a political football in many ways, but it was truly fun and rewarding to be part of something so important. Who knew that the real program, combined with the TV show, would prove to be so life-saving, so important, make so many inroads into the whole new world of pre-hospital care?

Carol Bebout opened the second County paramedic school (at USC) and was in charge of the paramedic unit of the Emergency Medical Services Division for the County. At the end of her career with LA County, she was responsible for all paramedic provider agencies, base station hospitals, and EAP ambulances, countywide. When she left the County in 1978, she went to Daniel Freeman Memorial Hospital in Inglewood, which is also a paramedic base hospital as well as a trauma center and paramedic training facility (under the direction of Dr. Michael Graf, medical director of training), where she was director of the emergency department. She is currently the research nurse in the General Clinical Research Center at Cedars Sinai Hospital in Los Angeles.

Peggy Stoker

Peggy Stoker was an RN at Harbor General and later became one of the paramedic instructors. After the decision was made to incorporate the character of Nurse Dixie McCall into the series, actress Julie London (who played nurse Dixie) approached Peggy and asked to spend time with her in the MICU and for Peggy's assistance in making her character more realistic and believable.

Stoker was the Emergency Medical Services Association data specialist for the State of California in Los Angeles as well as the trauma emergency medicine information system head for the Emergency Medical Services Agency, County of Los Angeles. She retired in 1994 and now resides in Bigfork, Montana.

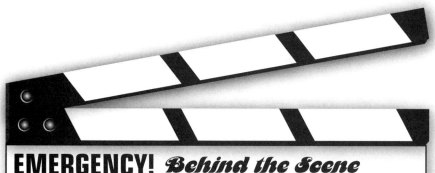

EMERGENCY! *Behind the Scene*

CHAPTER 8

Squads, Engines, and Equipment

Squad 51

The First Squad 51

The squad used in the 2-hour World Premiere and various other early episodes was in-service as Squad 36—a 1969 D-300, Dodge 1-ton truck with round, magnetic-backed plastic disks on the doors and rear covering the real squad numbers. The Rescue Squad 10 in the *Emergency!* World Premier was an in-service unit, RS8, a 1970 Dodge 1-ton D300 truck with the platter setup for the lights on the roof and the magnetic disks covering the real numbers.

Rented Squads

Early in season 1, Universal was able to rent other in-service squads from the Fire Department reserve fleet before obtaining a TV squad. For the most part, there were two Dodge models of squads used in the program, and sharp eyes will note in the stock footage that sometimes "new" Dodge shots are interspersed with the "old" Dodge in the same episode. There was also the "real" squad used in the pilot and stock footage, other rented vehicles, and the 1972 Dodge that was used for the completion of the series and two later *Emergency!* TV movies.

TV's Squad 51

The Chrysler Corporation provided the chassis for TV's Squad 51, and Universal Studio craftsmen constructed the utility body based on LA County specs. Nameplate data indicate that it is a 1972 Dodge Fargo DeSoto, Model number D30, VIN number D31BD4S066256. It was not registered by Universal until 1974, thereby causing the misconception that it was a 1974 model. It is powered by a 440-cubic-inch gasoline engine. It features an automatic three-speed transmission, power steering, four-wheel disk brakes, and air conditioning. The fire department did not have any 1972 Dodge models, which made this squad unique to the department. The previous series of vehicles purchased as squads were 1969 models.

This squad was registered to Universal Studios as a commercial vehicle. The studio transportation department was responsible for getting it from the studio to wherever they would be shooting on location each day. Firefighter Alan Barbee, who worked at Station 127 during some of the filming, stated, "The Union rules were so strict, that when the squad was driven out of the station by the actors and "Cut" was yelled, Universal's union driver had to drive it back into the station and reposition it for filming the scene again."

This vehicle was issued a commercial license plate number of 70324H by the California Department of Motor Vehicles. However, it often appears with another commercial plate, 19542W, or the Hollywood prop, tax-exempt license plate, E999007, on the vehicle before filming began. On rare occasions, the prop department forgot to switch the plates and nobody noticed until after the scene filming was complete.

The "E" within the diamond or octagon shape on California license plates does not denote emergency vehicles but signifies a government vehicle that is exempt from state and local taxes. City and county exempt vehicles were issued plates with an "E" within an octagon, and state exempt vehicles had an "E" within a diamond. With the large number of tax-exempt vehicles now registered in California, the "E" is no longer used so that an additional number may be included. Instead, the words "California Exempt" now run across the top of the plate.

Sharp eyes may notice different lettering schemes used on the squad during the series and movies. Lettering on the doors and the rear of the squads varied with the model of the Dodge. The word "Paramedic" on the doors of the squad replaced "Rescue Squad" and was put on after series completion when it went into reserve status for the County. "Rescue Squad" has since been reapplied during the squad renovation, putting it back to 1972 specifications.

In 1978 as the TV series and movies were completed, the LA County Fire Department (LACoFD) requested that Universal Studios donate TV's Squad 51 to the LACoFD. It was placed into reserve status and given an LA County Shop number of 49030. The commercial plate was turned in and a "real" tax-exempt plate number, E727413, was issued by the Department of Motor Vehicles and used through 1999. It was actually put into service on occasion to replace Squad 3 in the East LA area. The paramedics knew that they were driving the famous Squad 51 and complained that it was not in good condition. Mostly, the squad sat outside at the LA County train- ing center. In 1998, the County of Los Angeles Fire Museum Association requested that the County of Los Angeles donate Squad 51 to the Museum Association. The county's board of supervisors approved a resolution au- thorizing the transfer.

According to Captain Paul Schneider, LACoFD and Director of the County of Los Angeles Fire Museum Association, the squad had less than 5000 miles on it when the museum took possession of it, because most of the driving in the series was short and stock footage was often utilized. By April 2004, it had accumulated 56,655 miles on it, from limited in-service use with LA County and attendance at parades and fire musters (**Photo 8-1**).

A Stand-in Squad

A Dodge D100 was used as a "stand-in" for Squad 51 when it was crushed by a jet engine in the 1978 *Emergency!* TV movie, *Survival on Charter 220*. It was a retired unit and had not been inservice in quite some time. The visible differences were obvious because the D-100 has round side mir- rors, lack of chrome grab bars on the utility body, and squared-off chrome handles on the body cabinet doors. It also had a different lettering scheme than the TV squad. Surprisingly, not one tear was shed by the off-duty C shift medics from Station 51 or by Johnny and Roy at the site of their de- stroyed squad.

The D-100 is a half-ton capacity truck, usually with a small block V8 or inline 6. The half-ton truck was the truck of choice for light utility work and was a lightweight capacity truck with light-duty springs and suspension.

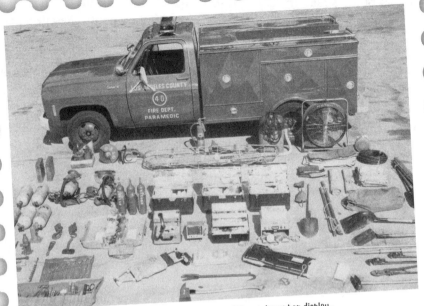

PHOTO 8-1   Squad 40 in 1975 with medical, rescue, and fire equipment on display.
Source: Courtesy of Los Angeles County Fire Department, Photo Unit.

Rescue Squad Storage Compartments[1]

Storage compartments vary due to utility body design and battalion preferences, but a few selected items were consistent across all of the rescue squads in the County. Generally, squads were outfitted alike to facilitate ease of removing the equipment from the cabinets if a firefighter was to pull an overtime shift at another station.

Most of the paramedics kept their turn-out gear wherever they were most comfortable with it. Usually this meant the drivers kept it in the compartment on their side of the squad and passengers kept it on the right-side compartment behind the cab, where the self-contained breathing apparatus air tanks and cutting torch were stored.

All the squads kept forcible entry tools (e.g., wire cutter, ram bar, pry bar, sledgehammer) in the forward upper compartment on the left side of the squad. The left middle compartment often held the rescue saw (circular or chain), gasoline, extra blades, hydraulic jacks, and Porta-Power. The

[1] Thanks to retired LA County Paramedic/firefighters and *Emergency!* Technical Advisors Bob Lee Hancock, Mike Lewis, and Joe Bartak, Jr.

cabinet over the left rear wheel was used for the defibrillator, scope, and second drug box. The compartment at the left rear was a supply cabinet containing IV solution, needles, and other similar medical necessities.

The rear upper compartment of the left side of the squad contained belts, block and tackle, and a tool drawer of small tools. An asbestos blanket was used for covering patients who were trapped in their vehicles while firemen used a circular saw to cut away vehicle body parts for extrication. (Asbestos is excellent in reducing the fire hazard from the sparks generated by the saw, but it was discovered to be a health hazard and is no longer used for this purpose.)

The recessed area in the bed of the utility body stored two rows of air bottles and a K-12, a gasoline-powered circular saw with changeable circular blades that are used to cut through steel. Gasoline-powered ventilation fans (smoke ejectors) may have been stored here as well.

The low storage cabinet at the rear of the squad, where it says "Los Angeles County Fire Dept," is where the stokes, rescue blankets, Miller boards, and shovels were stored. Some squads also kept their ropes in this compartment.

In the right front compartment, the drug box, defibrillator, scope, radio, charging equipment, resuscitator, and hare traction splint were stored. The right middle compartment housed two trauma boxes and a burn box. Up above on a shelf were splints and other equipment. In the right rear, additional miscellaneous supplies and tools could be found.

Emergency!'s Squad 51 equipment location depended on which side of the squad the crew was filming. The squad carried only the equipment necessary for a given episode due to weight and space limitations. The truck companies carried most of the heavy equipment, including the Jaws of Life.

Other models of Squads in LA County's fleet were Fords and Chevrolet Custom D30s. LA County recently ordered Ford F-350XL Super Duty Power Stroke Turbo Diesel V8s to begin replacing the current fleet. In some areas, "heavy squads" are inservice and carry Mass Casuality Incident equipment and other large tools. Every squad is a little different, depending on the area that it serves, proximity of the closest truck, local area needs, and paramedic preference. Extra equipment can include chain saws, rotary saws, fans, and various other heavy rescue gear such as the Jaws of Life®, etc.

Trauma and IV Boxes

Firefighter/paramedic Gary Davis recalls that the first IV box was a leather doctors' bag. "Pre-loads were unheard of at the time," he said, so "all the vials and ampoules were individually wrapped in cloth and packed into the bag, along with the syringes." Eventually, a nurse purchased a small fishing tackle box to replace the bag, and the paramedics labeled and organized equipment in the sections of the box. This was a vast improvement, Davis recalls, since "the ampoules were always breaking in the bags, no matter how well we tried to protect them." Later, firefighter/paramedic Rocky Doke saw the need for better boxes and designed the IV/trauma boxes now used on squads. Doke's brother owned a plastics company, and the two worked together to design the black boxes. Some of the trauma boxes were off-the-shelf units that Rocky purchased, ("Old Pal" tackleboxes that were manufactured by Woodstream) remodeled a bit, labeled with the company name, and sold to the County. In September 2004, the County of Los Angeles Fire Museum Association obtained from Doke a new old-stock trauma box that he found in his garage and donated to the museum for the Squad display. The "Old Pal" boxes were also used on *Emergency!*.

The Engines

Engine 60

One of the two primary Engine 51s was an in-service 1965, 1250 gpm, open-cab Crown Firecoach (Serial number F1400, model number CP-125-93), original LA County maintenance vehicle shop number FD215 (subsequently revised to 49215). In service as Engine 60, it was stationed at Universal Studios (LA County Station 60) and is now on display at the County of Los Angeles Fire Museum. This engine was used during filming on the Universal studio lot during the first two seasons. It was not able to leave the Studio grounds for filming, and this is when Engine 127 came into play.

Again, the magnetic-backed disk with "51" covered the "60" on the doors. Adhesive numbers covered the engine/station number on the front of the engine (because the cowling was made of aluminum so magnets would not stick). Universal Studios' Engine 60 mileage was quite low; as of October 2003, the original miles were 19,920. The original license plate number was E532714 (gold on black), and it currently has E656322 (gold on blue). Due to its age, it was never placed into reserve status and was turned over to the museum upon retirement in 1987. It was in fact the last open-cab Crown to be in service for LA County. Surprisingly, there was very little damage to the body, with just a few dents in the bumper areas and a badly faded paint job. The County of Los Angeles Fire Museum has plans to restore the engine and install two sets of doors that can be put on the rig. Two doors numbered as "60" and two as "51" will be interchanged as necessary for parades and other events.

Engine 127

Engine 127, sister to Engine 60 (one of seventeen 1965 Crowns) also portrayed Engine 51 and was utilized for stock footage for the World Premier and subsequent shots on location and at Station 127 in the Carson area (such as the refinery rescues) until it was replaced by the Ward LaFrance (WLF). The Crown's serial number is F1388, and its LA County shop number is 49214.

Although this Crown was cosmetically the same as Engine 60, it had a different motor and a few other minor differences. Engine 127 can be seen as Engine 127 in several later episodes and often heard being "toned out" to respond with Engine 51 on various alarms. The cab was enclosed and a Twinsonic light bar was later installed, replacing the gumball. It originally had a 935 Hall-Scott motor (as was typical of the Crowns) and was re-powered in the late 1970s with a Cummins NTF 295.

After leaving Station 127, Engine 127 went into reserve status and was housed at Station 10. Station 95 (137 W. Redondo Beach Boulevard, in Gardena, just north of Carson and 8 miles north of Station 127) had as first-out a 1981 American LaFrance (ALF). On an unrecorded date in the mid-1980s, the ALF was in the shop, and they were using the former Engine 127 brought over from Station 10 to be inservice as E95. The Crown was involved in an accident near its station with a semi-truck, which demolished the front of the apparatus. Squad 36 and Engine 36 (from 127 W. 223rd Street in Carson, 2 miles west of Station 127) and at least two private ambulances responded to the accident, but injuries to firefighters and the truck driver are unknown. "Big Jim" Allen, Repair 13, the Fire Department mechanic, also responded to assess the damage. Records are incomplete as to the ultimate disposition of the engine after the accident.

Other Open-Cab Crowns

A number of other Crowns were used for "on-location shots" in the program in other areas such as Malibu, where they put the "51" numbers on the closest available circa 1965 open-cab Crown. If a suitable engine could not be located—by this time there was very few open-cab Crowns left because most had been retrofitted—E127 would be driven to the location with another County engine filling in at Station 127. All this difficulty in locating and moving apparatus was resolved with the appearance of a "new" Engine 51.

There were other open-cab units in service, but they were not cosmetically the same as Engine 60 or Engine 127, so they could not be utilized as filming doubles. The Crown equipment at Station 8 was an example; both Engine 8 and Engine 208 were hose wagon/pumper combos.

Los Angeles County still has some Crown Firecoach engines in service, not the 1965 vintage but later mid-1970 manufactured apparatus. They are either reserve apparatus (Engines 559, 572, and 587) or call firefighter apparatus (Engines 112, 269, 279, 314, and 317). The last Crown purchased by LA County was a 1980 Crown 50-foot Telesquirt, shop number 49407. It began service as E89 in the City of Commerce, which later became E50, and it is now E559. The last remaining Crown Quint in service is at Station 104.

The Crown Firecoach Company began in 1904 as the Crown Carriage Company, manufacturing carriages and wagons. The Crown Firecoach was first off the line in 1951 and was considered to be the Cadillac of fire apparatus. The last Firecoach to be built was in 1985, with the factory finally closing in 1991. All in all, LA County purchased 141 Crown Firecoach apparatus from 1954 through 1979.

Offered as a factory option for the open-cab Crowns was a canvas top. Engine 209 was outfitted with one, and a photo can be seen in Captain Dave Boucher's book *Devil Wind Fire Wagons*. It is unknown how many other LA County Crowns had this rag-top.

The Ward LaFrance Engine

According to WLF documents, (March 25, 1971), LA County ordered 42 WLF P-80 engines, beginning with spec number 80-591 with delivery completed by November 30, 1972. Eight more WLFs were ordered and delivered in 1974. Underbidding Crown Firecoach, the engines cost the department $44,000 each and were delivered over a 3-year period. The Wards sat a crew of five and would eventually become one of the most popular models that the company ever produced, mainly as a direct result of *Emergency!*.

Early in 1973, with all these Wards coming to LA County, the company realized just how visible this new TV program was and wanted its engine to be showcased on *Emergency!* rather than the Crown. Arrangements were made to obtain a WLF for the show that would be Engine 60's and Engine 127's replacement. The model delivered was a 1973 WLF Ambassador with the Ultra-Vision windshield, model number P80-1000D-5,[2] spec number 80-811, on a 178-inch wheelbase; it was donated to Universal Studios by the manufacturer. Its assigned California license number is E999058.

The distinctive Ward P-80 body and cab first appeared in 1961 as a demonstrator, Spec# 8000, that later sold to Ripley, West Virginia in 1962. The cab at that time was known as the Mark 1 CFE cab. Later refinements brought that cab to what is now known as the "Ambassador" or P-80 cab.

---

[2] P=Pumper, 80=Cabstyle, 1000=Pump size in GPM, D=Diesel engine, 5=500 gallon booster tank.

Four members of the LACoFD flew back to New York at NBC's expense to pick up the engine. After a series of required pump tests and inspections at Ward's facility in Elmira Heights, New York, WLF officially turned the engine over to Universal City on April 13, 1973. It was issued a New York commercial license plate of 7131-GM. The crew began a 26-day journey to Universal Studios in the new Engine 51 (see Chapter 17). The engine made its first appearance in episode 3.2, "The Old Engine." Ironically the episode title had nothing to do with the "old" Crown being replaced but referred to an even older fire apparatus that Johnny and Roy had purchased.

Just as different model squads appear throughout the show in various stock footage, the same is true with the engines, although more rarely. For example, in an early third season episode, the guys get into the squad next to the Ward engine, the station rollup doors open, and the Crown is visible as the squad pulls out.

The WLF representative on the West Coast, George Ashley, said, "The only agreement made with Universal was that WLF would get the benefit of the rig's exposure on the show as long as the show was filming, and then the rig would revert ownership to LACoFD. I do know that once the show started airing with the Ward as E51, the sales of the P-80 series almost tripled. There was no way that WLF could have afforded that kind of advertising exposure on a nationwide basis."

However, Engine 51 was not built to LA County specs, because it had a smaller pump and engine. "The LA County spec Wards have 1500-gpm Hale pumps, derated to 1250 gpm, but on a test we were able to get 2000 gpm with a slightly higher engine rpm," according to George Ashley. Engine 51 had a 1000 gallons per minute, two-stage Hale pump (at 150 pounds per square inch)—the same as LA County's Forester and Fire Warden rigs. LA County Ward engines are Cummins Diesel NHTF-295 and NTF-365 HP turbo charged; E51 is a Cummins Diesel NHF-265 HP and not turbo charged (265 horsepower at 2300 rpms). LA County spec Wards and Engine 51 both have 500-gallon booster tanks. Engine 51 came with an Allison HT-70, 6-speed automatic transmission. E-51 has the same outside body appearance as the LA County Consolidated District rigs.

This particular model of the Ward (Engine 51) was classified as a "stock" engine by WLF and, as such, was usually a bit cheaper for smaller departments to be able to purchase. In fact, the engine delivered to Universal to become Engine 51 was originally ordered by the Lake Park, Florida, Fire Department and was already on the production line at the factory in Elmira, New York, designated as Lake Park Engine 24. Universal needed to start filming for the third season, and the engine designated by WLF for Universal would not be ready in time. WLF contacted Lake Park Fire Chief Larry Joyce by phone to inform him that the show's engine would not be

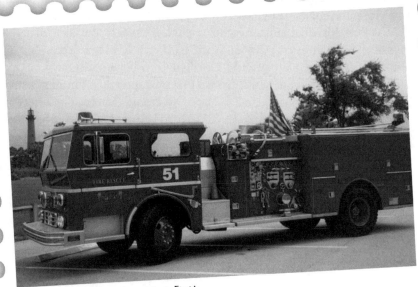

PHOTO 8-2   Fire Rescue 51 in service in Florida.
Source: Courtesy of Keith Campbell.

ready in time and asked if a trade would be acceptable. Chief Joyce consented, and the show's WLF went to Lake Park after it was completed. Lake Park's WLF (the next engine that came off the line) was sent to Universal right away **(Photo 8-2)**.

Eventually Lake Park received a 1973 Ward, spec number 80-922, on October 18, 1973, which was originally destined to be Universal's Engine 51. Lake Park's original engine cost the department only $24,000, which was remarkably lower than LA County's fleet. Their replacement engine arrived with extra "chrome, bells and whistles," according to former Lake Park firefighter Bryan Fields, gratis from Ward. It came with a Detroit Diesel 265-horsepower engine, with an Allison HT-70, 6-speed automatic transmission with a chrome bumper, chrome tow eyes, extra window trim, and a 1250-gpm, single-stage Hale pump.

The Lake Park WLF, which was painted red at the factory, was repainted in 1986 to conform to Lake Park colors—white with a red stripe. It was restored and repainted red in 2000 and numbered as Engine 51. It was in service until June 29, 2002, when Lake Park merged into Palm Beach County. The engine was later sold at auction to Keith Campbell, an engine operator with Palm Beach County Fire-Rescue. Campbell restored the engine, which had been stripped of all its equipment and required major pump work. The engine was used for parades, charity functions, and other special events. A beer tap plumbed into the engineer's panel and a Kool-Aid dispenser on a hose reel made it quite popular at musters. Its Florida license plate read FOOLS-51 (FOOLS being the acronym for Fraternal Order of Leatherheads Society, a reference to leather helmets).

In early 2006, Campbell sold the engine (with 36,000 miles on it) to the Canouan Fire Department, located on Canouan Island in the West Indies. It was the first engine on the small resort island. They kept the beer tap and the Kool-Aid dispenser.

Universal's Engine 51 Is Not Ready for Filming

"When E51 first arrived from back east after the tour, the Universal camera department complained that the rig came from the factory with tinted glass all around and that had to be changed to clear glass so as not to screw up the color shots from inside the cab. So I had to replace all the glass," states George Ashley, WLF rep, who later became Repair 10 for LACoFD. The windshield was the four-pane, Ultra-Vision, double-slant glass area that allowed the driver an unobstructed view of the road.

Universal's E51 original paint was Dupont Dulex #936744-Red enamel, a Chrysler red color, which was a different color red than the squad and LA County specs. This caused a few moments of concern for the show's producers, but as producer Ed Self commented, "We looked at the engine and the squad and back again. True, they weren't exactly the same color but would anybody at home notice? Everyone was staring at me and after a moment I decreed that they were close enough."

After the Ward was delivered, and in service, Webb's Mark VII Productions would contribute to the house fund at FS60 where it was stored because the firefighters cleaned, washed, and changed hose if needed when it came back to its "quarters" in the studio shop after the day's shooting. Additionally, at the end of each filming season, Mark VII Productions wrote $100.00 checks to the house funds of all the LA County Fire stations, and $500.00 to the Department's Benefit & Welfare Association. Webb called it his payment for "creative ideas" submitted by station personnel each year.

During the off-season and after the series shut down, the *Emergency!*'s Ward saw service at Universal Studios Fire Station 60, as Engine 260. It would be assigned LA County shop maintenance number 49353, which can be clearly seen below the pump panel in some season 6 episodes.

Because the vehicles used in the show (both the Squad and engines) were dressed as actual LA County emergency vehicles, both the Ward and the squad had to display "out of service" placards in the front windows while driving on the city streets while en route to and from filming sites. The Ward also had a magnetic placard on the door that covered "LA County" and read, "*Emergency!* NBC Saturday 8 PM, A Universal Mark VII Production."

Other WLF units can be seen in the series, most notably as Engines 73 and 114 and as Engine 18 in the *Charter 220* movie and as Engine 110 in the *Steel Inferno* movie. These units were actual LACoFD engines. Hollywood Fire Authority, a film car rental company based in LaVerne, California, east of Los Angeles, has one of the original LA County 1972 Wards, shop number 49495. In the engine log book it is written that it was sent to the *Emergency!* set about a dozen times for "large fire scenes," not as Engine 51, but as one of the background and additional responding units seen in the series. In later years it saw service as Engine 168 in El Monte and had other various reserve engine assignments throughout the County, lastly as Engine 587 in the City of Industry up to April 1999 when it was sold.

As of 2006, LA County still has a few of the Wards in service. Three were at the Headquarters Training Center as Training Engines 3, 4 (formerly E535), and 5. One was stationed in the desert community of Lancaster at Station 117 as Engine 5117, as a reserve apparatus (shop number 49316). Another was located at Station 129 also in Lancaster as Engine 5129 (shop number 49311). However in 2007, most if not all of the remaining Wards were sold at auction.

Explorer 10

One other Ward, shop number 49513 (or 613), was operated by the LA County Fire Explorers as "EXP 10." The rig was fixed up by the Battalion 10 Post—they reupholstered the seat in cloth, replaced the engine cover and headliner, refinished numerous items on the rig, and added tinted windows and a stereo system. Unfortunately, when last seen at the LACoFD Training Center, it was filthy inside and out, had a broken window, several missing pump panel handles, and faded paint. Its current status is unknown.

LA City Wards

The City of LA purchased twenty-two 1500-gpm Ward Ambassadors in 1976 (shop numbers 60282 through 60288, and 60308 through 60322. Eleven City stations each received two of the new Wards, one outfitted as a Pumper and one as a Wagon. They were all open-cab Wards; some were later retrofitted. All were powered by Cummins NTA-400 diesel engines with manual transmission and fitted with Hale 1500-gpm pumps and 500-gallon water tanks. At least one is still in service, at LA City station 26, with several in reserve status. In mid-2005, the City auctioned off ten of the WLFs, some with almost 200,000 miles on them.

The Ward LaFrance Corporation

The Ward LaFrance Truck Corporation ceased operation in 1979 because of major financial problems and was reformed under a new name, Ward79, which closed down ten years later. The Ward LaFrance Truck Corp. had no corporate connection with ALF but did have a family connection. Addison Ward LaFrance, who founded the Ward LaFrance Truck Corporation, was the son of Asa Willis LaFrance, who, along with his brother Truxton Slocum LaFrance, founded ALF some years earlier.

The History of Engine 51 in Los Angeles County

In 1924 Los Angeles took delivery of thirty-six new, right-hand drive ALF engines. The first mention of an *Engine 51,* an ALF, appears in the LACoFD's 1939 annual report. The date of this report corresponds with the replacement of Engine 1 and Engine 3's ALFs with new Seagrave apparatus.

Engine 1 (now a relief engine) was lettered, "Los Angeles County Fire Dept" on both sides of the hood and now numbered "Engine 51" on the body just behind the pump outlets. All lettering was in white paint.

Relief Engine 51 was eventually placed in reserve status in 1948, completely stripped of equipment. (The Department used to have relief and reserves.) The difference was that a relief was fully equipped and a reserve had no equipment; this terminology has since changed. As a designated relief engine, Engine 51 saw service at several locations throughout the County.

As a relief engine, it would actually have been referred to as Engine "five-one" not "fifty-one." Today, this reference system is used for reserve engines such as engine 5-163 or 5-16. When the department had more than fifty engines in service, they referred to engines using a zero between the five and the old assignment number of the apparatus, or the station number, where the relief apparatus ended up being assigned.

When Dick Friend was 14 and an auxiliary fireman up in Rolling Hills, he and the other volunteers trained on, what else, a 1924 ALF which was at that time Lomita's Engine 6.

The County of Los Angeles Fire Museum has a 1924 ALF in its collection. Paul Schneider states, "The ALF is currently in storage and under its battered exterior, from sitting several years in a children's park in South Gate, is a complete and well-preserved power train, frame, and suspension!"

Engine 51 at Station 51

However, the first "real" engine in service as Engine 51 would be a 1949 General-Pacific fire engine, assigned to newly built Fire Station 51 located in the 4500 block of Arlington Avenue (cross of Atlantic Avenue) in 1951.

The General's license plate was E36402 (the "E" within an octagon), gold numbers on a black plate. The number "51" in gold leaf was within a gold circle on the doors of the apparatus, and "Los Angeles County Fire Dept." was in gold leaf on the hood.

The "General," as such engines were commonly called, had its roots in St. Louis, Missouri, and has gone the way of the Crowns, WLFs, and many other fire engine manufacturers. The company began as a carbon-tet fire extinguisher company in 1918 as the General Manufacturing Company. By 1926, the General Fire Truck Corporation was formed and began producing fire apparatus. A few years later, the company moved to Detroit, where it put its "shell" on a chassis from Chevrolets, GMCs, Fords, and others with a Packard V-12 or a Super V-8 motor. In 1937 a West Coast subsidiary was established in Los Angeles, known as the General-Pacific Corporation. This is where Engine 51 was built. The last General came off the line in 1957.

Other Apparatus

Repair 14

This vehicle was seen only in two episodes in season 6, but "Charlie the Mechanic" made an impression. It was a 1974/1975 Dodge 1-ton, D-300, with a service truck body. It is very similar in appearance to the rescue squads of the day. On the doors it had the County seal affixed with the word "FIRE" underneath. The "R14" identification was affixed on the fender cowling just above the D-300 model identification. It did not have a light bar because it was not an emergency vehicle, but it sported two amber, forward-facing spots. Throughout the series, two different vehicles portrayed Repair 14. In "Breakdown" (episode 6.15), there is a rear-facing speaker mounted behind the cab, but in "The Boat" (episode 6.19), the speaker is gone.

Dennis "Ace" Pump Escape

Johnny and Roy purchased a British Fire Appliance in "The Old Engine" (episode 3.2); they responded with it in "The Parade" (episode 4.13) and then sold it in "The Old Engine Cram" (episode 5.2).

It is first identified on *Emergency!* as a 1932 Dennis, although in reality, this model was produced only between 1934 and 1939. However, the information/press release sent out by Universal to the newspapers and weekly television magazines identified it as "a 1920s vehicle" for "The Parade" episode. In "The Old Engine Cram," it is mistakenly identified altogether, once as a "1925 or earlier Paige fire engine" (in the newspaper want ad), then by John as a "Twenty-three Paige" (per the script). The same vehicle appears in all three episodes.

This particular model Dennis fire engine seen in the program is known as an "Ace." The Ace was mainly supplied to the British market, although some engines were exported to New Zealand, Australia, and India. According to Dennis records, none appear to have been sent to America for actual in-service use. In the 1930s, the Ace engine cost between 500 and 1000 British pounds ($2500 and $5000 in 1970s U.S. dollars), depending on what type of equipment the customer desired and size of pump installed.

The Dennis Ace was originally fitted with a 4-cylinder, 3.7-liter gasoline engine with a maximum of 60 horsepower. The gross running weight under guaranteed conditions was 4 tons 16 cwt (9600 pounds), and the chassis weight (less fuel, spare wheel, equipment, and tools) was approximately 1 ton 16 cwt (3600 pounds). The overall chassis dimensions were 17 feet 7/8 inches in length and 6 feet 4.5 inches in width, with a wheelbase of 9 feet 6 inches. The vehicle used on *Emergency!* had a Braidwood body and was fitted with an Ajax ladder. By 1935 Dennis introduced the Ace "Light 6," which came with a larger 6-cylinder engine.

"Pump escape" refers to the appliance having a pump and a 30-foot extension ladder that was pulled off from the back of the engine. The early 30-foot ladders were made of laminated wood with manufacturers (besides Ajax) being Bailey and Dewherst. This model could also come with a 50-foot extendable ladder with large wheels attached, positioned at the back of the appliance; removing the ladder facilitated maneuverability in tight alleyways and made it easier to get close to the buildings. This appliance would then be known as a "wheeled escape."

A larger appliance, the Dennis Big 6, by way of comparison had an inline, 6-cylinder engine with an 850-gpm centrifugal pump. It was also manufactured during the 1930s and had more power. The cost of a Big 6 in 1939 was £3184, purchased directly from Dennis Brothers Pty. Ltd. of Guildford, England. Diesel engines were offered but most brigades opted for more speed with the petrol (gasoline) engines. The Big 6 could be fitted with a pump escape or wheeled escape ladders.

The manufacturing of Dennis fire appliances began in 1908, and they were long a staple of the British Fire Service, including service in countries such as New Zealand, Hong Kong, and Australia, where the New South Wales Fire Brigade was the biggest user outside of the United Kingdom. Other fire services included Singapore, Athens, Brisbane, Barbados, Cairo, Penang (Malaysia), and Shanghai. The company was sold in 1972, with the primary concentration on the export market by the new owners. By 1984 the company, Hestair Dennis, concentrated on chassis building only because of the rising costs of complete body building of fire apparatus.

In 1985 John Dennis, grandson of one of the founding brothers, decided to start his own fire apparatus, body-building company. Primarily a Coach builder before this (nothing to do with fire engines or Dennis the fire engine manufacturer), he took over the company, renamed it Dennis Specialist Vehicles, and in 1986 a true Dennis fire appliance once again rolled out. Dennis Coachbuilders not only continues to manufacturer the Dennis Saber and Dennis Dagger fire appliances, but continues to provide fire chassis for the Volvo, Mercedes Benz, and Scania companies.

Unfortunately, it is unknown what museum or private collection the Dennis was obtained from that was utilized on *Emergency!*. The year of manufacture, original customer, and exact date the vehicle left Dennis Works are also unknown.

Engine 382

Engine 382 appeared in the *Emergency!* World Premier and "Brushfire" (episode 1.4). It is a 1957 four-wheel drive Yankee/Cavalier brush rig, chassis number C80235 and model number 367 COE, LA shop number N-539. It was originally assigned to Station 73 then later to Station 82, where it saw service from Malibu to Gorman. It was sold to Big Bear in 1973, where it was repainted ALF safety lime-yellow and renumbered BE291 (Brush Engine 291). Through the efforts of David Boucher and Jim Page, who at one time was the rig's engineer, it was returned to Los Angeles in 2000 with plans for restoration of its original appearance. Its California exempt license plate of E110881 was turned in, and it was issued a Historical Vehicle plate, HV 841K. It is now on display at the LA County Fire Museum in South Gate.

Safety Color Lime-Yellow

ALF developed the safety color "lime-yellow" in the early 1970s and named it "American LaFrance Safety Lime Yellow." WLF developed its lime-yellow paint and introduced it in 1971. A lot of money was spent via scientific studies, advertisements, and surveys in the early 1970s in trying to convince fire departments of the safety feature of this color. Many departments across the country did order the lime-yellow paint for their engines, regardless of the manufacturer. The color, although indeed proven to be a safer color to the eye, especially at night, was never popular with firefighters, although it is still in use in several departments. Other apparatus manufacturers developed "lime" paint colors as well.

LA County Engine 505/Universal Studios Engine 260

Reserve Engine 260 at Universal Studios also appeared in several episodes of *Emergency!*. It started out in 1953 as a Huntington Park Fire Department engine and came to LA County in 1970 when Huntington Park was absorbed into the County Fire Department.

At the time of its retirement from County service, it had been assigned as Engine 50 and then Engine 505. In the mid-1970s, Assistant Chief Paul Schneider (uncle of the current County of Los Angeles Fire Museum director, Paul Schneider) convinced Universal Studios to keep the engine for movie and TV work, and it became Engine 260 at Universal Studios Station 60.

Built by Coast Fire Apparatus Company of Martinez, California, on an International chassis, this 1000-gpm fire engine is powered by a 935-cubic-inch Hall-Scott engine. The LA County shop number is 49277, VIN number is 481009, and body number is 859; there are currently 39,242 original miles on it. It was donated to the County of Los Angeles Fire Museum in 1995 and is currently on display.

Squad 209

Squad 209 was seen only briefly in "Honest" (episode 2.17) and "Propinquity" (episode 3.20), although actually it is the same footage. It is seen off to the right as the ambulance enters the tunnel at Rampart (Harbor General Hospital) followed by Squad 51. It is parked near the emergency department entrance at Harbor General during filming of an on-location scene. It was also referred to often on Squad 51's radio—"Squad 209, 10-7 to St. Francis"—and in "Honest" (even though they are sitting at Rampart) as well as in "Dinner Date" (episode 2.10) and "Rip-Off" (episode 2.20).

Los Angeles County Fire Museum

All these apparatus and more, including Jim Page's restored Rescue 11, with the exception of Squad 209, Repair 14, and the Dennis Ace, are currently property of the Los Angeles County Fire Museum. The engines are housed in a warehouse located at 8635 Otis Street, South Gate, California. The Museum does not maintain operational hours and is only open to the public twice a year during open houses.

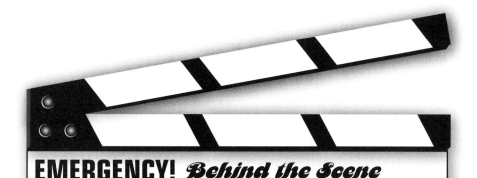

EMERGENCY! *Behind the Scene*

CHAPTER **9**

Filming Locations

Fire Station 106

LA County Fire Station 106 in Rancho Palos Verdes, California, was thought ideal to depict the fictional Station 51: it was new and on a relatively quiet street, and, at least then, it had good access. However, Station 106 was impractical for the series for several reasons—the building faced east, so it would have sun and shadow problems for filming, and it was too far from the studio to transport all the required equipment.

The studio eventually located Station 127, which was similar in construction to Station 106. More importantly, Station 127 faced south, which was ideal for filming. Station 106, Battalion 14 headquarters, currently runs a paramedic squad, an engine, a patrol unit, a quint, a utility unit, and has two Battalion Chiefs.

Fire Station 127

LA County Station 127, at 2049 East 223rd Street in Carson, became Station 51 in the program. At the time, this was a fictional County station number. This station is located 15 miles south of LA International Airport (LAX) off I-405. The station opened up February 15, 1967. It is built in a drive-through style, although the narrow side drive on the east side of the station and lack of turn room in back result in the engines always backing in. There are several stations in the County with this same floor plan and exterior, designed to save money in architectural fees.

Station 127 has never been a paramedic station (the closest paramedic station is FS36, just about 2 miles away). At the time, it had a 1965 open-cab Crown Firecoach at the station as Engine 127, with a 1968 Crown truck with an 85-foot Pittman-Snorkel (shop number 49248) as Truck 127 (replaced in 1990), and Foam 127, a 1967 Ford F-250 with the platter light setup. All three of these apparatus appeared in several episodes of *Emergency!*. In November 2006, 127 received a new KME Predator as "Engine 127" (shop number F1495). Also in the station are a 1998 KME Renegade Aerial-Cat 75 Tiller (shop number F0617) as "Light Force 127" and a 1984 Mack MC686FC Foam as Foam 5127 (shop number F0376). It is a reserve unit that came from the Shell refinery when it closed.

Since 1985, Station 127 has been known as the Robert A. Cinader Memorial Fire Station. A plaque is affixed to the station wall near the front door. Station signage, installed in 1985 creating the memorial to Cinader, was changed in 2006 to reflect the current lettering and design, conforming to Los Angeles County Fire Department (LACoFD) standards. On the inside of the station in the apparatus bay, plaques on the wall state "Fire Station 127—Home of the Show "Emergency!," flanked by two helmet shields indicating Station 51.

For the crews working at Station 127, the location was not ideal. Immediately across the street is the British Petroleum refinery, formerly the Atlantic Richfield Company facility. Immediately behind it is the Conoco/Phillips refinery, which was formerly UNOCAL, and the Royal Dutch Shell refinery. And in the late 1960s, a HazMat (hazardous materials) incident at the chlorine factory across the street sent a chlorine cloud drifting toward the station. Firefighters were not able to start Engine 127, but they were able to start the truck and drive out. This accident damaged vehicle paint, killed the grass in front of the station, turned pennies green, and even damaged the station's television. The station was uninhabitable for 3 days. As a result the station had small breathing apparatus (BA) sets attached to the walls next to the beds. The same held true for Station 10 on Del Amo Boulevard in Carson with the installation of the small BA sets. Station 10, actually located on the Shell Oil refinery site, had a 4" Sulfate line running underneath but experienced no problems.

Firefighter Bob Hoff was assigned to Station 127 just after the incident happened:

> The guys that were there told me about it….In the late night or early morning hours there was a leak that caused a gas cloud to form and drift toward the station and surrounding buildings….Truck 127 happened to be returning from a canceled run and was backing into the station when they saw the cloud heading for the station. They were able to warn the other guys still at the station. As I remember none of the guys on duty was seriously injured.
>
> When I arrived there we had small 5-minute [oxygen] bottles that we could put on and get to the rigs where our regular BAs were. I also remember we drilled often on how to change our air bottle in a nonbreathable atmosphere.

The BA bottles are no longer there because they have since been removed. FS 10 removed theirs when Shell stopped being a refinery about ten years ago. FS 127 did the same after they dismantled the Chlorine factory across from the Chevy Dealer.

An insight to working at FS 127 and FS 60 according to Captain Vernoie Steele, FS 56:

> I most certainly watched *Emergency!* before I joined the department. I thought it was a great show. I worked at FS 127 for only 6 months back in 1989. I was a boot firefighter then and it was my second fire station out of the academy. I was studying hard as I really was trying to get off probation so I really wasn't too privy to people coming into the station inquiring about Johnny and Roy. It was a little tough for me back then being an African American and a woman. Again I just wanted to get off probation. A few years later, I worked a few times at Fire Station 60 at Universal. I actually got inquiries about Johnny and Roy when working there. A new station, and a new number, in honor of *Emergency!* was built and Johnny actually came out during the dedication ceremony.

Captain Steele has been with the department for seventeen years and was promoted to the rank of Captain in 2000.

The following was remembered by retired LACo firefighter/paramedic Jeff Brum:

> I was sixteen when I first watched the show. At that time *Adam-12* was my favorite show but *Emergency!* took its place. The show did steer me in the direction of becoming a firefighter. It was the work they did and the lifestyle they led that influenced me. It was a long process becoming an LA County firefighter and once I was there it didn't seem real.

I was assigned to Station 127 and it was funny the first time I saw the station, it still looked liked it did in the TV show. I didn't realize there was an oil refinery right across the street. Little has changed inside the station. We had visitors almost everyday and from all over the world. I didn't realize the show was so popular outside the United States. Fans of the show ranged from just a simple tour to please show me Johnny's locker! Some fans would show me areas of the station that had changed. One female fan was so giddy when she saw Johnny's locker she couldn't stop laughing. One guy in the military almost missed his flight overseas just so he could see the station; we got him a cab to the airport just in time.

Bob Hoff was working at 127 just as the series began, and waiting for the next paramedic class to start. He said people would come around and just wanted to see the station, what it was really like. When people inquired about a Paramedic Squad, they would send them to 36s, just up the street from them. Bob would later become a paramedic and a TA for *Emergency!*.

Fire Station 60

LA County Station 60 was based on the grounds of Universal Studios at the time series was filmed. As luck would have it, similar open-cab Crowns were in service at Stations 60 and 127. Engine 60 was an in-service unit, and an alarm system was set up on the soundstage at the interior set of Station 51 in case Engine 60 was required to respond to an actual alarm. The fire equipment was not permitted off of Studio property for fire calls or filming outside their area. The station was in service until a new station was built on Studio grounds and old Station 60 was torn down during studio expansion. Part of the *Jurassic Park* ride now occupies the former site.

LA County opened new Fire Station 60 on October 30, 2003. The station number has been unused since Universal Studios opened its new Station 51 at the studio. The station, located in Signal Hill, is equipped with a KME four-person paramedic engine and responds only within the city of Signal Hill. It can leave the district for emergency automatic aid and mutual aid responses, where the station will be immediately backfilled, but all training and other activities must be handled within the district.

Fire Station 51

As indicated earlier, LA County now has a real Station 51, again. Station 60 on Universal Studio grounds was replaced by a new, modern LA County Fire Station 51 in November 1998. The Universal tram tour goes in front of Station 51, about 200 yards uphill from where FS60 was located and is on the former site of the "burning house" prop (a seemingly appropriate location), which closed in 1992. Station 51 currently houses a 1999 KME Renegade as Engine 51 (shop number F0594), a 1999 GMC 2500 Sierra Pickup as Paramedic Squad 51 (shop number F0625), and a 1992 Ford F-350 Standard Cab as Patrol 51 (shop number F0143).

This was not the first "real" Station 51 serving the LACoFD. There was an LA County Station 51 located in the unincorporated area of the county along the east side of Lynwood that opened in 1951 with a 1949 General-Pacific fire engine. The station was a single-story, single-bay station in a residential area on Arlington Avenue, located on the south side of the 4500 Block of Arlington Avenue, just east of Atlantic Ave. (just a bit north of the intersection of Atlantic and McMillan Street), in what was then called the Lugo area. The words, "Eng. Co. 51" were over the wooden, barndoor-style doors of the apparatus bay.

The station was closed sometime in the late 1950s as a result of dwindling areas of responsibility and annexations by Compton, Lynwood, and Paramount. The old station sat vacant for several years until it was demolished. The former Station 51's area is now served by the LACoFD Engine 148 district.

There has been some confusion regarding the fact that there was a Station 51 in Los Angeles during the time of filming the series. This was, and still is, an LA City Station 51, not a County station. It is one of three stations that serve the LAX Terminal area.

Rampart Hospital

Stock footage, aerial shots, and long shots for Rampart Hospital utilized County of Los Angeles Harbor–UCLA Medical Center at 1000 West Carson Street in Torrance, California, known as Harbor General Hospital prior to affiliating with the University of California at Los Angeles. It is located about 4 miles from Station 127. This is where many of LA City and County paramedics, other fire department firefighters, ambulance company emergency medical technicians, and mobile intensive care nurses actually went through their training. The exterior ambulance entrance to Rampart for the "tight shots" and the hospital interior were built on Universal's lot.

The name for the Rampart Hospital came out of Jack Webb's *Adam-12*. The Los Angeles Police Department (LAPD) station building where *Adam-12* was based was actually the Rampart Division before transferring to the Wilshire Division. Rampart was northwest of downtown Los Angeles. It is where *Adam-12* Officers Malloy and Reed worked, and it is a real division of the LAPD.

Fictional Rampart Hospital phone number was 555–4667. Rampart's radio room (later episodes) phone extension was #3112. Dr. Brackett's office at Rampart Hospital was room number 127, and his hospital beeper/ pager number was 162. The hospital was often referred to as the "Rampart Emergency Hospital."

While Harbor General has a Torrance mailing address, it is actually located in a narrow strip of unincorporated area between Carson and the Los Angeles City strip. There is a stretch of landscape less than a mile wide that connects the central portion of LA with the Los Angeles Harbor.

Originally, Harbor–UCLA Medical Center was a station hospital at the LA Port of Embarkation. The army sold it to the LA County Department of Charities in 1946 as war surplus, and UCLA's School of Medicine became affiliated 2 years later. The basic structure of the building has not changed much since the eight-story replacement facility opened in 1963.[1] It is one of several trauma centers in the LA area, and it offers both physician training and research programs. However, due to rising costs, the number of trauma centers in Los Angeles is shrinking. In the 1980s there were more than twenty trauma centers in the LA area; today there are just fourteen.

Fire Stations Utilized During the Filming of *Emergency!*	
Station	**Episode**
LA County Station 8 7643 West Santa Monica Boulevard Los Angeles, CA	*Emergency!* World Premier, 1972 "Equipment," episode 5.4, 1975 *Emergency!* movie, The Steel Inferno, 1978
LA County Station 127 2049 East 223rd Street Carson, CA	*Emergency!* 1972–1977, 124 60-minute episodes
LA County Station 110 4433 Admiralty Way Marina Del Rey, CA	*Emergency!* movie, The Steel Inferno, 1978
LA County Station 65 4206 North Cornell Road Agoura, CA	"Isolation," episode 6.20, 1977 "Inferno," episode 3.21, 1974
LA County Station 68 24138 Calabasas Road Calabasas, CA	"The Camera Bug," episode 4.10, 1974 *GO*, September 7, 1974. an NBC kids program

---

[1] http://www.ladhs.org/ Health Services of Los Angeles County.

Fire Stations Utilized During the Filming of *Emergency!* (continued)

Station	Episode
LA City Station 36* 638 Beacon Street San Pedro, CA	"Not Available," episode 6.2, 1976
LA County Station 43 921 S. Stimson Avenue La Puente, CA	"Insomnia," episode 3.8, 1973
LACo Fire Department Headquarters 1320 N. Eastern Avenue Los Angeles, CA	*Emergency!* movie, *Greatest Rescues of Emergency!*, 1978
Barton Heliport LACo Air Operations Headquarters 12605 Osborne Street Pacoima, CA	Excellent overview in "Right at Home," episode 5.17, 1976
Fire Camp 9** Santa Clarita Truck Trail Sylmar, CA	"Right at Home," episode 5.17, 1976

*This facility, San Pedro Municipal Building, housed the Fire and Police Departments, including the jail, from 1928–1972. This facility now houses a Fire Museum, in the area of the former fire station, operated by the Los Angeles Fire Department Historical Society. http://www.lafdmuseum.org/.

**Former pilot for LACo, Gary Lineberry, says of the fire camps, "Camp 9 is still in use today as a paid camp, as opposed to several of the inmate camps in the county. It was originally established as a base for the air attack helicopter because it is at the 4000-foot level and provided a good jumping-off spot for fires in the north end of the county. The other paid camps in the county are Camp 2, the headquarters camp next to JPL in Pasadena, and Camp 8 in Malibu. Both of those camps also have a helicopter assigned at various times during the fire season. All paid camps are staffed by fire suppression aides (FSAs), who are young guys and gals who have an eye on the fire service and use it as a way to get a feel for the work. It is hard, back-breaking work on the fire line for these folks, and, unfortunately, service in the camps does not give them any extra credit with respect to getting on with the LA County Fire Department. But it does give them experience, and there are graduates of our camp system on departments all over the country."

EMERGENCY! *Behind the Scene*

CHAPTER **10**

Supporting Equipment

Ambulances

A film rental company (California Hearse & Ambulance Sales Company or CHASCO, a division of Snyder Ambulance) provided many of the ambulances used on *Emergency!* and *Rescue 8*. Magnetic signs were affixed with either "J & R" or "Miller's" logos by the Universal Studios property department. On rare occasions, the signs were left off and "Snyder" would be providing the transport. The fictitious "Mayfair" logo was the primary name utilized throughout the series. CHASCO film car units, along with Schaefer Ambulance Company in LA, were regularly used in *CHiPs* and many other popular series of the era, including the popular 1976 movie, *Mother, Juggs, & Speed*.

One ambulance utilized in *Emergency!*, Snyder Unit 33, was a 1968 Chevrolet 3500 series panel style vehicle. Snyder Unit 33 would be driven to various locations or to the Universal lot for the ambulance shots by two off-duty LA City paramedics. They would act as extras in the load-and-go scenes, also known in the trade as "swoop & scoop" and "scoop & haul." Other units of Snyder's were a 1969 National Suburban and a 1968 Miller-Meteor Cadillac; Ford Super-Duty Econoline vans were used in later episodes. The "Miller's" ambulance vans showed up again after series end in the *Emergency! Movie, Survival on Charter 220.*

The Modular Ambulance used in the first few episodes was provided by Goodhew/LA and was purchased from Texas. It originally was used in a Fort Worth, Texas, funeral home. By the mid-1970s, Modular Ambulance Corporation was providing the ambulances (as noted in end credits) and ran with the fictitious "Mayfair" logo. Modular Ambulance of Dallas, Texas (Modulance), built its chassis on Ford F350 one-tons and cost approximately $3500.00.

Other ambulances used in the series were a 1968 Cadillac Fleetwood 75 (low-boy) manufactured by Miller Meteor, a Chevrolet Suburban, 1969–1971 Ford Econoline and SuperVan model vans, a Chevrolet C-30 Cheyenne (modular), and the 1975 F-350 Chevrolet C-30.

Apparatus Numbers

Universal's property department made the numbered adhesive and magnetic disks for all the apparatus used in the program, matching the number for the fire truck in the script. Unlike the fictitious "'51," the apparatus numbers used were real station numbers. Dick Friend, who assigned the numbers during script review said, "I purposely used engine numbers that probably never really would respond together because of distance. Our guys got a kick out of it when they saw units from, say, Glendora, responding to a fire in the Marina over 30 miles away." The additional responding apparatus were mostly reserve apparatus with off-duty firefighters. Reserve apparatus were numbered in the 600 series, and the crews were able to keep their newly assigned engine number such as "29" or "82," for example, as a souvenir.

Lights

Beacon Ray or "Gumball"

Federal Sign & Signal Corporation is the manufacturer of the familiar revolving light called the "Beacon Ray." The Beacon Ray came in various mounting configurations, lens colors, and in either two- or three-bulb configuration. The rotator, nicknamed the "Gumball" because of its shape, could be mounted on a flat plate or pedestal, as seen on Crown Engines 60 and 127, or on the roof of the cab of the Ward LaFrance Engine 51. This particular Beacon Ray is the Model 17, a two-bulb model, which revolves at 40 revolutions per minute (rpm) and produces 80 flashes per minute. The late 1960s price has the Model 17 ranging from $75 to $82, depending on how it was mounted. Earlier models had a glass lens; the multicolored lenses were made of plastic and were used primarily in Midwestern and Eastern communities.

The Light from Mars

The forward-facing, oscillating Mars Light™ was original equipment on the Crowns delivered in 1955–1958. However, this light did not meet 1960s California Highway Patrol (CHP) regulations stating that a light must be visible in all directions, a full 360 degrees. Nevertheless, it appeared on various responding Crowns and other equipment on the show.

LACoFD Platter

Prior to the purchase of the Twinsonic light bar, Los Angeles County Fire Department (LACoFD) had its own emergency lights setup. Made in County Shops, it was a metal plate upon which were two red lights facing forward (the right one flashing, left one steady burning) and an amber light (which was flashing) facing to the rear. Between the two forward-facing lights was a mechanical Federal Signal G66 model siren. Mounted on a post was a large flashing "lollipop," side-facing, intersection light. Above that (on squads, including Squad 10 as seen in the *Emergency!* World Premier) was a white light. The white light indicated to helicopter pilots that the vehicle displaying such a light was a rescue squad.

TwinSonic

Federal Sign & Signal also manufactured the famous TwinSonic Light Bar, which became available in the early 1970s. The TwinSonic featured a two-bulb rotator on each side of the unit. The two rotators were moved by a chain and sprocket connected to a small 12- or 24-volt motor. The rotators were on the far side of each lens unit. Next to them were mirrors that provided an additional burst of light outward when the rotator directed light to the mirrors. In the middle of the unit, covered by polished silver plating, were the turning motor and speakers for the electronic siren. On the left side of the California Model CTS-12 TwinSonic (California TwinSonic, 12-volt) on Squad 51 was a fixed, steady-burn, red light facing forward and a flashing amber light facing rear. This was fitted to conform to CHP and California Vehicle Code regulations regarding lights on all emergency vehicles.

On top of the TwinSonic's center chrome speaker housing was a beacon light that burned white to indicate to helicopter pilots that the vehicle below was a paramedic/rescue squad and not a repair unit or other similar-looking vehicle. The lens was manufactured by the Do-Ray Lamp Company in Chicago, Illinois, and it was installed on a chrome base fabricated by County

Fire Shops at the time the light bar was installed on the new squads. The beacon was activated when the light bar was turned on.

Do-Ray was long a manufacturer of automotive lights for civilian vehicles and emergency lights for police and fire vehicles. Technical specs for the lens were Do-Ray marker light stock number 1130 (also available as AutoLite 666); the bulb in the fixture was an 8-watt GE 67.

Sirens

The Growler

Federal was also the manufacturer of electronic sirens popular across the country and the Q electromechanical siren, nicknamed the "Growler," is on Engine 51 (Ward LaFrance). It was designed to be hidden in a front bumper or the face of an apparatus with just the face of the siren showing. In the case of Engine 51, it was recessed just above the grill. A foot switch used by either the driver or captain operated the siren. Once the siren peaked in its pitch cycle, the operator took his foot off the foot switch and the siren cycled down. The siren put out an ear splitting 123 decibels at 10 feet. A brake switch, usually mounted on the dashboard, was used to quickly stop the siren. Other models could be mounted on the front bumper area or a roof mount.

Air Horn

The air horn on Engine 51 (the Ward) was a Grover 1510 model. This is a 24.5-inch-long horn with a 6-inch flared bell. Grover Products Company is still in business supplying horns for marine vehicles, emergency vehicles, and trains.

Electronic Sirens
PA20 Siren

Federal Sign & Signal also manufactured the siren assembly mounted in the squad and engine, which was the PA20A electronic siren. However, the sound heard during the show was a sound effect developed at Universal Studios by recording various siren functions available on the unit. The same siren sound can be heard on many Universal productions such as *Adam-12, Kojak,* and *McCloud.* The same siren sound effects were used in the post-series movies filmed in Seattle and San Francisco. The PA20's speakers were fitted into the TwinSonic light bar for Squad 51 or in the grill area for other apparatus. These priced out at $250, including speakers.

Hi-Lo Siren

In some later episodes, including the movie *The Steel Inferno,* a distinctive European type "Hi-Lo" can be heard from the squad. This two-tone air horn sound originating in Europe was developed electronically into the Federal Siren system, which was used by several departments, including the LACoFD, for a short time. Later the tone was considered to be unreliable and was no longer allowed to be used. It was also not approved for use by the CHP. It is still part of the siren package for use in other parts of the country. The PA-15a siren came without the Hi-Lo and was on earlier equipment.

Tools

Hurst Jaws of Life® Rescue Systems

During filming for the second season, the manufacturers of the Jaws of Life rescue system (Hurst Performance Inc.) contacted *Emergency!*'s set director Mickey Michaels and asked him if they could loan him a set of Jaws to use on the show for the publicity. At the time, the Fire Department did not have this expensive (almost $7000) tool, and Robert Cinader advised that no equipment not in regular use by the Fire Department could be used on the program.

When Michaels informed Hurst, it donated a set of Jaws of Life to the LACoFD. With that out of the way, *Emergency!* obtained a set, complete with compressor and Jaws, and two Hurst representatives provided the training for Randy Mantooth and Kevin Tighe for use on the show. "Peace Pipe" (episode 2.5) is the first time it is used on *Emergency!*.

The Jaws of Life was originally developed in 1972 for the racing industry and is now found in virtually every fire and rescue service throughout the world. Since 1984 the Jaws of Life has been a registered trademark of Hale Products Inc., an IDEX Corporation. The Jaws of Life was used in several episodes featuring trapped persons in vehicle accidents.

The product name of "Hurst" was initially used at the scene but that was quickly abandoned in favor of the more appropriate "Jaws." The implications to the accident victim of "Get the Hurst" sounded too similar to "Get the Hearse." There are now several different makers of hydraulic spreading tools, such as Amkus and Lukas, but Hurst was the original.

The Jaws of Life is not one, but actually a collection of several tools. The actual Jaws of Life are two titanium arms fitted to a hydraulic cylinder. The movement of the arms has a force of up to 9 tons. The Jaws Model 32 used on the program weighed more than 70 pounds. The "32" is in reference to the inches of spread at the tip of the jaws.

The power comes from a hydraulic piston that, when moved within the cylinder, works a rod and gears connected to the two arms to spread the arms apart when hydraulic fluid presses against the piston. The power comes from two hoses connected to a portable hydraulic pump powered by a 5-horsepower Briggs and Stratton pull-start, air-cooled, 2-cycle gasoline engine. The hydraulic fluid inside is antistatic and nonflammable, although it is toxic. It will also eat through a polycarbonate helmet.

Another tool that was used is the Hurst cutting tool, which has a cutting force of 15 tons. The Jaws were not carried on the LA County Squads in "real life" but on the truck companies. Today, in a few instances, depending on location in the County, squads will carry a set of Jaws.

Jet Ax

Explosive Technology sent Jet Ax to *Emergency!*'s set decorator Mickey Michaels, along with a film about the device in an attempt to gain free publicity from the show.

This product from Explosive Technology was basically a shaped charge of explosive materials. When detonated, the product actually cut a thermal opening right through the material it was placed against. It simply blew a hole through the door, wall, roof, etc. The company, now known as OEA Aerospace, manufactures explosive-activated components, ordnance systems, and aircraft escape systems, including systems for the Space Shuttle. However, Johnny Miller, assistant prop master and stuntman, says that he does not remember using this device on any of the 110 episodes he helped film. Remember, if it was not in use by the fire department, it could not be used on the program.

Porto-Power

The Porto-Power was carried on all the squads, including 51. It is a hand-pumped hydraulic tool with a single piston with a snapped-on attachment used for a variety of tasks similar to the Jaws, such as separating steel plates or acting as an hydraulic jack. The Porto-Power can handle lifts of 2, 4, and 10 tons depending on the model. Nontoxic mineral oil or other type of oil can be used for filling the hand pump.

K-12 Circular Saw

The squads also carried a Partner model K-12FD Fire Rescue circular saw and used it in several episodes. The saw was first invented in 1958, originally as a rescue tool for airlines. Because of its ability to cut through walls, doors, floors, and roofs, many fire departments made the K-12 standard equipment aboard rescue units. The K-12 has gone through many design revisions since it was shown on *Emergency!*, but it is still one of the principal pieces of rescue equipment carried aboard LA County Fire apparatus.

The saw is made up of a 6-horsepower, two-stroke, air-cooled, pull-start engine (which means pulling on the pull cord turns the flywheel, which cranks the engine, like a gas lawn mower). It has interchangeable circular saw blades 14 inches in diameter. The K-12 will cut to a depth of 5 inches, sufficient for most pipe- and steel-cutting applications. The K-12 has a nominal weight of about 22 pounds (without fuel or blade attached).

Kennedy Probe

The Kennedy Probe as used in "Botulism" (episode 1.2) and "Syndrome" (episode 2.16) is/was a real listening device with a microphone attached to one end of the expandable pole and the other end plugged into a receiver unit. There are four, 3-foot poles that screw together in the kit. The ear phones were also plugged into the receiver unit, amplifying the sounds heard by the microphone. Squad 51 carried several items that were used in the series that in actuality only the trucks carried; this device was one of them, and the Probe was carried on only a few of the trucks. Several of the technical advisors were asked about this device, but none had seen it or knew how it worked.

Radio Equipment

BioPhone

The BioPhone Model 3502 was a UHF multichannel radio set into a portable case. There were two units provided by Biocom Inc. of Culver City, California, to the producers of *Emergency!* in 1972. These were actual units, like much of the equipment in the program, but neither of them was operational. The heavy batteries were removed to make them easier to handle. The voice dialogue between the paramedics and Rampart was dubbed in later. The electrocardiogram telemetry seen from the cardio scope and from the corresponding unit at Rampart was also a simulation. The BioPhone unit was first demonstrated in January 1970 at a press conference at Harbor General Hospital, which, along with LA County Supervisor Kenneth Hahn, was to show it to the new Los Angeles County mobile intensive care units as well as to the television newspaper critics and writers. The Model 3502 commenced production soon after.

The BioPhone 3502 featured a General Electric PE series radio embedded into the case, which had a "gain" antenna, with 50 watts of transmitting power. This power was sufficient to reach most LA County repeaters. The antenna used on the BioPhone was a one-quarter wave UHF antenna that provided the most portability, but it could not be used while in an ambulance. A setup was used to connect the BioPhone to an antenna on the ambulance, much like a magnetically mounted CB antenna. In one episode, ("Problem" 2.1) the magnetic mounted antenna was knocked off as the ambulance moved out with Roy attending to the patient **(Photo 10-1)**.

The 22-pound unit was made of laminated fiberglass with aluminum trim. It was powered by a fast-charging nickel-cadmium (NiCad) battery,

INTEROFFICE MEMORANDUM
FORM 2022

DATE | 5/16/72
TO | R.A. CINADER
FROM | MICKEY MICHAELS
SUBJECT | PARAMEDIC UNIT FOR HOSPITAL-MOBILE CAR&&STUDIO
COPIES |

1-HOSPITAL EMERGENCY TELEMETRY AND COMMUNICATIONS SYSTEM

BIO-COM HOSPITAL BASE UNIT TWO STATION SET UP
$9,000.00

2-MOBILE UNIT FOR STUDIO

TRUCK STUDIO TRANSPORTATION
BIO-PHONE...................$3,900.00 EACH
DATA SCOPE-EKG.............$2,000.00 EACH
DATA SCOPE-DEFIBRILLATOR...$2,000.00 EACH
SPECIAL SMERGENCY OXYGEN RESUSCITATOR
WITH CART. $500.00

MICKEY MICHAELS

MM/stb

PHOTO 10-1   Purchase order for medical radios to be used on *Emergency!* at Rampart.
Source: Courtesy of Rozane Sutherland, author.

which could recharged to full power in just 15 minutes. Once charged, the battery would allow 1 hour of continuous transmit time. Spare batteries and a charging unit were kept at the station so a new battery could be placed onto the unit as necessary. It was part of the morning routine for the paramedics to check the battery output to make sure it was fully charged.

The BioPhone had various options available; the base model was priced at $2560. Duplex operation was an option at $450 extra. Enhancement to 120 watts of transmitting power was $250. Additional frequency operations were $150 per each frequency.

Motorola developed a version of the BioPhone in 1972 called the AP-COR (Advanced Portable Coronary Observation Radio). Although similar in appearance, including the orange box, it did have a bit of a different layout and a few more options than the Biocom model. Some agencies had both units. According the vice president of Biocom, Carl Van Cott, Motorola mistakenly thought the orange color was part of LA County specifications.

BioPhones have long since been retired from use in LA County, even as backup. The paramedics now use a combination of cell phone, the squad's mounted radios (MED 9 is used to contact the base hospital by radio), and the ASTRO handheld portable radio to contact the base hospital.

Telemetry is no longer sent to the hospital. The paramedics read the heart rhythms themselves and let the base station know what type it is.

Squad Radio

Squad 51 originally had the VHF Motorola Motrac 75 Mobile FM two-way radio installed, much like what was used in the *Adam-12* cars. It was mounted over the PA20A Interceptor siren (see earlier discussion). It was later replaced with the General Electric Mastr II. It would be later replaced with the GE Mastr II Executive Series, which is still in the squad today.

Handi-Talkie

When out of the engine and squad, the crew used a Motorola Model HT-220 Handi-Talkie portable radio. The portable radio is indicated "in use" between other units on scene by saying, for example, "Copter Fourteen, this is H-T Fifty One."

This particular model was introduced in 1969 and could be ordered with up to six transmit and six receive channels. The HT-220 could transmit with up to 5 watts of power on VHF. The radio operated on rechargeable NiCad batteries. Because there was no onboard charging unit in the vehicles, the HT-220 was recharged at the station after returning from an incident. The recharging process took about 10 to 14 hours to complete, so spare batteries and radios were at the station. It originally was issued with a long extendable antenna that frequently was bent or broke off completely.

Later, a "rubber duck" VHF antenna that was only about 6 inches long was issued. More than one station captain closed the door of the engine or truck, with the antenna extended, breaking it.

Motorola Quick-Call Dispatch

Since 1995, no stations have been dispatched using the station control unit tones as heard on *Emergency!* as the primary means of dispatch. The tones when received at the station would activate the lights and open the apparatus bay doors. They have since gone to a computer-aided dispatch system with mobile data terminals in the stations and apparatus.

There has been some confusion over the tones used on the show. It has been proposed that they used FS50's tones, FS50's tones reversed, FS32's tones with the klaxon that was heard at the station (TV's FS51), or FS22's tones. Regardless, the tones were real, and not something Universal made up, and were representative of the system that was in use at the time.

Uniforms

Turn-Out Gear

Fire coats and pants worn by the crew of Engine and Squad 51 were authentic Body-Guard® Turnouts as issued by the LACoFD. The only changes made to the coats because of filming was to paint out (somewhat) the reflective strips so that they would be subdued and not flash back into the camera with all the lights and reflectors being used even during daylight filming. The world's leading manufacturer of fire and EMS gear, Lion Apparel Inc., headquartered in Dayton, Ohio, now produces the Body-Guard® Turnouts, as well as Janesville®, Paul Conway™ Helmets, and other familiar brands. It was not until the late 1980s or early 1990s that LACoFD started wearing full turn-outs around the clock of yellow Nomex©. Until this time they were still wearing the Transcon non-nomex pants at night (see Station Wear). Currently, Morning Pride supplies the LACoFD with its turn-outs.

Spanner Wrench

The tool on the turn-out coat in the leather pouch is a Spanner wrench. The wrench is made for $^3/4$-inch to 3-inch rocker lug and pin lug couplings on fire hoses. The all-purpose wrench, Style 10, features a belt hook eye, hammer head, and a gas cock shutoff. The wrench, about 11.5 inches long, is still being used by many departments and is available from the manufacturer, the Akron Brass Company, through several distributors.

Self-Contained Breathing Apparatus (SCBAs)

According to Mike Norell, the actors on *Emergency!* generally used real air tanks, weighing close to 40 pounds each, not lightweight props. "Randy and Kevin did have some prop air tanks on occasion," says Norell, in which the yellow bottle was made of balsa wood. "They only weighed 5 pounds or so and were no problem to wear. Except, of course, when there was real smoke, which we had pretty often. They mostly made white smoke from bee smokers, which aren't too bad, but once in awhile, they had to make black smoke, which choked you pretty good and it was funny to see Randy and Kevin bail out of the shots and run for the real air tanks." According to Marco López, "Just about everything we used was real because the producers wanted us to have authenticity....Those air bottles were real and weighty." Tim Donnelly recalls, "All the Breathing Apparatus I used were 'real.' We did work in a lot of special effects; the smoke was not good at all. In fact, we complained about the black smoke when they had to use it; bad stuff."

Tim Donnelly insists that he always used a real tank, although TA Bob Hoff says that there were lightweight wood air tanks for use by some of the actors—mainly used by those in the background, around the engines, or on the outside of the fire building because they were easier to carry.

Contrary to popular belief, these are not oxygen tanks that the firefighters wear, but rather compressed air. At the time, the steel tanks contained 1800 to 2300 pounds of compressed air, depending on the bottle manufacturer. Although they were meant to last 30 minutes, firefighters could go through a tank in 15 minutes or less, depending on their activity level. Today, lightweight tanks of aluminum and spun fiberglass hold up to 4500 pounds of compressed air.

Helmet

MSA (Mine Safety Appliance) Topgard helmets were in service between 1950 and 1983 in Los Angeles County. They were standard black issue for all ranks up to chief officers, who were issued white helmets. A white painted stripe on the raised crown of the black helmets designated captains. These were nicknamed "skunk helmets" for obvious reasons. When a man was promoted to captain, his crew would paint the "skunk" stripe on his helmet. This was done out of respect and tradition.

The front piece was divided into two sections. On the top, on a blue background, was "L.A County" in white lettering. The bottom section had adhesive reflective white station numbers on a black background for the ranks of firefighter and the apparatus driver (engineer, firefighter/specialist), red numbers for truck company firefighters, and gold for chief officers. The only difference on the captain fronts was that on the lower section, the numbers and background colors were reversed. Later, orange numbers would be added to identify the HazMat units. The public information officer's helmet front would have black letters, "PIO," on a white background in the lower section.

During season 4, on the firefighter/paramedics helmet fronts, the station numbers were changed to reflectorized green. This change was in keeping with the LA County changes to the helmets to identify paramedics. The helmet fronts, including the lettering and numbering, were made in the graphic arts section of the department.

Los Angeles Fire Department (LAFD) began wearing the black MSA Topgards in 1940, which replaced the aluminum helmets that were manufactured by Cairns, Pettibone, and Forker. The black helmet color went out in the 1960s when they adopted the following color scheme, still utilizing the Topgards: yellow for firefighter and engineer/apparatus operator; orange for captain; standard white for chief officer. LAFD kept the same rank color coding when switching over to the Phenix Technology 1500.

LACoFD, upon obtaining the Phenix in the 1980s, adopted the LAFD rank color coding scheme. It is a helmet that is loved or hated by the wearer. Although available in red, the typical color for a captain's helmet, they (LAFD and LACoFD and a few other departments) have chosen to utilize the orange color. They, along with many other departments in California, around the United States, as well as several foreign countries are using the Phenix Technology 1500 series helmets.

During the transition from the MSA to the Phenix in 1983, the blue-over-black reflectorized helmet shield, similar to the MSA design, was adopted. This shield was unique because it was a low shield, and the clear face shield would rise over the helmet shield when in the up position. LACoFD later abandoned the clear face shields for goggles, and the taller leather helmet shield was created. Firefighters are not issued the leather shield; they have to purchase their own. Most of the time, the crew buys the new shield as a gift when someone is promoted.

MSA, headquartered in Pittsburgh, Pennsylvania, still makes a Topgard helmet but only in a safety hardhat/construction version. The fire helmet line was discontinued because it no longer meets National Fire Protection Association specifications.

The Bulls Eye

It would not be until season 6 that two, 2.5-inch circular, adhesive-backed, reflectorized stickers, also designed by the graphics arts division and later nicknamed the "Bulls Eye," would appear on each side of the paramedic helmets. A white border with a red half circle on top and a green half circle on the bottom was separated by a white bar with the word "Paramedic" in black. This was also in keeping with the LACoFD changes to identify paramedics at the scene of incidents.

A 5-inch patch identical to the circular sticker was worn on the turn-out coats, but the patch was never used on the TV program. The idea at the time was to easily identify who and where the paramedics were at the scene of an emergency. Remember, LACoFD paramedics did fire suppression work also. With the identifying patch on the back, the medics could be taken away from the firefighting and directed to EMS as needed. The use of SCBAs covered the patch, thus negating its purpose.

The circular sticker on the helmets was discontinued when LACoFD switched to the Phenix Technology 1500 First Due Firefighter series helmets around 1983. The helmet fronts are now leather with the rank inset across the top with LACoFD inset along the bottom. Station assignment is shown with reflectorized numbers on the sides of the helmets.

Station Wear

The light blue uniform shirts, dark pants, and dark jackets the cast wore were authentic LA County issue. The utility uniforms were manufactured by Transcon Manufacturing in Los Angeles, still in business supplying gear for fire, EMS, police, and military. The pants were also available in flame-retardant Nomex® but were not required for the program. Prices for the uniforms in the 1970s prices were: pants $8.90, a jacket $10.45, and the short-sleeve blue Poplin shirts were $5.90.

Uniform Badges

The badges worn on the program were authentic LACoFD badges and were collected each day at the end of shooting by the Studio property department, stored for safekeeping, and reissued the following day as needed. Johnny Miller, the assistant prop manager, advised, "Badges were given to us on a loan from County each season, numbers recorded for permanent cast members. Guest firefighters got fake ones."

Johnny's badge number is 330. Roy's preliminary "official" badge number was to be 174. However, Roy is seen wearing badge number 141 in several photos. Marco López remembered that his badge number was 125. Of the other cast members contacted, none recall their badge number. Mike Stoker advised that he did not wear his department-issued uniform or fire gear on the set. He was issued gear from Universal's property/costume department like everyone else.

V. H. Blackinton in Attleboro Falls, Massachusetts, manufactured the badges for the department in the 1970s; then the Entemann-Rovin Company took over. The Sun Badge Company in Ontario, California, currently holds the contract, as they do for the LAFD. Because the badges are essentially identical from each of the companies, often, upon promotion, someone will be given a recycled Entemann-Rovin badge. LA County uses the same basic design for all of its badges, with the California walking bear on top. A variation of this badge is used for the LA County Lifeguards and a variation of the design for the LA County Police Department. The change is in the center, where a seal or some other defining mark would be placed.

In one instance during the course of the series, regarding the issuance of badges as required, Mike Stoker, in uniform and waiting for the scene in which he would appear, was not wearing a badge on his uniform shirt. The scene at a gas station fire in "Insanity Epidemic" (episode 6.14) called for him to be wearing his turn-out coat and thus the badge was not required.

The badge number in LA County is not significant in relation to the person wearing it. In fact, badge numbers change each time a firefighter changes rank because a new badge is issued.

Belt Buckles

The belt buckles are authentic LA County issue, also once supplied by the Entemann-Rovin Company in Commerce, California, and now manufactured by the Sun Badge Company in Ontario, California. The buckles, considered "badges," although part of the uniform package, are issued by the LA County Firefighters Union 1014.

Not station wear nor LA County issue, but often seen in several of the episodes where Gage is off-duty in civilian clothes or Mantooth is seen wearing it when not working is a 1960s vintage brass Caterpillar belt buckle, about 2 by 3 inches. It has an early version of the D9 bulldozer over the word, Caterpillar.

Name Tag

The nametags the paramedics used on the show are two-ply engraved plastic, white on the surface with blue underneath, $3/4$ inch by 3 and $1/2$ inches long. The name was etched onto the white surface to show the dark blue underneath so that the name would stand out. John Gage's name tag, for example, read: J. GAGE, PARAMEDIC on the top line and underneath the name: MOBILE INTENSIVE CARE UNIT, all in capital letters.

In one instance, wardrobe forgot to properly outfit Kevin Tighe's uniform shirt; he is not wearing his name badge or his paramedic pin in a scene from "I'll Fix It" (episode 4.2), in the scene in the hospital emergency room with Dr. Brackett treating an injured juvenile.

Nametags for the firefighters were two-ply engraved plastic, black on the surface with white color underneath. They were slightly smaller because they only had the last name of the individual engraved.

Paramedic graduation pin

The small, round, half-inch pin that Roy DeSoto is wearing over his name badge is an authentic paramedic graduation pin from Harbor General. The gold-colored pin is identical to the logo seen in closing credits except that "Harbor General Hospital" arcs across the bottom of the logo on the pin completing the circle with "Los Angeles County" arcing across the top. Gage is also seen wearing the pin, although he technically graduated from Rampart.

The "Emergency Paramedic" emblem was designed for the County Health Services Paramedic Training Unit. All graduates received the pins from whatever hospital paramedic program they graduated from. The emblems were also placed on private ambulances staffed by certified paramedics. A small version of the Los Angeles County Paramedic seal is centered on the LA County paramedic badges, although not officially. It is a gold pin with red and white enamel for the various symbols.

It is said that California Senator James Wedworth and Assemblyman Larry Townsend, the men responsible for the Paramedic Act, had a hand in designing it. Originally it was going to be a Pueblo Indian holding a baby in her arms as a sign of nurturing. At the last minute, Supervisor Kenneth Hahn stepped in and changed the sign to the caduceus.

The logo as seen in the closing credits is from an actual seal that paramedics could put on their private cars. It is a 4-inch diameter decal, the old dip-in-water style. They were made by the Lacquer-Graph Company in Los Angeles, and several were sent to Universal's property department by the company and then on to Mickey Michaels for use in the program.

Helicopters

During the course of the series, LACoFD helicopters were utilized in several episodes, all flying out of what is now known as Barton Heliport at 12605 Osborne Street in Pacoima. During the time of the filming of *Emergency!*, it was simply known as County of Los Angeles Fire Department Air Operations. The heliport is located adjacent to Whitman Airport at the southeast end of the field. Some filming for the 1957 TV program *Whirlybirds*, starring Kenneth Toby (who also appeared in *Emergency!*), was filmed at Whitman Airport.

At least three different helicopters were consistently used, and Copter 10 and Copter 14 (FAA number N8192J) are of the same design, Bell 205s. Copter 15 was a Bell 204 (FAA number N148JC). They are the civilian version of the UH-1 Iroquois (Bell "Huey," the helicopters used by the U.S. Army in Vietnam).

The water tank under the helicopter can be taken off or put on by a crew of three in 5 to 10 minutes. Copter 14 appeared with and without the tank in the series. If not shooting a brush fire segment, or if not required for actual use, the tank was taken off because it removed 340 pounds of dry weight. The tanks are built by the Sheetcraft Company, which is located at the Santa Paula Airport. Owner Bill Mensing has been manufacturing these tanks since 1971, and they are used all across the world, including Canada, China, and Australia, for brush firefighting.

The tanks, called SkyHydrants™, are designed to carry from 100 gallons to 375 gallons of water, depending on helicopter capability, in two compartments, allowing for two drops of about 190 gallons each or one drop of 375 gallons (about 3000 pounds of water, or 1360 kilos). The tanks primarily drop water with Class A Foam, which is basically a liquid soap, commonly called "wet water," which is injected to the water tank just prior to the drop. Wet water gives the water a penetrating ability for greater saturation of the brush. The treated water penetrates more quickly, extinguishing the blaze with only one-third as much water.

According to an LA County spokesman, the chemical Phoscheck has also been used, which is the pink-tinged fire retardant more commonly seen dropping from fixed-wing aircraft. It is actually an ammonium/phosphorus-based fertilizer that is quite effective; it is also nutrient rich, which promotes regrowth. Borate has not been used since the 1960s; although effective, it sterilized the ground and killed everything it touched.

Newer tanks have been redesigned and weigh about 100 pounds less than the older models. LA County has some tanks that are more than 30 years old and still in service with only minor repairs necessary. The tanks currently cost $85,000 each. The tanks can be fitted with hoverfill snorkels or landfill capabilities. The large tanks can be filled in about 30 seconds.

Color Scheme
Gary Lineberry, former pilot for the Fire Department, advised that the red and white color scheme seen in *Emergency!* was replaced in the late 1970s with the current black, yellow, and white. He says, "It was a good, high-visibility paint scheme and it helped distinguish between our aircraft and those of LA City Fire Department. So, gradually over the years, we changed to that color pattern as the other aircraft needed new paint jobs." The LACoFD fireboats have also adopted this color scheme.

U.S. Coast Guard Helicopters
These helicopters appeared in five episodes of *Emergency!* and the *Emergency!* movie, *Steel Inferno*. Although the paramedics from fictional Station 51 responded on cliff rescues and calls to Catalina, that work was actu-

ally assigned to LA County Station 38's paramedics. The paramedic rescue squad was later relocated to Station 58, where they still responded to the Coast Guard Station at Los Angeles International Airport when needed. By 1984 Station 18's paramedics had been assigned the duty because of their closer proximity to the Coast Guard station. Later, other County paramedic squads would be utilized.

The U.S. Coast Guard (USCG) approached the LACoFD about providing paramedic service for medical transfers from Catalina Island as well as from other Channel Islands to the mainland of California. This working relationship also involved the USCG for boat, surf, and cliff rescue assistance.

The type of aircraft seen in episodes of *Emergency!* was the Sikorsky S-62 (HH-52A Sea Guard) helicopters. They were in service from around 1962 through 1985. They were replaced by the HH-65A Dolphins, which are still in service.

The USCG Air Station seen in "Election" (episode 5.3) and "The Boat" (episode 6.19), when Squad 51 arrives to be picked up to go to Catalina for a rescue, is not what it seems. What is seen as the squad drives up is the air control tower at Long Beach airport (Daugherty Field). The tower is still in service today. According to Commander Jim Sommer, executive officer of USGC Air Station Los Angeles, emergency patients may land at Long Beach or be flown directly to the helipad across from Torrance Memorial Hospital. In keeping with LA County protocol of a paramedic being on board with the patient(s) and as seen in "The Boat," they were raised to the Coast Guard helicopter in the basket and everyone went to Rampart. The same was true for the episode "Election," but in this case the medics were raised by flotation collars.

Personal Vehicles

Randolph Mantooth
Mantooth appeared in a few episodes driving his own 1969 Land Rover. It is a Series II, 88-inch wheelbase, U.S. model made by British Leyland. This was actually Randy's personal vehicle, California registration, 591DWV. This vehicle has a 2200-cubic centimeter engine, mated to a 4-speed manual gearbox.

Mantooth's Land Rover is seen in both "Snake Bite" (episode 3.6) and "Welcome to Santa Rosa County" (episode 6.10), among other episodes, parked out back of the station. It is also seen in the opening scene of the *Sierra* crossover, "Urban Ranger," filmed in Yosemite National Park. Unfortunately, the Land Rover was destroyed, along with Mantooth's home, in a 1978 brush fire in Agoura Hills, in the Santa Monica Mountains, west of Los Angeles.

In the "Unlikely Heirs" (episode 6.3), Johnny arrives at the station in a pickup truck, not his Land Rover. He's driving a new 1976 AMC Jeep J6 Honcho 4 × 4 pickup. It is seen only once.

Kevin Tighe

Roy's car was Tighe's own Porsche model 356 Cabrio Speedster convertible. This vehicle was a two-seater built, as he says, "for speed and handling." The Speedster was fitted with an engine up to 2000 cubic centimeters, which generated up to 130 horsepower. The Speedster came as both a coupe and Roy's convertible Cabrio model.

Tim Donnelly

Donnelley's off-white VW van was seen on the show a few times, most notably when he sat at the rear of it to put on those human fly shoes in "Inventions" (episode 3.22).

Dick Friend

The LA County Public Information Office's Chevrolet, an official fire sedan, was used in one episode, when a script change called for a chief's car and Dick's was the only one on the scene. According to Friend, the car was only 3 or 4 days old:

> I brought it to the bottom of a hilly road on Universal's back lot and gave it to a transportation driver. He got in, floor-boarded it and roared it backward up the dirt road with clouds of dirt and sand flying as the wheels dug into the soft roadbed.
>
> The Transportation Captain was also at the bottom of the incline, and I walked over toward him. He was waiving his arms and shaking his head. He walked up the dirt road and I followed. Up top, I stayed clear while he confronted the driver. Several minutes later the driver started walking back down the hill. The Transportation Captain had fired him on the spot. My car was nicely cleaned when I got it back.

Jim Page

Page's light blue Ford Country Squire station wagon with faux wood paneling is parked across the street from the station and is seen in *Emergency!* stock footage—before the Ward arrives and as the apparatus turns left out of the station. It is seen with the shots as taken from the Crown overhead and from inside the station as the engine and squad are exiting the station.

EMERGENCY! *Behind the Scene*

CHAPTER **11**

Special Effects and Stunt Work

Special Effects

Special Effects Team

This team included, among others, Greg C. Jensen, Jr., Dave Lopez, Frank Pope, "Uncle" Don Hathaway, and Paul Hickerson.

Emergency! Survival on Charter 220

This film includes an impressive plane crash scene. Mark Thomson, former stunt pilot, owned a prop and stunt work company called Aviation Warehouse in El Mirage, California, that supplies airplanes, airplane mock-ups, and what are called "airplane cadavers" for TV and motion pictures. The producers of the movie "bought an area that had a few single family homes that were to be torn down in Compton, then bought an old [Boeing] 707 that I was cutting apart and literally dropped it into these homes. During the production they set it on fire, big time: the whole complex, broken airplane parts, jet engines, and everything."[1]

Mike commented, "*Emergency!* was one of my favorite shows," he stated in a 1997 interview with *The Business Press*. Looking back, Thompson believes he never would have been able to get into the film prop business if he hadn't pitched his services to *Emergency!*. Thompson supplied the jet passenger liner that was blown up in the movie *Speed* and supplied airplane parts for the TV program *LOST* filmed in Hawaii.

Mark Thompson's Aviation Warehouse was featured on the History Channel's *Modern Marvels* July 21, 2005 in the episode titled, "The Junkyard," The promo for the episode states "It's the place where old machines come to die. But for some people, it's also a treasure trove of possibilities."

Nearby mobile radio station field units were reporting a major disaster in Compton, and, according to Hannah Shearer, one of the film's writers, "It was possibly the biggest explosion we ever did—so large that pilots flying into LAX reported a plane down; somebody screwed up and forgot to tell somebody!"

> Dave Lopez and his special effects crew used, I can't even imagine how much, explosives. We broke a few windows with the concussion, and several homeowners a couple of neighborhoods over put in for repairs. I'm sure we complied, even though we doubted that the effects were felt that far away. It was pretty stunning: loud and big and very, very exciting. No homes to rebuild. Our location manager found a neighborhood of abandoned homes that were going to be torn down. We fixed them up inside to use for interiors. The crew used old plane parts and scattered them through the area before the explosion.

The Compton Fire Department assisted LA County in this movie and appeared on camera. Charles Coleman, who was working on the set at the time, said that nearby Compton High School had not been notified in advance. After the explosion the students were evacuated from all classrooms to the gymnasium. LA County firefighter/paramedic and TA Bob Hoff was on one of the LA County Fire Department (LACoFD) engines responding to the scene. The explosion, he said, was "stunning, impressive, and loud. A group of pre-schoolers that brought their chairs out to watch a movie being made literally scattered when the fireball erupted."

"The Promotion" (Episode 3.7)

This episode contains a multiple-vehicle accident on the San Diego Freeway (I-405). There is an illusion that the engine and the squad are moving, when they are actually stationary. This illusion was created by fog (smoke)

---

[1] Mike Hodgkinson, "Your Choice: Plane or Fancy," *Los Angeles Times,* October 12, 2003.

being blown across the scene toward the parked engine and squad. This segment was not filmed at Universal but at the old RKO Studios outside lot, which later became the Desilu Studios and is now part of the Paramount lot. In another episode, a fog filter was used on the camera to give the illusion of filming through fog and smoke.

Licensing

The LACoFD issues special permits to licensed pyrotechnicians for each show or program.

Greg C. Jensen, Jr., prior to forming his own special effects company, The EFX Shop, worked with other special effects people on *Emergency!* such as effects coordinator Dave Lopez and Frank Pope (now one of the big time powder men [explosive experts] in the industry), who was one of the four regular special effectsmen on the show. Along with "Uncle" Don Hathaway and Paul Hickerson, they produced fire effects as called for in the script, whether they were in a house or a vehicle. Jensen, who was being trained to join the team at the time, also worked on two episodes of Cinader's *Sierra* that called for fire effects. Jensen, as special effects on-set supervisor, would again work with Kevin Tighe in 1997 on a firefighting television pilot titled *The 119*, where Kevin portrayed an LA City battalion chief. The show was not picked up and the pilot never aired.

After 40 years in the business Jensen retired in April 2005. One of his last projects he worked on was the popular sit-com *Two and a Half Men* starring Charlie Sheen for an earthquake stunt.

Stunt Work

Many of the below comments were taken from the *Emergency!* Convention in 1998.

Regarding a question on stunt work, Randy Mantooth stated that the actors did most of the stunt work during the first few seasons, but stuntmen were employed to do the dangerous work. Mantooth recalls shooting a scene in which he and Kevin Tighe were sixteen or seventeen stories high on an exposed crane with fierce winds. Tighe was frightened at the height, and Mantooth was joking around, waving his arms and pretending he was falling to give Tighe a hard time. Kevin literally would grip the thing and try to become part of the paint of the structure that we were on, and all I could remember him saying as his eyes were averted from me was, "Randy, you're an a* *hole."

Tighe recalls, "I never had a problem with [heights] until one episode, I think it was the third season, where we were trying to get a crazy guy off a ledge. I wasn't tied off and we just sort of did it on the ledge; it seemed relatively safe, it was controlled, and we had stuntmen watching us. We finished the stunt and the director yelled cut and I just froze. I don't know why, I just was scared to death. They had to come out and lead me by the hand back in. Since that time, it's always been a little difficult doing the high stuff." Tighe says that the show had "fabulous stuntmen" and that after all of the special effects and stunts in the show each week, there were very few injuries.

Mantooth recalls one of them in which he burned his leg. After that accident, the actors were not involved in dangerous fire scenes for fear of safety concerns, since "flames are the only things you can't really control," says Mantooth. The actors would get close to the fires, but stuntmen would be used to run through the flames or other dangerous stunts. The actors weren't trained in stunt work, said Mantooth, "We were just young and stupid." The stuntmen would tell the actors what to do, and as time went by, Mantooth said, their stunt skills improved a great deal. However, the general rule, says Mantooth, was, "If you can see our faces, we're doing the stunts. If you can't see our faces, we did not do the stunts."

The only other major injury was caused by a jolt of electricity, which knocked Kevin Tighe to the ground in the first season and put him in a brace for 6 weeks.[2]

Stuntmen

Many stuntmen appeared throughout the series, most of them uncredited. The list that follows is by no means all-inclusive.

Howard Curtis

Curtis appeared in several *Emergency!* episodes, although seemingly unnoticed doing his stunt coordination or doubling for another actor. He appeared in the "The Boat" (episode 6.19) as a guest star and played a firefighter in "The Mouse" (episode 4.20). In that episode, Curtis is on fire after a jet aircraft crashed into a three-story apartment complex, and he became doused with jet fuel as a result of a secondary explosion during firefighting operations. The stunt also called for him to fall from the first floor balcony while on fire, then to be hosed down by firefighters on the ground.

Curtis also appeared in *Firehouse* (1973) as a firefighter and performed *Towering Inferno* (1974) stunt work. Incidentally, there were sixty-eight stunt people that worked *Towering Inferno*, all of whom were uncredited in end credits.

[2] Richard Warren Lewis, "Saturday Night Celebrity," *TV Guide*, August 3–9, 1974.

George Orrison

Orrison had been a stuntman since 1960, working as a double and performing stunt work for Clint Eastwood since 1973 in all his movies through 2002 in *Space Cowboys*. Orrison worked on *Emergency!* as a stunt double for Kevin Tighe in more than 98 episodes. He also appeared as an extra in at least ten episodes, most often as an ambulance attendant or orderly. His only credited role was in "Propinquity" (episode 3.20).

Angelo De Meo

De Meo was Randy Mantooth's stunt double and stunt coordinator for the series. He also appeared in nonspeaking roles such as an accident victim or an ambulance attendant. He portrayed a firefighter in at least three episodes and a SWAT officer.

Johnny Miller

Miller was both a stuntman for the show and the assistant prop master. He worked on almost the entire run of the series and appeared in many episodes. His face was usually not seen, or he wore disguises so he could appear in many episodes without being recognized. Miller says that he never doubled for firefighters and was usually an accident victim. Miller credits the special effects team for their pre-stunt work for making the stunts come off as well as they did.

Miller appears in the stokes basket in "Above and Beyond...Nearly" (episode 5.20) during the cliff rescue. He was on the side of the cliff, about 250 feet up, for 3.5 hours in a safety harness, while they shot the scene and helicopter sequence. Mantooth and Tighe, he says, were only a few feet off the ground.

Miller worked on many other movies and television shows such as the James Bond movie, *Diamonds Are Forever*, *Earthquake*, *Star Trek—TNG*, *Simon and Simon*, *Mad about You*, *Knight Rider*, *Colombo,* and many others. He was the stunt coordinator for American Movie Classic's *Behind The Scenes* programs. But he says that *Emergency!* was "the greatest show I ever did because it put the paramedic program on the map. A fun show, a fun time."

Scott Gourlay

Gourlay was a stuntman and was seen in many episodes, usually as police officer Scotty or as a hospital intern. He also appears being thrown out of doors and windows in many of the fiery explosions.

Harold "Hal" T. Frizzell

Kevin Tighe's stunt double performed other stunt work throughout the series and occasionally appeared as a far-away double for Tim Donnelly. He could be seen as an ambulance attendant or an orderly in close to forty episodes, mostly uncredited. Frizzell stated that the reason they used contract stuntmen for ambulance personnel was "because the driving was mostly stunt work."

Frizzell got his start in stunt work on the 1971 TV series *Alias Smith and Jones.* It was here that Randy Mantooth worked with him (episode 1.9) and requested Frizzell for *Emergency!*.

Thomas Rosales, Jr.

Rosales was Marco López's stunt double and, like other stuntmen, appeared in several episodes of *Emergency!* as various background extras including hospital orderlies. Rosales began his stunt work on *Emergency!*, and it was Marco López who was responsible for having Rosales be the first Latino stuntman to be accepted in the Stuntmen's Association. He is proficient in "fire burn" stunt work, among other things. He also appeared in *Towering Inferno* as a stuntman and in more than 200 films and TV shows as a stuntman or actor.

EMERGENCY! *Behind the Scene*

CHAPTER **12**

Episode Guide

Introduction

Filming Sequence

Shooting schedules for most episodes usually ran 6 to 8 days (or nights), depending on the locations and action. Not all episodes were shot on a Monday through Friday schedule; some started on a Thursday or Friday. Final script revisions were typically done at the production meetings the week before shooting was scheduled to begin. However, additional revisions could be made after shooting began if unforeseen problems occurred on the set; when known, such instances are reported in this chapter.

Often, segments scripted and filmed for a particular episode may be cut and end up in a different episode if story lines run too long. As a result, actors may receive credit in a particular show for roles that they play in future episodes. Most notable are the season 2 episodes that Jamie Farr did and did not appear in. In this case the end credits were not corrected prior to airing to reflect which episode he actually appeared in. This occurred several times throughout the series and with always the same clothing being worn, his or her uniforms, no one notices. This has been noted in several instances where certain scenes for episodes have been utilized elsewhere, and in one case, not used at all. When possible, instances where scenes have been cut from previous episodes are noted.

Episodes were not necessarily aired in order of filming becasue of issues such as network preemptions, scene editing, scheduling issues, unavailable filming locations and various other reasons. Nowhere is this more evident than in seasons 5 and 6. Shooting schedules, when known, have been provided for the episodes.

With continuing story lines rare for *Emergency!*, and no end-of-season cliffhangers or holiday episodes, this rescheduling of episodes usually made no difference. There is one exception to this in season 6; see if you can spot it. Continuing story lines are always a problem with serialized TV series, especially in syndication, but because *Emergency!* was a close-ended episodic series, viewers could miss an episode without losing the plot line.

Continuity

Whenever possible, continuity issues were caught before filming, during cast read-through or rehearsal, when it was still possible to make changes without reshooting an entire scene. However, sometimes these mistakes were not caught before it was too late and the film was already "in the can." An example of this was Johnny's locker, which moved several times from the one on the end to the locker next to it to one across the aisle ("The Smoke Eater," episode 4.16). In one episode, he even used Roy's, and Roy used Johnny's ("Syndrome," episode 2.16). Roy's locker moved around as well, from behind Johnny's ("Dealer's Wild," episode 1.5) to up against the wall. With Roy's locker up against the wall, same row as Johnny's, this makes for better filming and ease of conversation.

Filming Locations

Filming locations are noted where known, although many of these sites have changed greatly since the time of filming. Some episodes were filmed entirely on Universal's lot; various soundstages and outdoor scenes are noted. Filming on the backlot was cost effective and frequent.

The classic suburban street, "Colonial Street," appears in many Universal shows including *Leave it to Beaver, Hardy Boys, Providence, CSI:NY,* and *Desperate Housewives.* All the homes on Colonial Street are mostly two- or three-sided buildings and are on wheels so that they can be easily moved. A few are completely enclosed and are used for storage. When a person opens the front door, an L-shaped wall provides the interior background. When a series uses one or more of the houses consistently, additional interior props will be built so that the move to the soundstage is seamless. Universal's New York Street was also used on *Emergency!* for downtown or business street scenes. Throughout the series, Universal portrayed other movie studios (World Studios, Mammoth Studios, or World Pictures) but never appeared as itself. A map of the Universal Lot showing all the buildings and filming sets including all those mentioned in this book can be found on the Universal Studios site "The Filmmakers Destination."

Video and DVD Release

Often, in syndication, some scenes from the original episodes have been cut to make more time for commercials. This is due to the time required for additional commercial time being sold for a 60-minute program. An episode in the 1970s ran usually 48 to 50 minutes long with the remainder being taken up with commercials. Today an hour script is only about 42 minutes on average with 18 minutes of commercials. Thirty-minute programs today are only about 22 minutes long with 8 minutes of commercials. The *Emergency!* VHS tapes sold by Columbia House and JEMS Communications were original and uncut episodes, including the original music and opening scenes with no voiceover. The NBC/Universal-authorized DVDs beginning in 2005 contained all the so-called lost scenes and were full and complete episodes as originally aired.

Episode Titles

Episode titles are not seen during opening credits, which is standard operating practice industrywide in the United States. For the most part producers and series creators did not want their series to be seen as mini-movies; therefore, series titles never ran. The titles would, however, be used in the various television guide listings as the episode title, along with the synopsis and guest star information sent out by the studio to the weekly magazines and network affiliates. Titles were utilized in the post-series *Emergency!* movies.

A Typical Script

A script for a 60-minute program usually runs 50 to 60 pages, depending on amount of dialog and/or action sequences. The following is not a page out of an actual *Emergency!* script because the scripts remain the property of Universal Studios. The scene numbers are typed in both the left- and right-hand margins. Dialog is centered on the page, with the name of the character speaking, above the lines. Scenes, camera shots and angles, and other inflections appear in capital letters. The page number of the script is in the upper right corner of the page.

Pages may be different colors, beginning with white. The script is usually revised several times prior to filming (and sometimes even during filming) with revision number and date noted along with the page number. Each revision would get a different color paper with the first revisions on blue paper followed by pink and other colors to follow (usually yellow, green, goldenrod, buff, salmon, cherry, then tan). Final scripts would often look like a rainbow.

104 INT. BASE STATION—DAY   104
FEATURING Brackett listening at the speaker.

> GAGE'S VOICE
> ...weight about 130; Victim of a fall.
> She has a dislocated shoulder. The vital
> Signs are normal.
>
> BRACKETT
> (into speaker)
> Any other injuries?
>
> GAGE'S VOICE
> Negative. She is in considerable pain.
>
> BRACKETT
> Give her 30 milligrams Talwin I-M and
> bring her in as soon as you can.

CUT TO:
105 EXTERIOR—ACCIDENT SCENE—DAY   105
Where DeSoto is already reaching for a hypodermic.

> GAGE
> (into radio)
> Ten-Four. Thirty milligrams Talwin I-M
> and bring her in.
> (to DeSoto)
> I'll get an ambulance.

Gage walks out of the shot.

> DESOTO
> I'm going to give you a shot
> for the pain.
>
> ERIKA
> You'll have to get the cat.
>
> DESOTO
> What?
>
> ERIKA
> It's up the tree where the dog chased it.

(CONTINUED)

The following episode guide was constructed from a consensus of existing information including, but not limited to, weekly television guides, script call sheets, and shooting schedules. Every attempt was made to ensure the accuracy of airdates and related information. Most notably missing, unfortunately, are the Technical Advisor names for many of the episodes. An alphabetical listing of the episodes with episode number is included at the end of the chapter.

SEASON 1

Emergency! World Premier

Episode #0.1

Production #31317

Filming began: November 22, 1971

Airdate: January 15, 1972

Writers: Harold Jack Bloom and R. A. Cinader

Executive producer: Jack Webb

Associate producer: William Stark

Director of photography: Jack Marta

Art director: John J. Lloyd

Film editor: Warren Adams, ACE

Set decorator: Mickey S. Michaels

Director: Jack Webb

Assistant director: Phil Bowes

Sound: Robert Betrand

Editorial supervisor: Richard Belding

Unit manager: Joseph E. Kenney

LACoFD Technical Advisor: Dale Cauble (PM0002)

Guest cast: Martin Milner, Kent McCord, Jack Kruschen, Ann Morgan Guilbert, Lew Brown, Art Balinger, Virginia Gregg, Herb Vigran, Don Ross, Colby Chester, Katherine Kelly-Wiget, Marco López, and dozens of off-duty LACoFD personnel

Synopsis

The two main fire/rescue events are a large warehouse fire and rescuing workers from a tunnel cave-in.

After graduating in the first paramedic class, Roy tries to convince Johnny to join the paramedic program during interviews held at Station 10. Johnny, seemingly uninterested ("All I want to be is a "Rescue Man") changes his mind after a fireman dies for want of proper on-the-spot treatment. Marco López turns up in Johnny's paramedic training class, although not until half-way through the class (when instructor Dr. Joe Early sends them home for the weekend after telling them that the "hip bone is indeed connected to the thigh bone"). He also apparently graduated despite having missed half the training, as his appearance in the graduation exercise seems to indicate. This is, however, the last we see of firefighter/paramedic López.

The paramedics have to deal with opposition from both medical and civil authorities, including one of their staunchest opponents—Dr. Kelly Brackett. Dr. Brackett, head of Rampart Hospital's Emergency Division, doubts the need for a paramedic program. Nurse Dixie McCall urges Brackett to support Assemblyman Wolski's (Jack Kruchen) bill to create the program.

Johnny and Roy's first response after arriving at Station 51 is for a vehicle accident, where they ultimately end up directing traffic, while Dixie treats the two injured passengers, because they, Johnny and Roy, "weren't doing anything else." The only crew of Engine 51 who appear in station are two firefighters (uncredited) who suddenly come out of the kitchen and hover over Roy as he is answering LA County Dispatch (via Sam Lanier).

Brackett remains adamant until Dixie is injured at an auto accident while supervising Gage and DeSoto, who are not yet licensed to render medical aid. She nearly dies and is saved by the quick thinking of Johnny and Roy (filmed on the second day of shooting, November 23 on a hillside overlooking the San Fernando Valley). Eventually seeing the advantages of the program, Dr. Brackett goes before the legislative committee to testify in favor of passing the bill.

Before the vote, there is a tunnel explosion, and Gage and DeSoto are among the rescue units. They have all the life-saving equipment but cannot use it until the bill is passed. Dr. Brackett instructs the paramedics on scene via a two-way radio. At a crucial moment, Brackett places his career on the line to save a life.

Dr. Brackett's earlier testimony before the committee proved the key to getting paramedic legislation passed. Now the paramedics can practice their skills without having to respond to the hospital and pick up a nurse before responding to the scene of the incident.

Notes
This episode was filmed in 22 days. It was the only time that Katherine Kelly-Wiget (who plays Roy's wife, Joanne) actually appears on screen as Roy's wife. This is also the first of three *Adam-12* crossovers. Ron Pinkard

plays Dr. Tom Gray, not Dr. Morton, and Colby Chester has his first of three appearances in the series, this time as fireman Tony Freeman (Randy's partner on Rescue 10). According to Marco López, he knew that he was going to be a permanent cast member, but neither he—nor the producers—knew exactly what that role would be. One of the many uncredited actors in the movie is Rand Brooks, founder of Professional Ambulance Service in Glendale, California, who appears as an uncredited police officer at the scene of the accident; Brooks also appeared in *Rescue* 8 as a Senior Rescue Firefighter on Rescue 3.

Apparatus responding out of Station 10 are the actual vehicles assigned to Station 8. The rescue squad is a 1969 Dodge 300 1-ton engine, circa 1965 open-cab Crown (license E110857), and the Seagrave is used as Truck 10, with the obvious magnetic roundel on the front.

This 2-hour episode aired again in flashback format as "The Wedworth-Townsend Act" (episodes 5.15 and 5.16). See Chapter 2 for the primary filming locations for this movie.

"The Mascot"

Episode #1.1

Production #34401

Filming dates: December 23–31, 1971

Airdate: January 22, 1972

Writer: Preston Wood

Director: Lawrence Dobkin

LACoFD Technical Advisor: Roy Burlson (PM0020)

Guest cast: Patricia McAneny (Paula Slayton), Peanuts (the dog, Bonnie), Jock Mahoney (Lee Thompson), Jeff Davis (Peter Ballard), Susan O'Connell (Ballard's girlfriend, Louise), Candace Howerton (Genevieve McCurtain), Linda Watkins (Mrs. Leeds, Genevieve's mother), Beverly Powers, with Chief Pilot Roland Barton (LACoFD Air Ops Division, playing himself)

Synopsis

A woman (Patricia McAneny) involved in a car accident is concerned about her dog, so Johnny agrees to take care of the dog while she's in the hospital. Johnny and Roy treat an actor (Jock Mahoney) with chest pains and deal with his drunken party guests, a diabetic (Jeff Davis) and an emotionally disturbed woman (Candace Howerton). After Copter 10 picks the guys up at Rampart, they fly out to a remote area to rescue an injured hunter who fell off a cliff.

Notes

This was a 6-day shoot. Roland Barton was Chief Pilot for LA County at the time. The LACoFD heliport facility (Barton Heliport) located in Pacoima is named after him. The cap he is wearing has the patch of LA County Fire Camp 9, which is visited in "Right at Home" (episode 5.17).

"Botulism"

Episode #1.2

Production #34409

Final revision: December 9, 1971

Airdate: January 29, 1972

Writer: Michael Donovan

Director: Herschel Daugherty

LACoFD Technical Advisor: Michael Stearns (PM0011)

Guest cast: Calvin Bartlett, Anne Whitfield, Paul Langton, Virginia Vincent, William Stevens, Virginia Gregg (as Wilma Jacobs, RN), Susan Seaforth, Joshua Albee, Harlen Carraher, Bruce Powers

Synopsis

A cameraman (Calvin Bartlett) breaks his leg under unusual circumstances on a movie set and is taken to Rampart. Dr. Brackett's early diagnosis of botulism is the first indication of an outbreak. A search for contaminated food leads to Nancy Dickson (Susan Seaforth). A man breaks his back after he fell from the smokestack at the power plant and held on by a boson's chair. Johnny plots his revenge after being the repeated target of practical jokes. Roy and Johnny rescue a boy (Harlen Carraher) trapped in a collapsed building.

Notes

Technical advisor for this episode, Paramedic Michael Stearns, was one of the four members of the cross-country tour with the Ward LaFrance (see Chapter 17).

The Kennedy Probe, as used in this episode in the collapse building rescue, was a real listening device with a microphone attached to one end of the expandable pole and the other end plugged into a receiver unit.

There are also notable inconsistencies with Engine 51. Stock footage of the Crown is used for the roll-out from the station, but a different engine arrives on scene at the power plant incident, with a Mars light on the windshield instead of the familiar Gumball, a chrome strip on the cab above the siren, a painted red bumper, and no front intake (the 4-inch hose to hydrant cutout).

Locations
The power plant scenes were filmed at the Valley Generating Station, 11801 Sheldon Street, Sun Valley California, at a steam generating facility. It is located northeast of the intersections of I-5 and the 170, between Burbank and San Fernando.

"Cook's Tour"

Episode #1.3

Production #34406

Final revision: January 10, 1972

Filming dates: January 6–13, 1972

Airdate: February 12, 1972

Writer: Daryl Henry

Director: Christian Nyby, Sr.

LACoFD Technical Advisor: James Tollefson (PM0030)

Guest cast: Frank Aletter (Roger Mundell), Jacqueline Russell (Judy Mundell), Dennis Rucker (Jay Hooper), Dorothy Green, David Knight, Bill Henry (second captain), Barbara Sigel (checkout girl), Bobby Eilbacher (kid in handcuffs), Dorothy Konrad (Beatrice Stover), Virginia Gregg (Nurse), Patricia Mickey (Student Nurse), Tammie Shaw (nurse), Lew Brown (deputy), Scott Smith (deputy)

Synopsis
Johnny delivers his first baby, over protests from the infant's father (Frank Aletter), and it is cyanotic. Roy worries that the guys won't like his cooking and attempts to make beef bourguignon. At Rampart, Dr. Early treats a 10-year-old boy (David Knight) who got his hand stuck in an antique vase. John removes handcuffs from a kid who is brought to the station by his friends. The staff at Rampart revives a man who suffered a severe electrical shock while repairing his washing machine. A man is trapped on a crane.

Notes
The boy is not given a name in the script, but Dr. Early calls the boy by his real name 'David' in the episode. Dorothy Green (mother of boy David with hand in vase) was in an episode of *Adam-12* with Randy (Log 88: "A Reason to Run").

Scott Smith was a real LA County fire captain at the time and was later hired as the technical advisor for *Firehouse* (1973), a movie starring Richard Roundtree and Vince Edwards, in which Smith portrayed a battalion chief and provided his fire engine.

The beef bourguignon recipe calls for burgundy, but fire department rules and regulations forbid the use of alcoholic products while on duty, even when called for in recipes, so the burgundy was omitted.

Locations

The home used for the interior shots of the childbirth scene is a real home (occasionally rented out to Universal) located just outside the studio grounds. The exteriors for this segment were shot on Universal's "Cosmopolitan Street." The footage of the squad driving up to the house was utilized again (as stock footage) for "Propinquity" (3.20) as the exteriors of the poker player's home.

Note the "Roy Rogers" Roast Beef Sandwich fast food place outside the supermarket where John and Roy are grocery shopping. With franchises all across the country in the 1960s and 1970s, the once popular sandwich outlets are now located in just nine states in the Mid-Atlantic region. Many locations were taken over by "Bob's Big Boy," "Arby's," "McDonald's," "Hardee's" (in the East), "Carl's Jr.'s" (in the West), and others.

"Brushfire"

Episode #1.4

Production #34402

Final revision: January 12, 1972

Filming dates: January 13–20, 1972

Airdate: February 19, 1972

Writer: Robert C. Dennis

Director: Hollingsworth Morse

LACoFD Technical Advisor: Robert Ramstead (PM0006)

Guest cast: Gary Crosby (Fireman Conway), Ellen Moss, Bob Hastings (man in robe), Tony Dow (looter), Trent Lehman (Andy), Edith Evanson, Lillian Bronson, Vince Howard (Officer Vince), Art Balinger (Battalion Chief)

Synopsis

Station 51 is called up to assist at an out-of-control brushfire in Las Plumas Canyon where a firefighter (Gary Crosby) is trapped under a fallen tree that has shattered his leg. Stoker uses a saw to cut the tree back to free his leg. This is Gage's first brush fire. The fire also threatens the house of a pregnant woman (Ellen Moss) who is in labor and can't be moved; DeSoto delivers his third baby. The paramedics rescue the elderly Lenover Sisters (Edith Evanson and Lillian Bronson), a looter (Tony Dow) is injured in a motorcycle accident, and a man (Trent Lehman) breaks his arm and loses his dog.

Notes

The Fire Department public information officer (PIO) sitting at the Fire Information Center was originally slated to be portrayed by LACoFD's real PIO, Dick Friend. Friend did not have a Screen Actors Guild (SAG) card at this time so an uncredited actor played this role. Friend was also portrayed by uncredited actors in ("Show Biz," episode 2.3, and "Women!," episode 2.9). Friend got his SAG card by season 2 and appeared as himself in "Inferno" (episode 3.21) and "The Screenwriter" (episode 4.1).

This episode is the only time in the series that an erroneous ID is used for an LA County helicopter. The tail number for the Bell 204 helicopter dropping water on the squad was unidentifiable, but a voiceover done later in a Universal sound booth states it is Copter 2, which was a tail number used in the fleet for a Bell 47 (think *M*A*S*H*).

Stunt doubles were used for Johnny and Roy driving the squad through the water drop. Edith Evanson appeared earlier in another LA County firefighting drama, *Rescue 8*, in the episode "Trial By Fire."

Locations

The elderly lady's house used in this episode is a familiar one located on Universal's backlot; it was the house used in the movie *Psycho*. The fireman trapped under the tree was also filmed on Universal's backlot, this time on Colonial Street. The scene where the Chief is talking to the boys about the fire was filmed at Arthur E. Wright Elementary School, at 4029 Las Virgenes Road in Calabasas, California. The grass fire scenes were actually footage of a large acreage fire filmed in Malibu in 1970. The fire trail scenes with the motorcycle rider and the run-bys through the fire trail were filmed on the backlot in the area known as "Falls Lake" and "Falls Canyon."

"Dealer's Wild"

Episode #1.5

Production #34404

Final revision: January 19, 1972

Filming dates: January 20–27, 1972

Airdate: January 19, 1972

Writer: Carey Wilbur

Director: Lawrence Dobkin

LACoFD Technical Advisor: Charles Bender (PM0017)

Guest Cast: Lou Krugman, Coleen Gray (Mrs. Thompson), Marian Collier, Mitch Carter, Buddy Foster, Sonja Dunson, Susan Madigan, Peggy Drier

Synopsis
Johnny keeps losing at cards and being stuck "in-the-tank" doing the dishes at the station, so he creates his own card game. Roy talks down a 14-year-old boy (Buddy Foster) in a plane after the pilot (the boy's father) has a heart attack. A man (Lou Krugman) attempts suicide three different ways, infuriating Dr. Brackett. The station responds to an overturned gasoline tanker and rescues a trapped man. A teenager overdoses, and Roy and Johnny have to deal with disinterested bystanders.

Notes
Ron Pinkard joins the hospital staff in this episode for his reoccurring role as Dr. Mike Morton.

In many stations, the person "in the tank" is the one doing the dishes, which may be decided by various games of chance. In many stations, if the cook must participate, he or she gets an automatic win, and it usually takes two wins to get out. The last two players left in the game hold a playoff to determine who will be in the tank. The runner-up is usually saddled with light-duty work such as sweeping, emptying trash, and mopping the floor. The person in the tank empties the dishwasher and makes sure everything is cleaned and put away. Before dishwashers, everything had to be washed, dried, and put away by hand; air-drying was not allowed. Some of the varied card games played in the stations range from 357 (also known as No Spleen Dean), Mafia Low, Dr. Pepper, Drive-By, 214, Wild-Twos, West Hollywood, and many others, all with a storied history as to their origination.

Locations
Airport scenes were filmed at the San Fernando airport. Closed in 1985, the airport was located NW of Whitman Airport at the intersection of 8th Street and Aviation Place (between the I-5 and 210, north of the 118). The apartment exteriors of the attempted suicide victim were filmed on Universal's backlot in Courthouse Square. The residence exteriors of the girl in convulsions were filmed on Universal's Industrial Street.

"Nurses Wild"

Episode #1.6

Production #34405

Final revision: December 9, 1971

Airdate: March 4, 1972

Writer: Fred Frieberger

Director: Herschel Daughtery

LACoFD Technical Advisor: Gerald Nolls (PM0004)

Guest cast: Royal Dano, Ray Ballard, Kip Niven, Christine Dixon, Victor Izay, Chris Forbes (Ellen Bart, student nurse), Patricia Mickey (Nurse Sharon Walter), Scott Gourlay, Sarah Fankboner, with Vince Howard and Colby Chester (the deputies).

Synopsis

Johnny falls for a student nurse (Christine Dixon) while teaching lifesaving techniques. A liquor store owner (Victor Izay) who shoots a robber (Kip Niven) is filled with remorse and has chest pain. Dr. Brackett, Dixie, and the student nurse (Chris Forbes) try to save the lives of both the robber and owner. A dog delays the rescue of an unconscious woman. A black widow spider bites a man. Dr. Early deals with an alcoholic (Royal Dano) suffering from the DTs, and Dr. Morton assumes an unconscious hippie is on drugs.

Notes

In this episode, the foam unit from Station 127 assists Station 51, which is called to an industrial accident involving a chemical leak where a man is trapped under a beam on some overhead pipes. Firefighters from S127 kept a spray on the leak and helped with the lines as Johnny and Roy lowered the victim to the floor. The others from S127 operated the foam unit, and Kelly and López spread the foam to prevent sparks from the K-12 from reaching the floor, which was covered with the chemical.

The actual firefighters from 127's were seen in this segment. Foam 127 was and still is stationed at Station 127. They currently operate a 1984 Mack, shop number F0367, as Foam 5127. It is a reserve apparatus.

Locations

The chemical plant scenes were filmed at the Valley Generating Station, 11801 Sheldon Street, Sun Valley, California. This locale, used in an earlier episode, will be the scene of other rescues.

Note the Moorpark Pharmacy across the street from the shooting at the liquor store incident. Leonard Maltin (film critic for *Entertainment Tonight*) advises that this segment was filmed in Toluca Lake, on W. Riverside Drive. It's below the 134 and just west of the 101 and Universal Studios. The building is still there, but ceased being used as a pharmacy about 5 years ago.

"Publicity Hound"

Working titles: Celebrity; Publicity Mad

Episode #1.7

Production #34407

Final revision: January 17, 1972

Filming dates: February 3–10, 1972

Airdate: March 11, 1972

Writer: Michael Donovan

Director: Christian Nyby, Sr.

LACoFD Technical Advisor: Richard Neal PM0009

Guest cast: Gene Raymond (J. P. Dumont), Gary Crosby (Paramedic Tom Wheeler, station 110), Dolores Vance, Sallie Shockley (Penny Fortas), Barry Higgins (Andy Jason), Bill Baldwin (Carl Evans), Edith Diaz (Mrs. Diaz), Scott Allen (Paramedic Kirk, station 110), Steven Cassidy (Don Mathews), Ted Gehring (construction foreman), William Bryant (Captain Curtis, Station 110)

Synopsis

Tom Wheeler (Gary Crosby), from Squad 110, upsets Johnny by constantly making the news with simple rescues, thanks to a reporter's (Bill Baldwin) help. Roy and Johnny respond to Marina Del Rey, covering for Squad 110 which is on another call, in the rescue of a man trapped in ship's rigging. Dr. Brackett clashes with an affluent tycoon named J. P. Dumont (Gene Raymond) over a diagnosis. A horse is rescued from a pit, and a 5-year-old girl (Dolores Vance) is rescued from a construction site storm drain. Paramedic Wheeler again makes the news as Gage and DeSoto hand the girl up to Wheeler where the waiting TV cameraman is filming the action.

Notes

The 125-year-old schooner (at the time of shooting) used in this episode was owned by a member of the writer's family. Station 110's captain said that the two-masted schooner was named "Isabel" and was 90 feet long.

Locations

Station 110, where Johnny and Roy (supposedly) board the Harbor Patrol Boat, is in reality the Marina Del Rey Los Angeles County Sheriff Department's station located at 13851 Fiji Way, about a mile from 110's. Station 110, never seen in the series, would not be seen until the movie *Steel Inferno*. The Harbor Patrol boats appear at the dock in "The Professor" (episode 2.15) when boarding LACoFD Boat 110. The call sign used in this episode, "*Del Rey Harbor Patrol,*" is fictitious. Now as then the patrol boats use the call sign 'Bravo' and boat number, such as 'Bravo 2'. The lighthouse at Fisherman's Wharf and the lifeguard station are next to it. At the time, the Harbor Patrol and the LA County Sheriff were separate entities, but the two agencies merged in 1984. Besides currently housing the Sheriff and the patrol boats, it also houses Lifeguard Station 1 (Baywatch del Rey). Look for the Lighthouse at Fisherman's Wharf and the Lifeguard station next to it. This is only one of eight Baywatch stations that comprise the LA County Baywatch fleet, including two based on Catalina Island.

The storm drain rescue was filmed on the Universal backlot, and construction for Universal Theme Park appears in the background. This same site was used for the electrocution segment in the World Premier movie, where in the background some production trailers and other studio vehicles are visible on a side road and California Highway 101 is in the background.

"Weird Wednesday"

Episode #1.8

Production #34410 (formerly #34408, which was assigned to Hang-Up, filmed a week later)

Final revision: February 9, 1972

Filming dates: February 10–17, 1972

Airdate: March 18, 1972

Writer: Daryl Henry (revisions by Robert Cinader)

Director: Lawrence Dobkin

LACoFD Technical Advisor: William Roger Crow (PM0007)

Guest cast: Jeanette Nolan, Arnold Stang, Henny Backus, Sherry Bain, Helen Baron, Anne Collins, Chris Forbes, Patricia Mickey, Bob Hastings, Pam Peters, William Katt (Wally Lytton)

Synopsis

Johnny is convinced that weird things will happen on their shift. A female parachutist lands in a tree. A boy tries to cryogenically freeze himself, and a man (Arnold Stang) is suffering from uncontrollable hiccups. An 80-year-old woman (Jeanette Nolan) breaks her ankle while celebrating her birthday, and the party moves to Rampart. A man collapses with chest pains while jogging. A prostitute brings in a Navy seaman suffering from chest pains who doesn't speak English. A woman on a golf course suffers from a possible snake bite. A drunk in a car (Bob Hastings) goes over an embankment, which causes more problems for Johnny.

Notes
In this episode, Christine Forbes reprises her role as Student Nurse Ellen Bart for the remainder of the season.

Locations
The scene where the squad pulls up to the parachutist in a tree was filmed on Upper Tram Road at Universal.

"Dilemma"

Episode #1.9

Production #34411

Final revision: February 7, 1972

Airdate: March 25, 1972

Writer: Michael Donovan

Director: Christian Nyby, Sr.

LACoFD Technical Advisor: Roscoe "Rocky" Doke (PM0008)

Guest cast: Seymour Cassel, Benny Rubin, Rose Michtom, Patricia Mickey, Chris Forbes, Hal Baylor, Bill McLean, Scott Allen (Kirk), Robert E. Kline, Marylyn Hassett (Cynthia)

Synopsis
Johnny is not interested in a girl (Marylyn Hassett) who has a crush on him. Engine 127 assists Station 51 when an elevator gets stuck between floors and the brake drum fails, trapping several people. One man (Benny Rubin) breaks his leg, and another person (Rose Michtom) is suffering with chest pains inside the elevator. A man (Seymour Cassel) has a problem with methane gas at a junkyard. An industrial accident at a rail yard overcomes two men while cleaning tank cars. A nursing student (Patricia Mickey) forgets to take notes, ruins an electrocardiogram reading, and is in awe of Dr. Brackett.

Notes

One of the railcars seen in this episode is now part of the Portola Railroad Museum and Collection in Portola, California; it is the long, white LPG tank car behind the action, identified as DODX 11642. The Museum obtained this car in 1985, renumbered it FR&W 12107, and uses it to store diesel fuel.

The device Gage used at the junkyard is called a combustible gas indicator.

"Hang-Up"

Working title: Alpha-Beta-Gamma

Episode #1.10

Production #34408

Final revision: February 14, 1972

Filming dates: February 24–March 2, 1972

Airdate: April 8, 1972

Writer: Preston Wood

Director: Lawrence Dobkin

LACoFD Technical Advisor: Gary Davis (PM0003)

Guest cast: Mort Saul, Shelly Novack, Chris Forbes, Savannah Bentley, Lew Brown, Art Balinger, Vince Howard, Don Ross, Scott Gourlay, and John Smith as Station Captain John Van Orden

Synopsis

Johnny has a "hang-up" over an episode of *Adam-12* ("Ambush," original airdate November 10, 1971) to which he missed the end. The Station is called out to rescue a would-be jewel thief (Mort Saul) from an air-conditioning duct. Later the crew responds to a fire where a man is trapped and injured in a radioactive room. Gage is hospitalized overnight as a result of receiving light radiation poisoning. An interrupted barroom brawl resumes at Rampart. Dr. Brackett treats a woman suffering from a migraine. A surfer with a bad attitude ruins his cast by going surfing and makes an already difficult night at Rampart even worse.

Notes

This episode is directed by prominent actor and director Lawrence Dobkin. In the *Adam-12* "Ambush" episode, Ron Pinkard portrays Officer Walt Barrett as he did in an earlier *Adam-12* episode, "Log 76: The Militants." Pinkard is not seen in the clips shown on *Emergency!*.

The end credits list John Smith as a guest star in the role of Captain Hammer.

In this episode, Roy refers to his wife as 'Ann' and not 'Joanne'; this is confirmed by the final shooting script. While Ann may be a nickname for Joanne, this is the only time she is referred to as such.

The technical advisor for this episode, Gary Davis, insisted that the radioactive incident be filmed properly and informed the director that "some corrections need to be made." The director told Davis, "When you see the final product, you will love it." Davis was not satisfied, and he again advised Dobkin that, "This is not the way we do it," but was told to "leave it alone." Davis was frustrated and did not want the Fire Department to look bad, so he contacted Cinader. Cinader informed Davis to, "Just tell the director how it should be done, period." Davis went back to director and assertively told him that he had spoken with Cinader and that the scene should be "filmed properly," and it was.

The original title of the script, "Alpha-Beta-Gamma," as named by the scriptwriter Preston Wood, came from the different types of radiation and particles. There were two types of equipment used in the radiation scene. The first was a gray device that was held in the room, known as a Portable Air Sampler. This device samples for airborne particulates by drawing air through filters using a high-speed rotary motor. These air samplers were not part of civil defense radiation detection kits. The filters are usually checked with a Geiger counter (CD V-700) to estimate the total activity. The filters are taken to a laboratory in a clean envelope to prevent contamination and are counted using a multichannel gamma spectrometer to identify and quantify gamma emitters.

The small handheld yellow device is a CD V- 715 Ion Chamber Survey Meter, which was the most widely produced of all the Civil Defense radiation instruments. The incident shows firefighters in full respiratory protection checking the activity of a sample with the CD V-715 high-range instrument. As used in this episode, it has a high psychological impact but is not very accurate (in this instance) according to J. Carl Kee, Radiation Safety Officer for KI4U, Inc, in Gonzales Texas. "I always wondered why they used the 715 in that episode instead of a CD V-700" (Geiger counter), states Eric Green, Civil Defense Museum in Dallas, Texas. Regarding placing the CDV-715 up against the air sampler, "That picture was for effect, not accuracy," states J. Carl Kee. "[There was] very poor technique and would contaminate the instrument making it useless for further work." The Civil Defense kits, usually maintained at shelters and fire stations across the country, were set up as local monitoring stations. They contained two of the V-715's along with a CD V-700 Geiger counter, which measures Gamma radiation and detects Beta radiation; a CD V-750 Dosimeter charger, and usually six CD V-742 pocket Dosimeters that read Gamma Radiation. The dosimeters were worn by the personal when entering a 'hot' area and would measure the amount of exposure from 0–200 roentgens and had to be re-calibrated after each use.

Alpha radiation travels only a short distance through the air and is not able to penetrate the skin or able to penetrate turn-out gear, clothing, or a cover on a probe. However, Alpha-emitting materials can be harmful to humans if the materials are inhaled, swallowed, or absorbed through open wounds. Therefore, there is no eating, drinking, or smoking in a 'hot' area.

Locations
The jewel thief in the air-conditioning duct was filmed on Soundstage 44. The radioactive room scenes were filmed on Soundstage 12.

"Crash"

Working title: Torch Song

Episode #1.11

Production #34403

Filming began: March 3, 1972

Airdate: April 15, 1972

Writers: Michael Donovan and Gerald Sanford, with revisions by R. A. Cinader

Director: Christian Nyby, Sr.

LACoFD Technical Advisor: Robert Belliveau (PM0001)

Other technical expertise by members of the Sierra Madre Search and Rescue Team

Guest cast: Cicely Tyson, Gary Crosby (Tom Wheeler), William Bramley, Don Matheson, Francine York, Sandy deBruin, Edmund Cambridge, Eric Laneuville, Patricia Mickey, Buddy Lester, Ronne Troup, Chris Forbes, Scott Gourlay, John Smith (Captain Van Orden), Gene Thom, Larry Twedell, Bob Watkins, Jay Benson (Crew Chief), Kirby Furlong (boy in plane), Roland Barton (Chief Pilot of the LA County Fire Department Air Ops Division, as himself), with members of the Sierra Madre Search and Rescue Team. Two other Search and Rescue members in the episode were actors; unknown actor as Jay Benson the Search and Rescue Crew Chief, and the other member that appeared in the helicopter sitting next to John and Roy was an actor.

Synopsis

Roy and Johnny are air-lifted from Station 93 via Copter 14 into a remote area to assist the Sierra Madre Search and Rescue Team (SMSRT) in the rescue of the occupants of a light plane crash with the wreckage lodged high in a tree. A burglar has a heart attack. Dr. Brackett treats a young football player injured from a hard tackle. A babysitter (Ronne Troop) brings in a 4-year-old boy who has swallowed some pills. Johnny wants Roy to apologize for calling him "some kind of nut."

Notes

Gary Crosby again portrays fireman/paramedic Tom Wheeler in this episode. The technical advisor for this episode, Robert Belliveau, recalls Gary Crosby rooting his stunt double on to make him look good.

Bobby Troup's daughter Ronne appears in this episode as well as in "Saddled" (episode 2.6) and "Body Language" (episode 3.12), and four episodes of *Adam-12*. She nearly played the title role in the TV series *The Flying Nun*. The program had been created for Sally Field, who had recently completed her run as *Gidget* on TV. Field initially turned down the series, and the role was given to Ronne. A pilot episode was filmed with Ronne in the lead. Field had a change of heart and decided to take the part. It was after this that Ronne won the part of Polly on *My Three Sons* and later as Barbara on *Knots Landing* (1987–1990).

The plane crash scene (filmed near a ski resort in Wrightwood, California) involved a single-engine plane with three occupants that ran out of fuel and performed a crash landing 75 feet up in a tree. The close-ups of the incident were filmed on Stage 3 at Universal; the plane was about 12 feet off the ground. Long before the invention of the "blue screen," the production crew hung a large tarp, painted to match the sky and mountains behind the tree.

Robert Belliveau advises that "the Sierra Madre Search and Rescue Team was at scene and provided technical expertise (rope and hi-angle rescue) as well as their vehicle." "The vehicle used in this episode was our 1968 Dodge Crew cab model W300 4X4, with the 'Trio T-2' canister *Adam-12* type emergency lights on the roof long since retired," states Dick Sale, the SMSRT webmaster at the Web site http://www.smsr.org/.

The team members that participated in the *Emergency!* filming were not credited. "The Team has always had a policy of not identifying individuals when releasing information to the press. When talking to the press we refer to them as "crew chief," "team member," or "searcher," states Arnold Gaffrey, SMSRT.

SMSRT is an all-volunteer team founded in 1951, and it was the first such organization formed in California. It is affiliated with the Los Angeles

County Sheriff's Department as high-risk civilian volunteers and with the National Mountain Rescue Association. Their primary area of operation is southern California; however, the team responds to calls for help in an area extending from Baja, California, through the High Sierra and into northern California. When this episode was made, they had only this one vehicle, which was parked at a very small Sierra Madre City fire station.

The station for the SMSRT is the former LACoFD Station 108 on the corner of Grandview Ave. and Stone House Road in Sierra Madre, which was closed around 1975 or 1976. The station was built, over the objection of many neighbors, and was in service less than ten years. It was still occupied, however, as an office for an Assistant Chief and the secretary through the 1980s and 1990s. Arnold Gaffrey, SMSRT, stated:

> We actually started parking our vehicles at Station 108 when it first opened. The station was built with an apparatus bay large enough for two engines. The county fire department only had one stationed there and because we were volunteer members of the fire department at that time, there was room for us to store our vehicles there. We didn't have our meetings there or store any other equipment because there was a full time fire crew in residence. When the station was decommissioned as an active station, we leased it from the fire department. During the next several years we shared it with various fire department units ranging from an explorer post to the area division chief. When the county decided to get rid of it, we purchased it.

SEASON 2

"Problem"

Working titles: Decision; Pressure
Episode #2.1
Production #35701
Filming: July 11–18, 1972
Airdate: September 16, 1972
Writer: Preston Wood
Director: Christian Nyby, Sr. (in his last directorial role for *Emergency!*)
LACoFD Technical Advisor: Gary Davis (PM0003)
Guest cast: Lloyd Bochner (Dr. Sunderland), Jim Turley, Jessica Rains, Willard Sage (Dr. Eccles), Michael Richardson, Kevin Dobson (the Deputy)

Synopsis
Roy and Johnny rescue a man (Jim Turley) whose car engine has fallen on him while he was making repairs. While Roy accompanies the patient in the ambulance he discovers that their two-way radio is not working (the antenna has fallen off the ambulance). Without medical supervision, Roy treats the patient who is aspirating. When the man later dies, his doctor (Lloyd Bochner) blames Roy for his death and attacks the paramedic program. A man (Michael Richardson) narrowly escapes death from a Texas Longhorn bull after falling off his motorbike. Roy thinks about quitting the paramedic program but later, after rescuing a child trapped in a house fire, he decides to stay.

Notes
While filming this episode, Randy Mantooth actually drove the squad (though only about 10 feet so the crew could mop the floor of the apparatus bay).

Locations
The segment involving the house fire was filmed at 1847 Ocean Avenue in Long Beach (see Chapter 16, The Long Beach Fire incident.) The segment involving the car engine was shot on Universal's Colonial Street on the first day of shooting.

Yearling Row Ranch (28754 Mulholland Highway in Malibu) was used to film the bull scene; this ranch was a regular weekend retreat for Ronald and Nancy Reagan in the 1950s and 1960s before he became Governor of California and is now part of the Santa Monica Mountains National Recreation Area.

"Kids"

Episode #2.2

Production #35708

Final revision: July 18, 1972

Filming began: July 20, 1972

Airdate: September 23, 1972

Writer: Michael Donovan

Director: Georg Fenady

LACoFD Technical Advisor: Dale Cauble, PM0002

Guest cast: Roger Perry (Mr. Gentry), Anne Whitfield (Susan, Chirley Gentry), Christian Juttner (Frankie Stewart), Richard Jaeckel (attorney), Gary Clarke (Mr. Peters), Scott Sealy (Randy Peters), Stephen

Manley, Don Carter (Tim West), Victor Izay (Judge), William Bryant (Police Sergeant Pierce), John Travolta (Chuck Benson)

Synopsis
A number of kids get into trouble, and the station gets a new mascot—a dog Chet names Boot. A boy (Christian Juttner) injures himself falling down an 8-foot post hole, although Dr. Brackett thinks the injuries are a result of abuse and is warned by an attorney (Richard Jaeckel) that his pursuit of the matter could jeopardize his career. Dr. Early removes a boy's (Scott Sealy) stuck finger from a steering wheel. Roy and Johnny rescue a boy whose head is trapped in a crawlspace vent under a house. While at the scene of a wildland fire, Boot helps locate an injured hiker (John Travolta) and then leaves with Truck Company 43, which assisted in the rescue.

Notes
This was 18-year-old John Travolta's first television appearance.

Richard Jaeckel would later appear in the 1973 TV Movie *Firehouse* with Richard Roundtree and Vince Edwards. He would reprise the role in the TV series of the same name in 1974. Roundtree would become a firefighter again in 1999 as a Fire Captain in the short-lived series *Rescue 77*.

In the opening sequence where Boot first appears, a voice over the speaker says, "Squad 59, cancel your response." When the station crew run out of the kitchen to the apparatus, Johnny and Roy go to the squad with an unusual engine crew (not López, Donnelly, Stoker, or Norell).

Locations
The exterior shots, with John Travolta, were filmed at Falls Lake backlot, including the canyon roads and ledge, filmed on the first day of shooting. The first rescue in the episode was shot on the same hill as a rescue scene from "Publicity Hound" (episode 1.7). The 4th day shooting-exterior for the kid whose head is stuck was filmed on Colonial Street, the exteriors of what was then called the Parker House.

"Show Biz"

Episode #2.3
Production #35711
Final script revision: July 27, 1972
Filming began: July 31, 1972
Airdate: September 30, 1972
Writer: Daryl Henry

Director: Sam C. Freedle

LACoFD Technical Advisor: Unknown

Guest cast: Henry Jones, Christine Dixon, Joseph Kaufman, Ted Gehring, Monica Lewis, Joseph Perry, Ezra Stone (Boris Miller), Scott Gourlay, Lillian Lehman (Rampart nurse), Deidre Hall (Rampart nurse), with an unidentified actor as an LACoFD liaison (Dick)

Synopsis
There is a photo shoot at the station, and Johnny is picked as the "Ideal Fireman." When Johnny and Roy can't reach Rampart by radio, a country doctor (Henry Jones) assists them with an injured man pinned under a tractor and then becomes a patient himself when he develops heart trouble. Roy and Johnny rescue a woman and her drowning husband from a pool and later rescue two stuntmen trapped on a waterfall at a movie studio. After the Ideal Fireman photo shoot, the sponsor decides that Johnny does not look like a fireman and wants to use Roy instead.

Notes
Ezra Stone portrays the same character, Boris Miller, in "Syndrome" (episode 2.16).

Locations
The waterfall rescue was filmed on Universal's backlot, where scenes from the Old West and Amityville (*Jaws*) are visible. The pool rescue was filmed at a residence on Moorepark Street in Toluca Lake, North Hollywood.

"Virus"

Episode #2.4

Production #35702

Final revision: June 28, 1972

Filming dates: June 29–July 11, 1972

Airdate: October 7, 1972

Writer: Daryl Henry

Director: Lawrence Dobkin

LACoFD Technical Advisor: Roger Crow (PM0007)

Guest cast: Dennis Patrick (Mr. Hollister), Cathy Lee Crosby (Jenny Hollister), William Gray Espy (Tim Duntley), Skye Aubrey (Madi Duntley), Mitch Carter (Danny Loring), Vic Vallers (Deputy Pauling), Jean Allison (Mrs. Brydon), Philip Brown (Mickey Brydon), Vince Howard, Deidre Hall, Patricia Mickey, Koki (exotic monkey)

Synopsis

A sick lady (Cathy Lee Crosby) with a monkey provides the key to a mysterious, highly contagious, and deadly virus that strikes several people, including Dr. Brackett, Johnny, and another LA County firefighter (William Gray Espy), who eventually dies from the virus. Roy and Johnny rescue a 14-year-old boy (Philip Brown) with an inner ear problem from a treehouse. The station responds to a call where a man is injured on a scaffold.

Notes

Philip Brown and Randolph Mantooth would work together again in the late 1990s when they were both appearing on the ABC soap opera *The City* where Philip played "Buck."

Locations

Treehouse rescue was filmed on Universal's Colonial Street. The scaffold scenes were filmed at the F&M building (320 Pine Avenue, Long Beach), The long shots were stunt doubles for Gage and DeSoto. The building would be used again in "Peace Pipe" (episode 2.5). The scenes with the sick LA County firefighter were filmed in an actual residence near Agnes and Woodbridge in North Hollywood.

"Peace Pipe"

Episode #2.5

Production #35706

Final revision: June 16, 1972

Filming began: June 20, 1972

Airdate: October 14, 1972

Writer: Michael Donovan (revisions by Robert Cinader)

Director: Christian Nyby II

LACoFD Technical Advisor: Roscoe "Rocky" Doke (MP0008)

Guest cast: Kip Niven (Mr. Taylor), Brooke Bundy (Mrs. Taylor), William Campbell (Sam Jenks), Jennifer Lesco (Debbie Taylor), Vince Howard, Renee Lippin, Joe Pizzorusso, Ken Lynch (food stand owner), Tom Waters (construction foreman)

Synopsis

Chet constantly pesters Johnny about his Native American heritage and ultimately suggests a treaty. At night, a drunk driver (William Campbell) rams a parked car, trapping a 7-year-old girl (Jennifer Lesco) inside. John and Roy remove a child's hand from a gumball machine. A woman has a problem with her new girdle. The station must discover how dangerous fuel oil got into the water system and caused several fires. A sniper makes a roof rescue dangerous.

Notes
Many segments for this episode were based on real accounts. The fuel oil segment was based on a true story, although many viewers thought that it was too far-fetched. The girdle episode was also based on a real event in which a heavy woman's bra needed to be cut; once cut, the bra flung around and hit firefighter/paramedic Gary Davis in the face. The gumball machine story was also based on a true event.

This episode was the first time that the Jaws of Life® were used in the series (see Chapter 10).

Locations
Exterior house fire scenes were filmed on Universal's Colonial Street. The house scene in which Gage is hit with the fire was filmed on Soundstage 21, and stunt doubles were used for Gage and DeSoto. The scene with the hydrant and construction crew was filmed at the corner of San Fernando Road and Sheldon Street at the Valley Steam Plant (just north of Burbank and east of I-5 in the San Fernando Valley).

The car accident was filmed at the Stop & Shop at 12039 Ventura Place in Studio City on the sixth and final day of shooting but was the first incident in the episode.

The sniper and scaffold rescues were filmed at the F&M Building (320 Pine Avenue, Long Beach). The building, completed in 1923 as the Farmers and Merchants Bank Building, is still in business as such. The building where the sniper was shooting from, across the street, is the Willmore, own-your-own apartments at 315 W. 3rd Street. It was named in honor of the city of Long Beach's founder, William Willmore. The segment showing Johnny and Roy (stunt doubles), as looking down from atop the F&M building sign to the street with the F.W. Woolworth building visible, shows the intersection of Pine Avenue and 4th Street. The Woolworth now houses Gold's Gym, and across the street is the Walker building (401 Pine Avenue). Once a department store, it is now lofts.

The segment involving the kid with his hand stuck in the gumball machine is a true event as relayed by firefighter/paramedic Gary Davis. Although used in this episode, it was scripted for *KIDS*. It was to be shot in North Hollywood on Lankershim Boulevard on July 27th (the exteriors of the Hot Dog Stand). Although in earlier scripts, the final draft of the *KIDS* script didn't have the scene, it was pending. The script said " To be written." It was later filmed on the Universal lot and inserted in this episode.

"Saddled"

Episode #2.6

Production #35707

Final revision: August 7, 1972

Filming began: August 9, 1972

Airdate: October 21, 1972

Writer: Herb Purdum

Director: Georg Fenady

LACoFD Technical Advisor: Bob Belliveau (PM0001)

Guest cast: Larry Storch (Ben Wesley), Elizabeth Baur, Ronne Troup (Lisa Hill), Kelly Troup (Debbi), Michael Rupert, Deidre Hall, Jay Hammer, Barbara Bosson (Timmy's mother), Charles Guardino (Timmy's father), Christopher Gardner, Edward Crawford

Synopsis

Johnny thinks he can make some extra money by riding in rodeos. The squad goes to a hole-in-the-wall restaurant when a soda bottle explodes in a girl's face. They return later for a gas explosion injuring a man (Larry Storch). After falling from a tree, a young boy (Christopher Gardner) with a rare blood disease suffers a head injury. A school bus with children and a nun (Elizabeth Baur) goes off an embankment. Dixie has a run-in with a portable X-ray machine and injures her toe.

Notes

According to Technical Advisor Bob Belliveau, the crew had to take precautions with Larry Storch, who had a bad back. The Los Angeles Archdiocese was consulted on this script for advice and approval for the school bus scenes where the paramedic assists a nun. Angelo De Meo (stuntman) is wearing a helmet from Station 110 even though 210's was toned out; the Captain's helmet is correct.

Two of Bobby Troup's daughters appear—Ronne (as Lisa Hill) and Kelly (as Debbi). Kelly is the daughter of Bobby Troup and Julie London. This is the only episode in which Kelly would appear. Ronne would appear in two other episodes.

Locations

The restaurant scene was filmed on Universal's Court House Square and was also used as the hot dog stand from "Peace Pipe" (episode 2.5). The school bus rescue segment was filmed on Universal's backlot.

Note that the same drive-by stock footage in this episode is used in "Peace Pipe" with the Squad passing the church and stopping at the apartment complex. The Faith Presbyterian Church of Valley Village (formerly First Presbyterian Church of North Hollywood) is located at 5000 Colfax Avenue (Valley Village, also called North Hollywood). The sanctuary seen with the tall bell tower was torn down in December 1994 due to earthquake damage from the 6.8 magnitude Northridge Earthquake on January 16, 1994.

The apartment building that the incident takes place in is just across the street from the church to the north and is still there. They are the Colfax Apartments at 5038-48 Colfax Avenue. This location is just off the 101 northwest of Universal. Apartment interiors were filmed on sound stage 41.

"Fuzz Lady"

Episode #2.7

Production #35712

Final revision: August 11, 1972

Filming began: August 18, 1972

Airdate: November 4, 1972

Writer: Michael Donovan

Director: Christian I. Nyby II

LACoFD Technical Advisor: Charles Bender (PM0017)

Guest cast: Paul Fix, Sharon Gless, J. Pat O'Malley, Ellen Moss, Nate Esformes, Drout Miller, Eric Server, William Durkin, Vince Howard, Meg Wyllie, Scott Barrett

Synopsis

Johnny falls for policewoman Sheila Thomas (Sharon Gless) when the squad is called to treat a mugger (Drout Miller) with a broken arm. Items are stolen from Rampart's emergency department, and Thomas is put on the case. Roy and Johnny rescue an elderly man (Paul Fix) with apparent senility from a fire. A grandfather and grandson sustain minor injuries in a model rocket explosion. A man is trapped and injured on a drilling platform crane when he tries to steal a boat. Boot returns to the station.

"Trainee"

Episode #2.8

Production #35715

Final revision: August 21, 1972

Filming dates: August 29–September 6, 1972

Airdate: November 11, 1972

Writer: Jim Owens

Director: Dennis Donnelly

LACoFD Technical Advisor: Gerald Nolls (PM0004)

Guest cast: Robert Pratt (Firefighter Ed Marlow), Jackie Coogan (Elmer Slifer), Charles H. Gray (Chief Sorensen), Vince Howard (police officer), Lillian Lehman (Carol Williams), Paul Nuckles (Robert McDonald), Ron Henriquez (sailor), Anthony Eldridge (Jerry Gamble), Iris Korn (old lady), Wynn Irwin (George Robinson), Craig Chudy (police officer), Don Pulford (police officer)

Synopsis

Former Vietnam medic Ed Marlow (Robert Pratt) is now going through paramedic training and thinks he knows more than Roy, Johnny, and the doctors at Rampart. His actions nearly cause the death of a victim (Anthony Eldridge) from a fall off a cliff, and he makes errors in both the treatment of a woman (Iris Korn) who has overdosed on pills and a man (Paul Nuckles) suffering from an insulin reaction. This former medic is considered a good firefighter and eventually gets reassigned to Station 41. Fire Chief Sorenson (Charles H. Gray) concludes, "The important thing we should remember is that not every one of us is cut out to be a paramedic."

Notes

This episode was the first of eighteen episodes directed by Dennis Donnelly, Tim Donnelly's brother. Battalion Chief Jim Page, the LACoFD technical consultant for the first two seasons, wrote the script under the pseudonym of Jim Owens. Robert Pratt appeared again (as a different character) in episodes 5.14 and 6.14. The Coast Guard helicopter utilized was unit #1375.

Locations

Carwash scenes were filmed at Academy Car Wash (13310 Sherman Way, North Hollywood). Auto wrecking yard scenes were filmed at Foreign Auto Wrecking (12537 Sherman Way, North Hollywood).

Cliff rescue scenes were filmed near Point Vicente Park between the old Marineland of the Pacific and the Point Vicente Light House/Coast Guard Station in Rancho Palos Verdes.

"Women!"

Episode #2.9

Production #35713

Final revision: August 31, 1972

Filming began: September 8, 1972

Airdate: November 25, 1972

Writer: Daryl Henry (revisions by Robert Cinader)

Director: Georg Fenady

LACoFD Technical Advisor: Lee Gustafson (PM0018)

Guest cast: Leslie Charleson, Ann Morgan Guilbert, Dick Van Patten, Joshua Bryant, Michael Richardson, Stacy Harris, Janie Baldwin, Randall Carver, Susan Damonte, Lillian Lehman

Synopsis
An attractive journalist (Leslie Charleson) accompanies the squad for a day and later accuses them of male chauvinism, especially Johnny. She covers the squad's rescues of a man trapped in a truck under live power lines, a man trapped in a sofa bed, and two victims in a bombed building. A man (Dick Van Patten) gets his arm stuck in a garbage disposal. Morton and Early try to save a boy who has eaten poison hemlock. The reporter also accuses Dr. Brackett and the Rampart staff of exploitation and discrimination against women.

Note
A quote from Johnny, "You know, I think we should call Dick Friend and tell him he's been conned by a women's libber who is completely freaked out of her mind." Dick, of course, is the LACoFD PIO and liaison to the show.

"Dinner Date"

Episode #2.10

Production #35705

Final revision: September 14, 1972

Filming began: October 9, 1972

Airdate: December 2, 1972

Writer: Dick Morgan

Director: Dennis Donnelly

LACoFD Technical Advisor: Wayne Nutt (PM0029)

Guest cast: Lynn Carlin (Mrs. Patterson), Jean Alison (Mrs. Conroy), Melissa Gilbert (Jenny Conroy), Emily Yancy, Michael C. Gwynn, Dawn Lyn, Laurette Spang, Drout Miller, Judy Farrell, Patty McCormack (Janet Caldwell), Deidre Hall (Nurse Sally Lewis)

Synopsis

Roy tries to set Johnny up with Joanne's cousin. A woman (Patty McCormack) almost hits a boy on a bike; she then starts choking uncontrollably and later has an epileptic seizure. A man (Drout Miller) is shot by his father-in-law while Dixie looks after his pregnant wife (Laurette Spang). A 7-year-old child (Dawn Lyn) has her arm trapped in a swimming pool drain. An obese man suffers from heart problems. Several drug-related victims are seen at Rampart, including a man with tetanus, a woman with gangrene, and a 16-year-old girl who took drugs laced with sodium hydroxide.

Notes

Laurette Spang (later star of *Battlestar Galactica*) also appeared in episodes 3.2 and 4.17. Patty McCormack also appeared as San Francisco Paramedic Gail Warren in the *Emergency!* movies *What's a Nice Girl Like You Doing...* and *The Convention.* Melissa Gilbert later starred as Laura in *Little House on the Prairie,* became president of the Screen Actors Guild, and is the youngest person ever to receive a star on the Hollywood Walk of Fame. Before this episode, Dawn Lyn Nervik portrayed Dodie Harper Douglas on *My Three Sons* with Ronne Troop.

  While Squad 51 is at the scene with the epileptic woman, a voice over the radio announces, "Squad 209, 10-7 to St. Francis." Squad 209 appears later in the season in "Honest" (episode 2.17).

"Musical Mania"

Episode #2.11

Production #35717

Filming began: October 18, 1972

Airdate: December 9, 1972

Writer: Kenneth Dorward

Director: Christian I. Nyby II

LACoFD Technical Advisor: David Phillips (PM0005)

Guest cast: Russell Wiggins, Kathleen Cackle, Katherine Kelly-Wiget (Betty Snyder), Scottie MacGregor, Lillian Lehman, Molli Benson, Deidre Hall, Stephen R. Hudis, Alice Hunn

Synopsis

After Chet cracks a joke about Johnny playing the squad's horn, Johnny takes up the bagpipes, trombone, and guitar and drives everyone at the station crazy. A nursery owner has fallen ill with tetanus, a teenage girl overdoses on illegal drugs, and a man in an ice cream truck is trapped under downed power lines. One man is stuck in a glider, and another is trapped and injured under a house. A boy is suffering from lead poisoning and a hormonal imbalance, but his father is too proud to accept "charity." Chet is studying for the Engineer's exam.

Notes

Katherine Kelly-Wiget portrays not Roy DeSoto's wife Joanne but Betty Snyder, daughter of the nurseryman. Fifteen-year-old Stephen R. Hudis portrays her nephew, Larry Snyder. Hudis is a renowned stunt performer, driver, and coordinator who teamed up again with Kevin Tighe in 1997 to film a TV pilot titled *The 119,* in which Tighe portrayed an LA City Battalion Chief (see Chapter 21). Katherine Scottie McGregor would go on to portray Mrs. Harriet Olsen, the school principal, in *Little House on the Prairie.*

"Helpful"

Episode #2.12

Production #35714

Final revision: September 15, 1972

Filming dates: September 19–26, 1972

Airdate: December 16, 1972

Writer: Preston Wood

Director: Lawrence Dobkin

LACoFD Technical Advisor: Robert Ramstead (PM0006)

Guest cast: Alicia Bond (doctor), Molli Benson (Nurse Gail), Jamie Farr*

Synopsis

Roy and his wife have a fight over Mike Stoker's spaghetti recipe, and Johnny just makes things worse by trying to help. A new doctor (Alicia Bond), who is emotionally upset and physically exhausted, makes some wrong judgments, and Dixie makes excuses for her. A man drives his car off a freeway on-ramp. A man falls off a ladder attempting to get a dog off a roof. Dr. Early uses psychology on a student of the occult. The station must find and rescue two children lost in a storm drain before it floods.

Notes
*Jamie Farr is credited in this episode although he does not appear until "Boot" (episode 2.19).

Locations
The freeway accident was filmed in Sylmar on an unopened stretch of freeway on the first day of shooting. The search and rescue of the two boys began at Falls Lake at Universal, and the storm drain portion was filmed in an alley off New York Street. The dog on the roof incident was filmed behind the *Marcus Welby, MD* (ABC 1968–1976) house on Colonial Street at Universal. The house was once identified by a Universal tram operator while driving on Colonial Street as "The Douglas house" from *My Three Sons*. In actuality that series was not shot at Universal, but at the old Desilu Studios that is now part of Paramount. Although, Fred MacMurray as Steve Douglas, the dad, worked, ironically enough, at the *Universal* Research and Development Corporation, it was revised/remodeled a bit for the Tom Hanks Movie, *The 'burbs* (1989), and further remodeled for other TV movies and TV programs including *Desperate Housewives*.

"Drivers"

> Episode #2.13
>
> Production #35709
>
> Final revision: June 8, 1972
>
> Filming dates: October 27–November 3, 1972
>
> Airdate: January 6, 1973
>
> Writer: Jim Owens (revisions by Robert Cinader)
>
> Director: Samuel Freedle
>
> LACoFD Technical Advisor: William Miles (PM0019)
>
> Guest cast: Dick Yarmy (football coach), Vic Mohica (Steve), Frank Maxwell (Captain Carter Engine 69), Lillian Lehman (Nurse Carol Williams), Molli Benson (Nurse Gail), Johnny Hartman (ambulance attendant), Jackie Russell (Mrs. Bond), James Beach (Police Officer Charles), Don Pulford (police officer)

Synopsis

Johnny is irritated by other people's bad driving habits and comes up with some interesting ideas. Roy and Johnny are teaching a CPR class to a group of women and are notified that their former paramedic instructor has died. A boy gets stuck inside a tree looking for an owl, and Squad 51 responds with Station 69. A star quarterback (Vic Mohica) collapses for unknown reasons. The station responds to a night call that turns out to be a dumpster fire and then responds to a hotel fire where a man is suffering from a heart attack.

Notes

Battalion Chief Jim Page, the LACoFD technical consultant for the first two seasons, wrote the script under the pseudonym of Jim Owens. Station 69 (the real station of engineer Mike Stoker) is toned out to respond "Engine 69 and Patrol 69" to the medical aid on the trapped boy in the tree.

Locations

The hotel fire was filmed on Universal studio streets and Soundstage 8.

"School Days"

> Episode #2.14
>
> Production #35703
>
> Final revision: July 13, 1972
>
> Airdate: January 13, 1973
>
> Writer: Kenneth Dorward (revisions by Robert Cinader)
>
> Director: Christian I. Nyby II
>
> LACoFD Technical Advisor: Michael Stearns (PM0011)
>
> Guest cast: Kip Niven, Ian Wolfe, Michael James Wixted, Ann Doran, Sandy deBruin

Synopsis

A new trainee (Kip Niven) appears to be lacking in confidence and is assigned to Squad 51. An elderly gentleman (Ian Wolfe) is trapped under a bookcase, a car hits an ambulance, a boy is injured by a chemistry experiment, and a man is trapped and injured at an auto salvage yard.

Notes

Firefighter/paramedic Michael Stearns was promoted to Captain shortly after working on this episode.

"The Professor"

Episode #2.15

Production #35721

Final revision: November 10, 1972

Filming began: November 28, 1972

Airdate: February 3, 1973

Writer: Michael Donovan

Director: Christian I. Nyby II

LACoFD Technical Advisor: Unknown

Guest cast: Hedley Mattingly (British official), Christopher Cain (Robert Bentley), Paul Picerni (Secret Service agent), Jane Merrow, Timothy Callahan (pilot), Frank Maxwell (Captain of Engine 113), Alma Lawton (English maid), Joan Pringle (pregnant mom)

Synopsis

A British official (Hedley Mattingly) shows signs of psychotic behavior for no apparent reason, and the Secret Service agent (Paul Picerni) won't give any clues. Roy has an admirer, yet Johnny accuses him of having no charisma. A man (Christopher Cain) is rescued while threatening to jump off a building. The medics deliver a premature baby. Johnny and Roy join Fireboat 110 and assist with a downed plane.

Notes

LA County Sheriff Department substation in Marina Del Rey again (as in season 1) substitutes for Fire Station 110, which are literally about $1^1/2$ miles apart. Johnny and Roy do pickup Boat 110, but at the Sheriff's dock.

Boat 110 has a jet propulsion unit mated to a Ford racing engine, which gave the vessel its distinctive growl sound. This particular boat, as Boat 110, has been retired and replaced at least three times since filming.

Current Boat 110 is nicknamed, "Blue Water Rescue." The boat was designed by Jensen Marine Consultants and was built by Kvichak Marine Industries in Seattle, Washington. The 38-foot boat is equipped with a 2400 gpm pump, 50-gallon foam tank, and a Stang fire monitor that can provide up to 1000 gpm of water flow. This is the same company that recently delivered fireboats to LAFD. Boat 110 is painted the same color scheme as the Helicopter fleet.

Locations

The Hi-Rise building used in this episode (the jumper) is in Glendale, California. It was built as the Glendale Center and is the now the Bank of America Building at 611 N. Brand Boulevard at State 134 Freeway, just east of Interstate 5.

The jetty where the plane crashes, visible from Station 110, is at the outlet of Ballona Creek separating Marina del Rey and Playa del Rey.

"Syndrome"

Episode #2.16

Production #35719

Final revision: November 9, 1972

Airdate: February 10, 1973

Writer: Michael Donovan (revisions by Robert Cinader)

Director: Dennis Donnelly

LACoFD Technical Advisor: Richard Neal (PM0009)

Guest cast: Jack Carter (Sy Kliner) Dub Taylor (old man at gas depot), Vince Howard, Ezra Stone (Boris Miller), Art Balinger (Battalion 14), Michael Morgan and Perry Castellano (boys on gas tank), Casey MacDonald (Janie), Barbara Brownell (Sandy), Kres Mersky (Gloria), Ta-Tanisha (Rosie)

Special Guest star: Robert Alda as Raymond Boyd

Synopsis

Johnny tries to convince Roy that he has tonsillitis, but Roy claims that his tonsils were removed when he was 5 years old. An actor at Mammoth Studios (Robert Alda), who is an old flame of Dixie's, is admitted to Rampart with chest pains. Two kids are trapped on top of a gas tank. Boot has a tick removed. Dr. Early treats a hypochondriac. A girl's college field hockey game turns violent. Station 51 responds to assist at a fire at Olive View Hospital, which has been abandoned since an earthquake the previous year. While entering an opening surrounded by rubble to rescue two suspected arsonists, Chet is trapped in shifting rubble and breaks his shoulder. Both Chet and Roy (who has his tonsils removed) room together at Rampart.

Notes

The Kennedy Probe is used in this episode (see "Botulism," episode 1.2). In the original script (see "Richter Six" in Chapter 13), the fire department responded to the hospital as if the earthquake had just happened. However, after scouting the area and noticing weeds several feet high, they revised the script. In the final script, the hospital was called Vallecito Hospital; it was changed to Olive Hill during voiceover taping.

Locations

The Mammoth Studios gates are actually the gates to Universal. The hospital establishing and interior scenes were filmed on location at Olive View Hospital and Sanitarium, 14701 Foothill Boulevard in Sylmar. Based on a true incident, Olive View was destroyed during the Sylmar Earthquake a year earlier on February 9, 1971. A year and a half later, Olive View, vacant and in shambles, was used for filming for the exterior and some interior scenes because rubble from the earthquake collapse for the filming crew to use was still present. The director advised that the building had shifted a good foot and a half, making the whole area tilted. The hospital, completed only months earlier in 1970, was ultimately demolished. It was rebuilt as Olive View-UCLA Medical Center and is now located at 14445 Olive View Drive, not far from the original location.

"Honest"

Episode #2.17

Production #35722

Final revision: December 15, 1972

Airdate: February 17, 1973

Writer: Daryl Henry

Director: Christian I. Nyby II

LACoFD Technical Advisor: Alfred Knight (PM0036)

Guest cast: Michael Lerner (newlywed male), Ann Whitfield (mother), Cheryl Lynn Miller, Beverly Saunders (newlywed female), Doug Rowe, Heidi Wynn, Vincent Perry, Vince Howard, Scott Gourlay (injured police officer)

Synopsis

Roy and Johnny argue over whether the truth should always be told; Johnny argues that one should be truthful regardless of the consequences, but Roy contends that the truth sometimes hurts. A young man attempts a high dive off a roof into a pool and misses. A newlywed couple (Michael Lerner and Beverly Sanders) is involved in a gas explosion. An elderly man concealing the fact that he is blind rescues his infant grandson who is trapped in a burning house; Station 9 assists. A boy with conflicting symptoms is brought into Rampart. The boy's mother (Ann Whitfield) does not tell the truth and withholds information from the doctors.

Notes
The real Squad 209 appears in this episode—it is the red van off to the right as the ambulance enters the hospital tunnel followed by Squad 51. Squad 51's radio announces "Squad 209, 10-7 to St. Francis" even though they are at Rampart. Stuntman Angelo De Meo appears as Johnny in this episode and takes the fall for him off the stairs.

Michael Lerner appeared as a newspaper reporter in the 1973 TV Movie *Firehouse* starring Richard Roundtree and Vince Edwards.

"Séance"

Episode #2.18

Production #35720

Final revision: November 12, 1972

Filming dates: December 7–14, 1972

Airdate: February 24, 1973

Writer: Preston Wood

Director: Georg Fenady

LACoFD Technical Advisor: Robert Forsythe (PM0034)

Guest cast: Charles Aidman (Harry Teal), Fintan Meyler (Dorothy Teal), Bruce Kirby, Jr., Suzanne Charny, Laurie Brighton, William Bryant (Captain, Squad 110), Angelo De Meo

Synopsis
The squad responds to a series of unusual emergencies after treating an injured woman at a séance. They respond to several calls at a house, where the wife (Fintan Meyler) is convinced that the bad things happening to her husband (Charles Aidman) are the result of her recently deceased sister who has come back to haunt them. An over-tranquilized teenager is brought to Rampart. The station rescues a man trapped and injured in a warehouse. A man is trapped under water (stuntman Angelo De Meo) in his car, and Johnny and Roy rescue him using the Jaws of Life.

Notes
Twenty-five stock footage shots of the squad were utilized in this episode: leaving the station, driving Code R, non Code R, tight shots inside the cab, the squad alone, the quad followed by an engine, etc.

The car-under-water sequences used the actual Engine 110, Boat 110, and Harbor Patrol boat. Five butane heaters were on site to warm up the cast and crew from being in the cold water, and stunt doubles were utilized for Johnny and Roy for some of the underwater scenes.

Locations
The warehouse sequences were filmed at Universal's Mill, just off New York Street. The séance house was on Colonial Street, and the interiors were filmed on Soundstage 6. The car rescue scenes were filmed at Marina Del Rey and in an underwater tank at Universal.

"Boot"

Working title: Duke

Episode #2.19

Production #35718

Final revision: October 20, 1972

Filming dates: November 7–14, 1972

Airdate: March 3, 1973

Writer: Preston Wood

Director: Christian I. Nyby II

LACoFD Technical Advisor: William Ridgeway (PM0010)

Guest cast: Vic Tayback (truck driver), Ann Prentiss (Fran), Zack Taylor, Susan Madigan, Jamie Farr* (not credited), Jock Mahoney

Synopsis
The station becomes concerned when Boot becomes listless and refuses to eat. They rescue a young woman whose sports car is pinned under a gasoline truck. A woman (Ann Prentiss) becomes the victim of multiple culinary disasters and requires Johnny and Roy's assistance. Dr. Early lifts a curse. There is an explosion and fire in a lab building at Rampart.

Notes
This episode was originally scheduled to air on January 27, 1973, but was preempted by news coverage of the Vietnam ceasefire. The episode title and the name of the mascot were originally "Duke," but this was rewritten after the dog was named Boot in an earlier episode.

Jamie Farr appears in this episode but is not credited. He was credited in episode 2.12, but did not appear.

Harold Frizzell was used for fire stunts. Doubles were used for Gage and Desoto. Johnny drove the squad in this episode.

Locations

The tanker/car accident was filmed at 13201 Sepulveda Boulevard and Old San Fernando Road in Sylmar. Some scenes were filmed at a newsstand where Gage buys a book on dogs. The newsstand was located at 10133 Riverside Drive in North Hollywood (Toluca Lake). This shooting did not make final cut.

Exteriors for Fran's apartment, the cook with multiple cooking disasters, were filmed at what was formerly known as "Bristol Court" on the Universal lot; a working apartment and bungalow complex with a pool area were used for multiple television and film projects. "Bristol Court" will again be used in episode 6.9.

Located on the grounds of Harbor General, Building K8 was utilized for some of the "lab" fire scenes. The 'K' buildings were technically not in the "line of sight" from Rampart's Coffee Room as observed by Dixie and Dr. Morton. Only the 'B' and 'D' buildings would have been. The 'K' building huts on the west end of South Drive were going to be torn down, and an opportunity was there for the special effects crew. Today there are no 'K' buildings listed because they have all been since demolished for a parking lot (near Research Park Drive and South Drive).

Jack Webb, although not involved in the daily production of the series, was on the set for the fire stunt at "Rampart." Other "lab" fire scenes were filmed behind Universal's New York Street near the Mill.

"Rip-Off"

Episode #2.20

Production #35723

Airdate: March 10, 1973

Writer: Michael Donovan

Director: Christian I. Nyby II

LACoFD Technical Advisor: Unknown

Guest cast: Regis Cordic, Maria-Elena Cordero (pregnant woman), Charles McGraw, Morgan Paul (Pauli), Harry Townes, Buddy Lester, Art Gilmore (battalion chief), Vince Howard, Iris Korn, Borah Silver (Sergeant Sommers), Charles Lampkin (airport employee)

Synopsis

Roy and Johnny are accused of stealing $500 from a heart attack victim's (Regis Cordic) wallet. The station rescues a pilot and co-pilot from a plane leaking liquid oxygen. A pregnant woman (Maria-Elena Cordero) and her husband (Morgan Paul) are involved in a car accident; Johnny and Roy deliver their baby.

Notes

Jo Anne Worley filmed a segment for this episode that later appeared in "Zero" (episode 3.10). Stock footage (filmed before the first season began) showing the Crown leaving station and heading to the airport does not have López or Donnelly in the jumpseats.

"Audit"

Working title: Advice

Episode #2.21

Production #35725

Final revision: December 29, 1972

Filming dates: January 25–February 1, 1973

Airdate: April 7, 1973

Writer: Preston Wood (revisions by Robert Cinader)

Director: Georg Fenady

LACoFD Technical Advisor: Thomas Douglas (PM0032)

Guest cast: James McEachin (construction worker), Kathy Cannon (pregnant woman), Robert Porter, Ray Ballard (con man), Ross Elliott, Kathleen King, Karen Philipp (Nurse), Mina Vasquez (student nurse)

Synopsis

Johnny is audited by the Internal Revenue Service. A professional medical con man (Ray Ballard) with two names shows up at Rampart. Dr. Brackett treats a pregnant woman (Kathy Cannon) with a heart defect. A man hit on the head wants to be treated by doctors and not by paramedics. A child is rescued from a locked car. The station struggles to free a construction worker (James McEachin), who is trapped and injured during a building collapse and wants Roy to amputate his leg before the rest of the building falls. He has a metal rod through his leg with 60 tons of rubble threatening to bury them both.

Notes

James McEachin appears in three other *Emergency!* episodes as Police Lieutenant Roy Crockett. Several stock footage scenes were used, including nine of the squad, two of the station, and two of the ambulance.

Locations

The child locked car in the car, filmed at the Lakeside Shopping Center at W. Oak Street and N. Pass Avenue in Burbank, just north of the Ventura Freeway (I-134), was filmed the first day of shooting.

SEASON 3

"Frequency"

> Episode #3.1
>
> Production #37401
>
> Final revision: January 3, 1973
>
> Airdate: September 22, 1973
>
> Writer: Kenneth Dorward
>
> Director: Dennis Donnelly
>
> LACoFD Technical Advisor: Michael Lewis (PM0037)
>
> Guest cast: Ron Kelly (Officer Drew Burke), Linda Kelsey (Pam Burke), Pamela McMyler, John Dennis, Cedric Wolfe, Ron Townsend, Mike Lane (biker), Karen Philipp (nurse), Heidi Wynn (Nurse Jeanette)

Synopsis

Four paramedic units have to share the same frequency for broadcasts to Rampart. It all comes to a head when all four units have incidents at the same time. Johnny and Roy respond to a call where a policeman (Ron Kelly), a friend of Johnny's, has been hit by a car. He is seriously injured and they are unable to make contact with Rampart. A man is trapped in a futuristic sculpture that he created. A man and his son are injured at a construction site. A biker gang rumble overloads the hospital staff at Rampart; Roy and Johnny help out. Johnny must deal with the death of his friend, the police officer.

Notes

In this episode, Johnny and Roy are working the B shift and not their usual A shift. Two different Crowns are used in this episode—the one leaving the station (Universal's Engine 60, as does 127's) has the distinctive gumball light on the windshield, while the Crown at the construction site has a forward-facing red light with mechanical siren on the windshield.

Technical Advisor Mike Lewis recalls,

> Frequency was one where I as TA was able to take a stand on one of the bit characters. In the show there was a meeting called of paramedics to discuss radio use when things were busy

and there were not enough radio frequencies for all the squads to work. When the actors were on set, there was a young man as a paramedic that had a very large Afro hairstyle and was way out of line for the dress code of the fire department. I told the director he would have to replace him, that it would not do. This actor was not real happy with the decision but was replaced.

Mike also worked on episodes 3.14 and 4.16.

Regarding the biker scene in the hospital, the director Dennis Donnelly recalls:

> The injured, from a motorcycle gang fight, all arrive at Rampart at the same time. One of the bikers is in the hospital corridor and spots an enemy on the table in the treatment room, he charges in to 'kill him.' The biker, played by Mike Lane, also played the 6' 6," 300 pound fighter in The Harder They Fall starring Humphrey Bogart. In staging the scene, Mike came up with the idea, "I'll charge in and go for his throat and you six guys try and stop me." The six guys are the two doctors, two orderlies, and two police officers who wrestled him to the ground breaking every piece of break-away furniture that was supposed to be broken. We used three cameras and printed on Take 1.

Dennis further stated that, "The hospital scenes from this episode made this my most difficult shooting day of all the shows I did, aside from weather and logistic problems." Dennis also stated that this was his favorite episode to direct because it had a very emotional scene with Gage informing his best friend's wife that her husband had died on the operating table after being hit by a car during a traffic stop on the freeway.

"The Old Engine"

Episode #3.2

Production #37402

Spec. run: March 2, 1973; revised May 24, 1973

Filming dates: July 6–13, 1973

Airdate: September 29, 1973

Writer: Preston Wood

Director: Christian I. Nyby II

LACoFD Technical Advisor: Harold Aronson

Guest cast: Ross Elliott, Michael Conrad, Laurette Spang, Regina Parton, Ann Doran, Raymond Man, Lorraine Baptist

Synopsis

Roy and Johnny buy an old rundown British fire engine (a 1932 Dennis) from a junkyard for $80. Station 51 gets a new engine, replacing the 1965 Crown.

Johnny and Roy ride on the tailboard. A woman overdoses on LSD, leading the two paramedics on a chase to the top of a building. Dr. Brackett treats a resilient gunshot victim. A politician suffers a heart attack, and the station responds to a warehouse fire where they rescue a firefighter who fell through the roof. Rampart gets a new look to the base station, including a cassette tape recorder and radio for transmissions by the fire department dispatcher.

Notes

Again in this episode, Johnny and Roy are on B shift instead of their usual A shift.

The episode title has nothing to do with the arrival of the Ward LaFrance as Engine 51 and the "retiring" of the Old 1965 Crown. The script, as written and titled, has to do with the Old British engine Johnny and Roy purchased and the script was written and titled prior to the arrival of the Ward. There were revisions to the script with the arrival of the Ward, and the cut scenes would appear in future episodes.

"Alley Cat"

Episode #3.3

Production #37407

Airdate: October 6, 1973

Writer: Charlene Sukins

Director: Alan Crosland

LACoFD Technical Advisor: Unknown

Guest cast: Brooke Bundy (mother), Sarah Brown (daughter), Virginia Gregg (actress), Lee Bergere, Nelson Olmstead, William Challee, George Ives, X Brands (Engine 81 Captain), Shirley O'Hara

Synopsis

A stray cat has kittens on Johnny's bed at the station. A family of three is trapped in a downed airplane, and Dixie must tell the daughter (Sarah Brown) that her father has died while Early and Brackett try to save the mother (Brooke Bundy). An old man gets his foot caught in a bear trap. A school develops a natural gas leak that renders a boy unconscious. Roy and Johnny rescue a man involved in a boating accident. The hospital treats an actress (Virginia Gregg) with a bruised ego.

Locations

The boating incident was filmed at the Castaic Lake Recreation Area in the Angeles National Forest, Castaic, California.

An English Visitor

Episode #3.4

Production #37416

Final revision: July 13, 1973

Filming began: August 6, 1973 (5th episode of the season filmed)

Airdate: October 13, 1973

Writer: Michael Donovan

Director: Alan Crosland

LACoFD Technical Advisor: William Hoke

Guest cast: Jamie Ross (Jason Channing), Lucille Benson (Martha), Craig Curtis, Judi Meredith (Nurse Sheila), Stanley Kamel (Harry Rivers), Mira L. Waters (Patsy), Barbara Boles (Shirley), Jack Bailey (Homer), Art Balinger (battalion chief)

Synopsis

A firefighter (34-year-old Jamie Ross) visiting from Coventry, England, pays a visit to Station 51 to observe American firefighter/paramedics in action and ends up saving Johnny's life. Rescues include a policeman who is badly burned by a Molotov cocktail and trapped in an elevator, a car accident and fire with intoxicating smoke, the wife (Lucile Benson) of a former sharp-shooter (Jack Bailey) with a gunshot wound, and a man trapped in heavy machinery. Dr. Brackett treats a singer (Mira L. Waters) in a diabetic coma with no help from her manager. The staff at Rampart deals with a defiant nurse (Judi Meredith).

Notes

An unidentified actor portrays PIO Dick Friend (the same one who played him in "Show Biz," episode 2.3, and "Women!," episode 2.9). Jamie Ross, who portrays the British firefighter from Coventry, was actually born in Scotland.

England's first paramedics came about in 1970 in the ambulance service. They were called "Miller trainer" (IV trained). Governed by the National Association of Private Ambulance Service, they have extended training in intubation and infusion, manual defibrillation, drug admininstration, and they can do chest needle decompression. In England, paramedics act totally independent of any hospital and have no direct (radio or cell phone) communication with a doctor, unless one arrives in a helicopter via Helicopter Emergency Medical Service in the London area or other Air Ambulance providers. Although Paramedics are trained to carry out a number of interventions, they are permitted to do so only "in an emergency" or "when assisting a doctor" and not as a matter of routine.

The English Fire Services are controlled by the department of the Deputy Prime Minister and, despite many attempts, there are no paramedic services within the Fire Service. Health organizations such as hospitals, doctors, and ambulance services are controlled by the National Health Service (NHS) and are two very different organizations. Only the NHS qualifies paramedics in England, and the title is strictly controlled.

Ambulance services in England have just been regionalized; every county or metropolitan area had its own independent service, and now many of the counties have merged. For example, in Sussex, which is located in the south of England, there was the Sussex Ambulance Service, but they have merged with Surrey and Kent to become the South East Coast Ambulance Service.

Community First Responders (CFRs) have also been established in England and are volunteers formed into local self-supporting groups to provide additional cover to areas where the regular ambulance service may experience delays. In England, ambulance response times for some areas can be up to twenty minutes. Because early defibrillation is the key to survivability following an arrest, the time delays are unacceptable. Therefore, CFRs are used. They are trained by the ambulance service and are equipped jointly by the Ambulance service and charity funding (British Heart Foundation).

CFRs are "toned-out" by cell phone and respond in their personal vehicles. Training is to First Person On Scene standard where the whole purpose is to provide early defibrillation and quality cardiopulmonary resuscitation (CPR). They respond to all emergencies except traffic accidents, disturbances, and police involvement.

With over 30,000 members in over 40 countries worldwide, the completely volunteer St. John Ambulance is strictly a nonparamedic "First Aid" provider, although they are trained in the use of semi-automatic defibrillators. They provide first aid, training, sales, and equipment and are England's leading first aid, transport, and care charity. Every town in England has a St. John ambulance division, at least two ambulances fully equipped, and most with a membership of about 20–30 people. They have a separate nurse section and an aero-med section with several of their own fixed-wing aircraft.

Locations

The heavy machinery rescue took place in a gravel pit in Monrovia, about 50 miles northeast of Station 51.

CHAPTE

EMERGEN

180

Synopsis
While
con

"Heavyweight"

Episode #3.5

Production #37405

Final revision: June 3, 1973

Airdate: October 20, 1973

Writer: Kenneth Dorward

Director: Dennis Donnelly

LACoFD Technical Advisor: Roscoe "Rocky" Doke (PM0008)

Guest cast: Barbara Sigel, Dennis Redfield, Pamela Peters, Sean Kelly, Rebecca Gibbs, Wayne Heffley

Synopsis

When Johnny pulls a muscle during a fire, he is teased about being out of shape. Roy and Johnny are trapped between battling neighbors. A young wife and mother (Barbara Sigel) is sure she is cursed when a series of bad things happen to her and her husband (Dennis Redfield). Johnny rescues an injured hang glider from a tree. Two men are injured in a fight, and their children want to finish what their fathers started. A boy is brought into Rampart after being electrocuted by a TV set.

Notes

Note that several instances of fireground file footage from the *Emergency!* World Premier movie were utilized in this episode.

"Snake Bite"

Episode #3.6

Production #37410

Final revision: June 6, 1973

Filming dates: July 26–August 2, 1973 (4th episode filmed of the season)

Airdate: October 27, 1973

Writer: Carroll Christensen

Director: Georg Fenady

LACoFD Technical Advisor: Tom Douglas (PM0032)

Guest cast: Richard X. Slattery (Hector), Reta Shaw (Nurse Ozella Peterson), Johnnie Collins III (Jake), William Bryant (Captain, Engine 85), Tony Haig (Dr Frick), Laurie Brighton (Karen), Don Carter (ambulance attendant), Jill Chandler (Joyce Varner), Sarah Frankboner (Joy)

returning from a fishing trip out of state, Roy, Johnny, and Chet ...e across seriously injured auto crash victims in a desolate area where ...nly a local doctor can authorize treatment. The station responds to a car of joyriding teenagers off the side of the road, and Johnny is bitten by a rattlesnake.

Notes

Special Note: During one of the many brainstorming sessions with Jim, I inquired about the writer of this particular episode because no one knew who he was. Jim sat back, chuckled a bit, and proceeded to tell me that due to the writers strike earlier in 1973 the "real" writer of this episode who was a Writers Guild member could not submit any scripts. The credited writer is actually Jim Page's daughter, Carolyn Christensen (not a Guild member), who used an altered first name and her married name to submit Jim's script.

The character name of Nurse Ozella Peterson is actually the name of Jim Page's aunt.

Character actor Richard X. Slattery, born in the Bronx and a 12-year veteran of the NYPD, is the bulldozer operator, LA County Tractor 2, a D-9 Caterpillar. He often portrayed a police officer in his roles on TV and film. Perhaps more recognized by viewers in the West as "Murph," the service station owner and spokesperson for an oil company known as Union 76. The new kid at the service station in the commercials was Larry Wilcox, who would later become Officer Jon Baker in 'CHiP's'.

The rattlesnake that bites Johnny is real. Although defanged, it had to be pulled off Mantooth's pants leg while filming. Robert Cinader advised the use of a rubber snake, but Ed Self went over Cinader's head to authorize using a real snake. In the original script, Chet was bitten by the snake.

LA County Copter 14 (a Bell 204-205/UH1 Huey/Iroquois) makes its first of several appearances on *Emergency!*. Randy Mantooth's own Land Cruiser also makes a guest appearance, with a California State Firefighters' Asssociation sticker on the front windshield.

This is the infamous episode with Captain Stanley and the backward mike.

"The Promotion"

Episode #3.7

Production #37413

Final revision: August 3, 1973

Filming began: August 24, 1973

Airdate: November 3, 1973
Writer: Preston Wood
Director: Christian I. Nyby II
LACoFD Technical Advisor: Harold Aronson
Guest cast: Tom Simcox, Michael Maitland

Synopsis

Roy passes the Engineer's test (scoring 9th on the written portion), but accepting the promotion would mean leaving the paramedics. A heavily fogbound freeway leads to a major traffic pileup during rush hour on the San Diego Freeway. While responding to an apparent suicide, Roy takes an unexpected swim in a backyard pool. Roy bails out a window at a structure fire just as fire explodes and knocks him into Johnny's arms on the ladder. They both fall to the ground where, although Roy is shaken up, Johnny is injured and must be hospitalized.

Notes

The original episode that aired included a segment with Roy walking alongside the engine, looking at the pump controls, getting into Mike Stoker's seat, and looking back at the squad. This important scene of Roy's consternation was cut in syndication.

Locations

The San Diego Freeway, otherwise known as 'Interstate 405' is visible in scenes shot on location out the back of Station 127.

The fog segment was filmed at the General Service Studios (old RKO Studios) (at Santa Monica Boulevard, and the corner of Las Palmas), later the Desilu Studios and now a part of Paramount Studios. Initial establishing freeway shots were taken in Glendale.

The scenes of the structure fire where Roy and Johnny are injured were filmed on the first day of shooting at the (unused) Hollenbeck Jail in Boyle Heights, East Los Angeles. Stunt doubles were used for Johnny and Roy. It was near the site of old LAFD station 2. They took down 2's a few years ago and just about everything on the block when they did expansions to Hollenbeck Division.

"Insomnia"

Episode #3.8
Production #37417
Final revision: August 6, 1973

Filming began: August 15, 1973

Airdate: November 10, 1973

Writer: Robert Hammer

Director: Dennis Donnelly

LACoFD Technical Advisor: Unknown

Guest cast: Ronnie Schell, Craig Chudy (marijuana victim), Dick Yarmy (truck driver), Hal Lynch, Stephen Manley (truck driver's son), Lee Farr, Joe Pizzorusso, Ron Burke (truck driver), Jim Nolan

Synopsis

Johnny's obsession about the lack of night runs leads to insomnia, which he and the station crew try to cure in various ways. A boat being trucked to the marina explodes. A truck driver (Dick Yarmy) and his son (Stephen Manley) are injured when the truck they are riding in swerves to avoid hitting a dog. A father and son are trapped in a gravel pit. A truck driver (Ron Burke) is pinned by his semi-truck. A friend (Ronnie Schell) brings a man (Craig Chudy) into Rampart in critical condition, and doctors race against time to save him after he smoked some marijuana.

Notes

Joe Bartak (Technical Advisor for episode 5.20) served as Randy's stunt double, riding the tail board in this segment filmed at Station 43. He further states, "I stood in for Randy in this episode where they filmed him riding the tail board, half dressed and half asleep. In the shot, only seen from the rear, it was really me. It was actually filmed at Station 43 in the City of Industry. I do remember them buying In-N-Out Burgers for everyone that night, now why would that stick in my mind? Almost everyone at 43's where I worked was in an episode at one time or another as an extra."

Stephen Manley also appeared in the *Sierra* crossover, "Urban Ranger," with Kevin Tighe and Randy Mantooth.

"Inheritance Tax"

Working titles: Inheritance and Money

Episode #3.9

Production #37421

Final revision: September 17, 1973

Filming began: September 19, 1973

Airdate: November 17, 1973

Writer: Arnold Somkin

Director: Dennis Donnelly

LACoFD Technical Advisor: Robert McCullough PM0038

Guest cast: Warren Berlinger, Michael Fox, Marion Ross (stockbroker's secretary), Mike McHenry, Art Balinger (battalion chief)

Synopsis

An elderly woman Roy and Johnny treated the previous year dies and leaves them a million dollars in her will. A child is trapped in a car under downed power lines. A stockbroker (Warren Berlinger) with heart problems is reluctant to be treated. A teenager (Mike McHenry) becomes ill after eating nineteen hamburgers in a contest that he loses. Station 51 responds to a three-alarm paint factory fire and treats a burned victim.

Locations

The exteriors of the stockbroker's office were shot at Universal's Lew R. Wasserman building just inside the Main Street gate.

"Zero"

Episode #3.10

Production #37412

Final revision: October 29, 1973

Airdate: November 24, 1973

Writer: Brian Taggert

Director: Christian I. Nyby II

LACoFD Technical Advisor: Unknown

Guest cast: Mariette Hartley (Vera Mannerling), Anthony Eisley (Jake Mannerling), Bobby Elibacher (Tommy Mannerling), Jo Anne Worley, Dick Enberg (TV host), William Bryant (Captain, Truck 85), Dick Whittinghill (news reporter), Scott Gorlav (police officer), Jan Arvan (hotel manager)

Synopsis

The squad responds to an early-morning call where a woman is screaming. The woman (Jo Anne Worley) teaches Johnny and Roy how to relieve tension. Johnny finds it takes a different kind of courage to face television cameras when the paramedics are interviewed by Dick Enberg on the TV program *Men in Action;* Johnny freezes in front of the camera, and Roy must bail him out. Roy climbs Truck 85's 100-foot aerial ladder to prevent a boy (Bobby Elibacher) from jumping from the seventh-story ledge of a high-rise apartment building. When the boy is taken to Rampart, the doctors suspect that he may be an abused child. His parents (Anthony Eisley and Mariette Hartley) resent the idea. Johnny and Roy rescue a worker from a doughnut machine. After Johnny rescues a boy from a burning warehouse, he again freezes up on TV and Roy comes to his rescue.

Notes

The screaming woman segment was originally filmed for "Rip-Off" (episode 2.20). Jo Anne Worley was the wife of Roger Perry, who made several appearances on *Emergency!*.

Dick Whittinghill was a morning disc jockey, on Los Angeles, California radio station KMPC, 1950–1979. Webb, an avid KMPC listener, had Whittinghill appear in several of his MARK VII Productions.

Dick Enberg, popular sportscaster, became NBC's top NFL play-by-play announcer. He also worked for ESPN and hosted *NFL on NBC*. Currently, Enberg is doing the play-by-play for CBS.

Jan Arvin also appeared in *Rescue 8*. She made two other appearances in *Emergency!*, in episodes "Transition" and "The Parade," both in season 4.

Locations

The burning warehouse segment was filmed near the old Terminal Island Bridge.

The segment on the child rescue from the building ledge was filmed in Long Beach and was a former Motor Hotel. Look closely and you will see the Queen Mary across the harbor. In 1982, the dilapidated and unused building, now with a fence around it, was also used in Charles Bronson's *Death Wish II* as the scene of his first vigilante revenge shooting. The building, just south of the former Pike, has since been torn down.

"The Promise"

Episode #3.11

Production #37424

Airdate: December 1, 1973

Writer: Dee Murphy

Director: Alan Crosland

LACoFD Technical Advisor: Unknown

Guest cast: Kip Niven (Bo Jensen), Patricia Hindy (Paula Slayton), Patricia Mattick (Kathy), Reva Rose (Edna Self), Russell Thorson (George Burke), Ted Gehring (Roy Nelson), Jean E. London (Nurse Anne), Hal K. Dawson, Fred Brookfield (Richard Allen), Gail Bonney (Martha)

Synopsis

Paula Slayton, who owned the dog that Johnny cared for in "Mascot" (episode 1.1), returns to keep her promise and presents Johnny with a puppy. Because Johnny lives in an apartment that doesn't allow dogs, he gives the dog to Edna Self, who is soon bitten by the dog. At the scene of a vehicle fire, a catatonic mechanic (Fred Brookfield) is brought to Rampart after his friend (Kip Niven) gives him a shot of heroin; he must later be rescued from a sixth-story ledge by Johnny and Roy. A young woman mixes bleach and ammonia and suffers from the resulting poison fumes. An elderly couple is trapped in their house by tumbleweeds.

Notes

The character "Paula Slayton" that appeared in "Mascot" (episode 1.1), was portrayed by Patricia McAneny.

Note Reva Rose's character name of Edna Self. Edwin Self is the Series Producer.

"Body Language"

Episode #3.12

Production #37418

Final revision: September 10, 1973

Filming dates: October 18–25, 1973

Airdate: December 8, 1973

Writer: Arthur Weiss

Director: Dennis Donnelly

LACoFD Technical Advisor: Frank Reavis

Guest cast: Ronald Feinberg (Donald Lompoc), Ronne Troup (Pam), Randy Boone (Bill Stagg), Kenneth Tobey (Doug Barton), Bill Williams (Pete), Frank Bonner, Julie Rogers (Betty Hall), Hank Jones (Stan Wilson), Joe Danova, Michael Campbell (Charlie Dent), Mary Angela Shea (nurse), Vince Howard (police officer), Scott Gourlay (police officer), Joshua Albee (youngster), Michael Morgan (youngster), Dick Berk (Archie Williams)

Synopsis

Johnny's girlfriend thinks that he proposed. A crop duster (Bill Williams) flying a Stearman (open cockpit bi-plane) makes a rough landing in a field and suffers a punctured lung; a bystander (Frank Bonner) is poisoned by the pesticides. A patient reports to Rampart with an ear infection caused by mothballs. A teenage couple hallucinates at Observation Park after eating daffodil bulbs. A weekend cowboy (Randy Boone) suffers a fractured skull and refuses treatment. Two drivers (Julie Rogers and Hank Jones) who are involved in an accident become friends. A rock band (The Delirium Three-men) goes over the edge, and one of its members suffers a heart attack.

Notes
The fictitious Mayfair Ambulance Company modular ambulance vehicle first appears. Frank Bonner later became Herb Tarlick on *WKRP in Cincinnati*. Bobby Troop and Julie London's daughter Ronne appears as a daffodil eater.

"Understanding"

Episode #3.13

Production #37425

Final revision: October 10, 1973

Airdate: December 15, 1973

Writer: Preston Wood

Director: Georg Fenady

LACoFD Technical Advisor: James Brewer

Guest cast: Phillip Pine, Kathleen Quinlin, Jock Mahoney (stable manager), John Russell, Benye Gatteys, Michael Vandever (bank robber), Mills Watson (bank robber), James Griffith, Robert Patten (police captain), Ray Fine, Anne Whitfield

Synopsis
Johnny and Roy treat a hostage with chest pains at the scene of a bank robbery and then become hostages themselves. A girl's (Kathleen Quinlin) horse is trapped in a burning barn. Johnny gives Chet his guitar. A man keeps forgetting his insulin shots. A girl (Anne Whitfield) calls the hospital, threatening suicide.

"Computer Error"

Working title: Checkmate

Episode #3.14

Production #37415

Airdate: December 22, 1973

Writer: John Groves

Director: Joel Oliansky

LACoFD Technical Advisor: Michael Lewis (PM0037)

Guest cast: Bonnie Bartlett, Mark Miller, Tani Phelps Guthrie, Audrey Landers, Joyce Jameson, Larry Storch, Don Most (Fred Wilson), Ellen Clark, Bing Russell, Hal Frizzell, Scott Gourlay (police officer)

Synopsis

After a dinner date, Johnny is overcharged on his bill and tries to get the mistake corrected. A young couple is rescued from a car accident, and the girl (Audrey Landers) may be pregnant. At Rampart, Carl Wilson (Bing Russell) tends to his son (Don Most) who was paralyzed in a car crash. Roy and Johnny respond to a call to rescue a pseudo-magician (Larry Storch) after he accidentally locks himself inside his safe. A woman (Tani Guthrie) is trapped in an abandoned well. Marco is injured at a hazardous junkyard fire due to phosphorus materials stored there.

Notes

Bing Russell is the father of actor Kurt Russell. Don Most (later Ralph on *Happy Days*) makes his first television appearance. This episode uses first season stock footage of the squad leaving the station—the Crown engine is still in the bay and Jim Page's car is visible across the street. During the crash scene, the radio announces, "Squad 59 cancel your response."

Technical Advisor Mike Lewis recalls;

> It took about eight days to shoot one show, the studio paid us about $1,000 for our time (up from the $300 the TAs first received). Jack Webb signed the first check I received, which looked like play money. His signature, as well as the rest of the writing, was all in different colors. The bank questioned the check and it took some time to cash it. They also filled our spot at the station while we were doing the shows. On the books the time was carried as a time exchange that we did not have to pay back.

"Messin' Around"

Episode #3.15

Production #37422

Airdate: January 12, 1974

Writer: Dennis Landa

Director: Richard Newton

LACoFD Technical Advisor: Clyde Cotner

Guest cast: J. Pat O'Malley, Ann Prentiss (Cindy's mother), Karl Swenson (Gus), Carol Lawson (Mrs. Wheeler), Joan Shawlee, Paul Bryer, Vince Howard, Tammy Harrington (Cindy), Paul Sorenson (Mike), Lance Kerwin

Synopsis

Johnny is besieged by the station's practical joker (Chet) playing 'The Phantom'. A child (Tammy Harrington) is trapped in a burning treehouse. A bulldozer drives off a cliff and lands on top of a garbage truck, injuring three men. A lovable old hypochondriac (J. Pat O'Malley) has a real illness for a change. The owner of a gas station has stomach problems. A man is speechless after his wife (Joan Shawlee) gives him sap from her houseplant. Roy and Johnny need help to treat a child (Lance Kerwin) who has swallowed ant poison.

Notes

Paul Sorenson is best known for his role of Andy Bradley in *Dallas*.

"Fools"

Episode #3.16

Production #37423

Final revision: December 7, 1973

Filming began: December 7, 1973

Airdate: January 19, 1974

Writer: Eric Kaldor

Director: Joseph Pevney

LACoFD Technical Advisor: Richard Neal (PM0009)

Guest cast: Bobby Sherman, Dennis Patrick (Dr. Kent Donaldson, Sr.), Carol Arthur, William Campbell, John Harmon

Synopsis

A new intern (Bobby Sherman) at Rampart who lacks compassion for people and trust in the paramedic program nearly makes a mistake. Brackett has him do a ride-along with the squad. A man is injured when his chimney explodes. A woman (Carol Arthur) gets her hand stuck in a mailbox. Johnny and Roy must rescue a man suffering from a heart attack who is trapped in a burning oil refinery tower.

Notes

The 1960s and 1970s teen heartthrob Bobby Sherman portrays the new intern. A qualified paramedic, Sherman joined the Los Angeles Police Department (LAPD) in 1988, attaining the rank of Captain where he taught CPR and life-saving techniques to incoming academy recruits. In 1999, Sherman joined the San Bernardino County Sheriff's Department in the same capacity he held with the LAPD.

Carol Arthur is the wife of comedian Dom DeLuise.

Locations

The mailbox scene was filmed, not on Main Street as the street sign indicates (a studio prop), but at the intersection of Lankershim and Cahuenga Boulevard, just down the street from Universal. The Universal "Tower" (Building 1280), now known as the Lew R. Wasserman Building, is in the background and ironically enough, on Main Street and Lankershim. The bridge, long since rebuilt, is the US 101 Freeway. Lew R. Wasserman was Chairman of Universal Studios from 1946 when it was known as MCA, retiring in 1996.

"Green Thumb"

Working Title: How Green Was My Thumb

Episode #3.17

Production #37426

Airdate: January 26, 1974

Writer: John Groves

Director: Christian I. Nyby II

LACoFD Technical Advisor: Gerald Smith

Guest cast: Will Hutchins, Eric Shea, Don Chastain (hospital chaplain), Leigh Christian, William Wintersole, Helen Clark, Donald Mantooth (Squad 95 paramedic), Pamela Hensley, George P. Wallace, Kim Richards, Vince Howard, Jack Kosslyn

Synopsis

Roy takes care of an elderly widow's (Leigh Christian) plants while she is in the hospital. Roy and Johnny assist a man who has breathing problems. A young girl's religious father (Will Hutchins) prevents necessary treatment. The station responds to a fire in a winery. Dr. Brackett and the paramedics perform backyard surgery on a man with an unexploded grenade in his abdomen.

Notes

This is the first of two appearances by Randy Mantooth's brother Donald. The unexploded grenade scenario was most recently utilized in episode 2.16 (February 5, 2006) of the medical drama *Grey's Anatomy,* but in this case the outcome was not as disastrous.

"The Hard Hours"

Episode #3.18

Production #37414

Airdate: February 2, 1974

Writer: Arnold Somkin

Director: Christian I. Nyby II

LACoFD Technical Advisor: Steven Jongsma (PM0035)

Guest cast: Dick Butkus, Nick Nolte (ER technician), Eve Brent

Synopsis

Dr. Early is diagnosed with a heart condition and undergoes bypass surgery. A pro-football player #55, the 'Animal' (Dick Butkus) is embarrassed to admit that his son tackled him too hard. A boy builds a life-sized rocket fueled by dry ice. Roy rescues a woman whose toe is stuck in the bathtub faucet. The squad comes to the rescue of an electric worker when he comes in contact with a live power line.

Notes

Dick Butkus was a former linebacker for the Chicago Bears from 1965 to 1973 (jersey number 51). The original script called for Butkus to be struck by a car while sprinting into the street to retrieve a thrown ball. Four stuntmen appear as hospital orderlies and ambulance attendants: Scott Gourlay, George Orrison, Tom Rosales, and Harold Frizzell (see Chapter 11).

"The Floor Brigade"

Working title: Big Business

Episode #3.19

Production #37403

Filming began: December 28, 1973

Airdate: February 9, 1974

Writer: Roland Wolpert

Director: Dennis Donnelly

LACoFD Technical Advisor: Robert Belliveau (PM0001)

Guest cast: Pat Buttram, Christopher Man, Don Diamond, Ray Ballard (floor cleaner), Stephen Colt

Synopsis
Johnny and Roy think about going into the floor-cleaning business on the side. A hermit (Pat Buttram) is trapped in his cave home. Johnny sustains minor injuries on a rescue on top of a water tower. The station battles a chemical warehouse fire. Dr. Morton treats a diabetic singer trying to make a comeback.

"Propinquity"

Episode #3.20

Production: #37429 (first draft numbered as 37428, which had been previously assigned)

Final revision: January 3, 1974

Filming dates: January 9–16, 1974

Airdate: February 16, 1974

Writer: Preston Wood

Director: Georg Fenady

LACoFD Technical Advisor: Robert Forsythe (PM0034)

Guest cast: Brendan Boone (Wayne), George Orrison, Gil Peterson, Don Hanmer

Synopsis
Roy stays at Johnny's place while his house is being fumigated, and it's a little too much togetherness for Roy. A woman is trapped in a burning car. A car hits the ambulance carrying Roy and the patient from the vehicle fire. A man having a heart attack (Don Hanmer) refuses to leave a poker game unless Johnny agrees to play out the hand. The station responds to an explosion at an abandoned refinery and rescues several people.

Notes
The title "Propinquity" (meaning nearness in time or place) refers to the situation with Johnny staying a bit too close to Roy.

Locations

The abandoned refinery scenes were filmed at the Shell Oil Cracking Plant near 190th Street and Vermont in Carson, south of the junction of the Harbor (110) and San Diego (405) Freeways.

The car versus ambulance accident was filmed just outside the back exit of Universal's back lot, the New Park Barham gate, located on the east side of the lot.

The burning car scene was filmed on Universal's New York Street.

A scene filmed, but not used (possibly for sake of time), is the outside of Frank, the poker player's house. The scene included a tight shot of the interior of the Squad driving up with Frank waiting outside the house for them. The tight shot of the three was at the "Berry Mansion" that was originally used in the 1938 Universal film *Little Tough Guys in Society*, located on Cosmopolitan Street. It is unknown if the house is still around, but Cosmopolitan Street is long gone, now replaced by offices. The only shot of the house we do see is a stock footage shot that was used in "Cook's Tour" in Season 1.

"Inferno"

> Episode #3.21
>
> Production #37420
>
> Filming began: November 7, 1973
>
> Airdate: February 23, 1974
>
> Writer: Brian Taggert
>
> Director: Christian I. Nyby II
>
> LACoFD Technical Advisor: Steven Jongsma (PM0035)
>
> Guest cast: Jack Hogan, Jack Manning, Beth Brickell, Wes Parker (reporter), Bill Andes, Angelo Gristani, Helen Page Camp, Art Balinger, Stafford Morgan, Buck Young, Alan MacLeod (LA County Helicopter 10 pilot)
>
> Special appearances by: Bill Welsh and Richard Friend as themselves.

Synopsis

At Rampart, Dixie gets her hand caught in a vending machine. Johnny and Roy are disappointed when they are not called to a major brushfire at Harvest Hills. Roy is preparing lunch when they finally get a call to aid Station 65. The LA County PIO (Dick Friend) gives a briefing to the media (Bill Welsh). Chet gets dirt in his eyes, and Johnny washes it out. A fireman (Jack Hogan) is trapped by an overturned tractor; Johnny and Roy go in for the rescue but are trapped by a fire and need to be rescued themselves. Back at Rampart, the doctors treat another injured paramedic (Stafford Morgan).

Notes

Watch for the *real* LACoFD PIO, and contributor to this book, Dick Friend to make an appearance as himself briefing the media covering the brush-fire. Also appearing is veteran Los Angeles news reporter for KTTV, KTLA, and KFI in Los Angeles and Emmy nominee, Bill Welsh.

Actual film footage of the Palos Verdes Fire that took place in July 1973 was utilized. It was a major fire that started in the late afternoon with heavy winds and burned all night; several large homes were lost. Dick Friend states, "I was all over the place, taking a strike team to the east side and putting them to work with structural protection."

Guest star Jack Hogan later appeared in *Sierra* as the Chief Ranger, which aired the same week in September 1974 that the first repeat of this episode aired.

Engine 60 in this episode is not a Universal Studios's engine because it could not leave studio grounds. If this was in fact shot on studio grounds, they would not have put their first response engine in this position. Several things make it a different engine, including the painted bumper, the license plate above the bumper, the "Mars" light on the engine instead of the dis-tinctive "Gumball," as well as the front siren is larger and not inset, and no cut out above the bumper for the hydrant suction hose, all things indicative of Engine 60. This Crown, portraying Engine 60, is circa 1962.

The overturned vehicle called "Squad 18" and "The Spryte" by the Bat-talion Chief is a Thiokol 1201a Spryte snow-cat fitted with 30" ATV tracks. It was an experimental but actual inservice vehicle in the 1960s and early 1970s by LACoFD for carrying large amounts of hose, as it was in this episode, into rough terrain during brush fires. With the wide use of the helicopters for carrying supplies into the field, the vehicle was considered impractical. LACoFD either had more than one of these Sprytes or the one they had was reconfigured with a roll-bar cab configuration model that is seen in Dave Boucher's book, *Devil Wind Fire Wagons*. The Thiokol Chemi-cal Company sold off its snow-cat devision to the DeLorian Motor Car Company in 1978 (Universal's *Back to the Future* car).

Real LA County Copter 10 and 14 are utilized in this episode.

Location

Station 65 used in this episode is located at 4206 North Cornell Road, Agoura. Just south of Interstate 101 near the Malibu Creek State Park. It was built in the 1930s as part of the Works Progress Administration (WPA) established in 1935. The fireplaces at FS65 are still in use. The 125-acre Presidential retreat known as "Camp David" was also built by the WPA.

"Inventions"

Episode #3.22

Production #37428

Shooting Date: Unknown, however note the Marine Corps "Toys For Tots" barrels behind the station, a December event.

Airdate: March 23, 1974

Writer: John Groves

Director: Kevin Tighe

LACoFD Technical Advisor: James Easley (PM0033)

Guest cast: Ross Elliot, Aneta Corsaut, Yvonne Craig, Zina Bethune, Reb Brown, Lorraine Baptist, Judd Laurence, Lillian Bronson (Norma), Robert Miller Driscoll (Norma's son), Hal Bokar (truck driver), Michael Richardson (cab driver)

Synopsis

The men at the station get excited about a competition for new firefighting inventions with a $250 prize. Marco and Stoker team up to try to create an entry for the invention contest, but things don't work out quite like they planned. Their invention, designed to put out fires, ends up catching on fire. Chet invents something of his own. The paramedics deal with crises involving possible radiation poisoning from radioactive waste in a wrecked truck and a cloud of sulfuric acid fumes. A mysterious illness befalls a businessman after a taxi ride. An overweight man steps through an attic floor and becomes trapped in the living room ceiling. A firefighter at Station 84 wins the contest with an invention originally thought up by Johnny and Roy.

Notes

This is the first of four *Emergency!* episodes directed by Kevin Tighe (including episodes 4.3, 5.4, and 6.5). Tim Donnelly's own Volkswagen van appears in this episode, when Chet tries on his newly invented shoes.

SEASON 4

"The Screenwriter"

Episode #4.1

Production #40607

Airdate: September 14, 1974

Writer: Eric Brown

Director: Georg Fenady

LACoFD Technical Advisor: Robert Forsythe (PM0034)

Guest cast: Shelly Berman (screenwriter), Larry Csonka (chemical worker), Carol Wayne (Renee), Brendon Boone (motorcyclist), Roger Perry, Kyle Anderson (admitting nurse), Terrence O'Connor

Synopsis

An insensitive screenwriter creates problems as he spends a day following Roy and Johnny's work with a tape recorder monitoring all their activities, which includes a motorcycle accident, an explosion and fire at a toy factory, and dealing with a chemical worker who is overcome by toxic fumes. Roy and Johnny assist in the delivery of a deaf couple's baby in a parking lot. Miss October, a friend of the screenwriter, causes problems.

Notes

Uncredited in this episode is Richard Friend, LA County PIO as the Fire Official introducing the screenwriter to the station. He advised that he kept blowing his lines with Shelly Berman and the director asked him, "Dick, I see you on TV all the time and you're great. What's the matter here?" As Dick explained to the director, "Those lines on TV are real, not rehearsed," and Fenady told him, "Forget the script, Ad-lib." One take and it was done. "Atta boy Dick," stated Bob Fuller who had come across from Stage 42 where Rampart sets were located. This scene was shot on Universal stage 31.

Larry Csonka, running back for the Miami Dolphins, portrays the factory worker. In the episode, Csonka, who was to act a bit delusional and wild in the scene, grabs Marco and throws him to the ground. At the time the episode was being filmed, Marco was recovering from a recent back injury, but no one informed Csonka. The filming began, and Csonka grabbed Marco and squeezed hard, Marco began to yell in pain. Csonka immediately dropped him and asked if he was OK. Marco replied, "Yes, you just popped my back into place. Thank you."

"I'll Fix It"

Episode #4.2

Production #40602

Written: February 19, 1974

Final revision: March 29, 1974

Filming dates: April 2–8, 1974

Airdate: September 21, 1974

Writer: John Groves

Director: Georg Fenady

Assistant director: Gene Law

LACoFD Technical Advisor: Unknown

Guest cast: Robert Bralver, Toni Laurence, Richard Kiel (Carlo), Randall Carver (deli clerk), Byron Nickleberry, Bing Russell (Richard Freeman), Eric Shea (Danny Freeman), Peggy Stewart, Savannah Bently (Missy), with firefighters from Station 85

Synopsis

Johnny and Roy respond to a call from Carlo's Deli and must remove a ring from a man's finger before the wife's jealous husband returns. A woman's (Savannah Bently) husband is trapped under their house, where an inactive oil well has erupted. A child is trapped in a pipe on a vacant lot. A 14-year-old hypochondriac (Eric Shea) challenges the doctor's diagnosis. Johnny and Chet try to put together a mini-bike for Dixie.

Notes

Richard Kiel may be better known for his role as "Jaws" in several James Bond movies.

Locations

Carlo's Deli scenes were filmed at this real-life restaurant at 6449 Lankershim Boulevard, North Hollywood. The house/oil well scenes were shot on Universal's River Road and Industrial Street. Dixie's mini-bike segment was filmed on Universal's Soundstage 35.

"Gossip"

Episode #4.3

Production #40601

Airdate: September 28, 1974

Writer: Preston Wood

Director: Kevin Tighe

LACoFD Technical Advisor: Unknown

Guest cast: Catherine Burns (Nurse Ann Ridgely), Zina Bethune (Ruth Johnson), Yvonne Craig (Edna Johnson), Ruth McDevitt (Mrs. Blaine), Ross Elliott (supervisor), Annette Cardona, (Mrs. Harrow), Reb Brown (victim), Lorraine Baptist (receptionist), Vince Howard, Judd Laurance, Anne Schedeen (Nurse Anne)

Synopsis

A nurse (Catherine Burns) spreads the rumor that Dr. Morton is having financial problems. Roy encourages Johnny to represent the station in the Fireman's Olympics. An armored car (Benjamin Armored Transport, #219) sideswipes a motorist, and Station 51 must break into the armored car to treat the injured guard. A man is electrocuted. The station responds to a chemical plant fire. A boy develops cyanide poisoning from eating peach pits.

Notes

At the beginning of this episode, before the introduction, Johnny is mopping the floor when two unusual calls come over the speaker—a child is stuck on an elephant and a fire alarm was accidentally set off by a Samoan firedancer's torch. These lines were unscripted and were perhaps a practical joke, but the clip made it into the final episode, probably because of Randy Mantooth's priceless reaction.

Locations

The Martel Industries Inc. chemical plant fire was filmed at Wilmington Bulk Terminal Inc. (401 Canal Street, Slip #5, Wilmington). The armored car incident was filmed at the intersection of Chandler Boulevard and Clybourn Avenue in North Hollywood.

"Nagging Suspicion"

Working title: Stocks & Bonds

Episode #4.4

Production #40614

Airdate: October 5, 1974

Writer: Joseph Polizzi

Director: Christian I. Nyby, II

LACoFD Technical Advisor: Bob McCullough (PM0038)

Guest cast: Robert Q. Lewis (Mr. Caldwell), Pamela Morris (Mrs. Caldwell) Cheryl Dunn (Jane), Lindsay Bloom (Suzy Clark), Jim B. Smith, W. T. Zacha (Go-Go club bouncer)

Synopsis

The men at the station find out that Roy can pick winning racehorses but never bets on the races himself, and they pester him to pick a winning bet. A lion bites a woman at the zoo when she falls into the enclosure, a go-go dancer collapses, a man's (Robert Q. Lewis) ego is bruised when he is punctured by cactus as he falls off his son's skateboard, and the squad rescues a police sergeant (Jim B. Smith) who was shot during an exchange of gunfire with a sniper.

"Fugitive"

Working title: Communication Gaffe

Episode #4.5

Production #40610

Airdate: October 12, 1974

Writers: Charlene Bralver and Robert Bralver

Director: Georg Fenady

LACoFD Technical Advisor: Lynn Seeley

Guest cast: James McEachin, Denny Miller, Brooke Bundy, John Elerick (Officer Sam Sterling), Paul Bryar (battalion chief), Jennifer King, William Bryant (captain, Squad 69), Brian Cutler (firefighter/paramedic Dwyer), Cliff Coleman

Synopsis

Roy and Johnny respond to a call where both a policeman (John Elerick) and a suspect have been shot during a liquor store holdup. The policeman's partner (James McEachin) demands that the injured officer, who is less seriously injured, be treated first and threatens reprisals if they treat the suspect first. Roy and Joanne go on a TV quiz show. A woman brings in her abused son for treatment. A pickup truck carrying kerosene collides with a station wagon and starts a brushfire. A boy suffers an allergic reaction to a bee sting.

"Surprise"

Episode #4.6

Production #40606

Airdate: October 19, 1974

Writer: Preston Wood

Director: Joseph Pevney

LACoFD Technical Advisor: James Brewer

Guest cast: Dena Dietrich (Nurse Betty Royers), Joe Kapp, Anne Schedeen, Bill Quinn, William Bryant (captain, Squad 95), Christopher Mears, Robert Bernard, Holly Irving, Ann Morgan Guilbert (motorcyclist), Celia Lovsky, Dub Taylor, Aneta Corsant

Synopsis

A surprise birthday party is planned for Dixie. A woman (Ann Morgan Guilbert) is thrown from a motorcycle into a cactus patch. A man (Joe Kapp) is trapped in his new sauna. Dixie breaks her ankle from kicking a shopping cart, falls, and suffers a concussion. Nurse Royers fills in for her. Two men are injured attempting to mount a sign on a building. An old woman (Celia Lovsky) refuses to leave her apartment during a gas leak, and the building explodes with Johnny still inside.

Notes

Joe Kapp played quarterback for the Minnesota Vikings and the New England Patriots football team. He is the only quarterback to lead teams to the Rose Bowl, the Canadian Football League's Grey Cup, and the Super Bowl.

Ann Morgan Guilbert did not receive credit for her role in this episode and is instead listed in the credits for "Daisy's Pick" (episode 4.7), for which this segment was originally scripted and filmed.

Locations

The building in which the men are injured was the Cenikor Foundation building, now the site of Long Beach Temple Lofts, at 835 Locust Avenue, Long Beach.

"Daisy's Pick"

Working title: Blind Date

Episode #4.7

Production #40617

Filming dates: July 3–10, 1974

Airdate: November 2, 1974

Writer: John Groves

Director: Don Richardson

LACoFD Technical Advisor: Gary Davis (PM0003)

Guest cast: Brit Lund (Daisy), John Caradine, Dolores Mann (Ruth Goldbert), John Carter, Francisco Ortego (Hernando), Steve Franken, Brian Cutler (firefighter/paramedic Dwyer), Ann Morgan Guilbert (credited but did not appear)

Synopsis

The bachelor members of Station 51 are in competition for the first date with the beautiful new nurse (Brit Lund) at Rampart. The station rescues a man frozen to the floor of an icehouse and a man in a theatre fire. Roy and Johnny help a man whose hands are glued to a model boat.

Notes

John Caradine also appeared in *Rescue 8,* the "Flash Flood" episode.

Blind Date was originally scheduled for filming April 1, 1974, but the date for filming ended up being in July, then was changed to the name of *Daisy's Pick* (same script).

"Quicker Than the Eye"

Episode #4.8

Production #40604

Final revision: July 25, 1974

Filming began: July 26, 1974

Airdate: November 9, 1974

Writer: Arthur Weiss

Director: Don Richardson

LACoFD Technical Advisor: John Laur

Guest cast: Mark Spitz (Pete Barlow), Suzy Spitz (Dora Barlow), Renee Tetro, Bill Sorrells, Paul Brinegar, Vince Howard, Michael Conrad

Synopsis

Tired of Chet's antics, the guys at the station get their revenge by playing some practical jokes of their own. A gun discharges by accident and injures a pregnant woman (Suzy Spitz). A construction worker trapped under a boat at World Studios refuses an IV. A man in a motorcycle accident who is unable to speak communicates with his thumb and directs Roy and Chet to assist his son.

Notes

Mark Spitz was a 7-time Olympic gold medal champion in the 1972 Olympics and appears here with his wife Suzy Weiner-Spitz. Mark won two medals in the 1969 Olympics and one gold medal in 1992.

The boat that traps a man is PT 73, which was used in the 1962–1966 TV series *McHale's Navy*.

Locations

The Barlow house (identified as 252 Eden Street) was actually located on Beck Street in North Hollywood. World Studios scenes were shot on Universal's lot and include Universal's Main Street Gate, soundstages, and Western Street, where the incident with the man trapped by timbers under the boat was filmed. The motorcycle incident and the scenes with the camper and unconscious boy were filmed on Universal's Laramie Ranch and Blair Canyon sections.

"Foreign Trade"

Working title: The Gasoline Crunch (April 30, 1974 draft)

Episode #4.9

Production #40613

Filming began: October 14, 1974

Airdate: November 16, 1974

Writer: Rick Mittleman

Director: James Gavin

LACoFD Technical Advisor: David Heath

Guest cast: James Shigeta, Kareem Abdul-Jabbar, Anne Seymore, Peter Halton, Reb Brown, Christopher Stafford Nelson, Donald Mantooth, Anne Schedeen, Rosemary Johnson, Joseph Perry (Engine 2 captain), William Bryant

Synopsis

Johnny and Roy consider trading cars. Dixie takes on hospital management after budget cuts affect her nursing staff, and she is offered the role of nursing supervisor. A victim chokes during pledge initiation at a fraternity party. The station (assisted by Boat 2 and Engine 2) rescues a woman (Rosemary Johnson) trapped in her car on the edge of an open drawbridge. A basketball player (Kareem Abdul-Jabbar) is involved in a fender bender. Dr. Early has uncontrollable hiccups.

Notes

NBA star Kareem Abdul-Jabbar was playing for the Milwaukee Bucks at the time this episode was filmed. He was later trained by Bruce Lee and starred in two movies with him where they fought on screen, *Goodbye Bruce Lee* (1975) and *Game of Death* (1978).

Randy Mantooth's brother Donald appears as the fraternity member who calls for help.

Identified as Boat 2 for LA County, the fireboat was actually Boat 2 of the Long Beach Fire Department. It was later renumbered to Boat 20 and was stationed at fire station 20, which is about 2 miles east and located at the eastern end of the Cerritos Channel under the Desmond Bridge. It will be seen again in "Simple Adjustment" (episode 5.10) identified incorrectly as LA County Boat 110.

It was of one of two Long Beach fireboats built in 1952 and 1953. They were both 56' 6" long and pumped 4500 gpm. Both of these vessels were replaced in 1986 and 1987 by the Liberty and the Challenger, which can pump 10,000 gpm each and are 88' 6" long.

LAFD station 49 with Boat 3 and Boat 4 is about a mile west of the filming location.

Locations

The drawbridge sequence where Marco shoots the "Bridger Line Gun" was filmed on the Commodore Schuyler F. Heim Drawbridge on the southern-most portion of Route 103, where it crosses over the Cerritos Channel. CA Route 47 starts on the south side of the bridge (Terminal Island), where it intersects with W. Ocean Boulevard. By going eastbound on West Ocean Boulevard, you will end up in Long Beach and by going westbound (State 47) it crosses the Vincent Thomas bridge to San Pedro and the I-110.

"The Camera Bug"

Episode #4.10

Production #40603

Written: February 20, 1974

Airdate: November 23, 1974

Writer: Rick Mittleman

Director: Richard Bennett

LACoFD Technical Advisor: Tom Douglas (PM0032)

Guest cast: Ron Masak (firefighter Bob Treborg), Dianne Harper (Trudy Benson), Peter Leeds (restaurant owner), Tyler Henderson, Adrian Ricard, Mary Rings

Synopsis

Johnny tries to put together a photo essay featuring his colleagues at Station 51 and distracts his coworkers in the process. The squad responds to a call at Fire Station 68, where a fireman (Ron Masak) is suffering from chest pains. A scorpion stings a flight attendant. A teenage arsonist suffers from smoke inhalation. The station must rescue an injured man trapped under an overturned truck full of dynamite. Dixie and Dr. Brackett deliver a baby at a restaurant where they are having lunch. Chet gets paid for a photo he submits to the newspaper.

Location

Station 68 scenes were shot at that real fire station (24130 Calabasas Road, Calabasas) located 41 miles from Rampart, where they responded from.

"Quartet"

Working title: Firehouse Four

Episode #4.11

Production #40618

Final revision: August 30, 1974

Filming began: September 4, 1974

Airdate: November 30, 1974

Writer: John Groves

Director: Joseph Pevney

LACoFD Technical Advisor: Alfred Knight (PM0036)

Guest cast: Lennie Weinrib (Fred Gibson), Charles Knox Robinson, Joanne Meredith, Linda Dano, Peter Colt, James Kline

Synopsis

The station (sans Roy) enters the Barber Shop Quartet competition to be held at the Fireman's Picnic. A portly man (Lennie Weinrib), trying to follow his doctor's orders to get some exercise, tests the squad's patience when he causes accidents while bicycling, jogging, and using an electric rowing machine. A woman overdoses on sleeping pills.

Notes

This episode was filmed prior to "Foreign Trade," which aired earlier. The incident involving Kareen Abdul-Jabar (Foreign Trade) was written and filmed for this episode but was pulled and inserted in the later filmed episode.

"Details"

Episode #4.12

Production #40615

Final revision: August 2, 1974

Airdate: December 7, 1974

Writer: Michael Norell

Director: Georg Fenady

LACoFD Technical Advisor: Steven Jongsma (PM0035)

Guest cast: Barbara Nichols (belly dancer), Walter Brooke, Tom Reese, Charles Quinlivin, Michele Noval (Nurse Mary), Erik Estrada (uncredited)

Synopsis

Johnny gets engaged to a woman (Michele Noval) he's known for only a few days and finds out there are a few things she didn't mention. While responding to a call, Johnny and Roy witness an accident in which a pedestrian is struck by a car. A woman is badly burned in a fire caused by improperly stored gasoline, and Dr. Early treats a man (Erik Estrada) with an eye injury. A belly dancer (Barbara Nichols) overdoses on diet pills, and a dog bites a boy. Roy and Johnny are trapped on a ledge of a burning building and must jump to safety.

Notes

This was the first of four scripts written by Michael Norell (Captain Stanley); the others are episodes 5.6, 5.21, and 6.22.

"The Parade"

Episode #4.13

Production #40612, #40611

Final revision: September 3, 1974

Filming began: September 13, 1974

Airdate: December 21, 1974

Writer: Preston Wood

Director: Georg Fenady

LACoFD Technical Advisors: William Hoke and Gill Gilespie

Guest cast: Laurie Burton, Stuart Nisbet, Timothy Blake, Yvette Vickers, Joseph Tatner, Sandy Balson, Phillip Pine, Stanley Adams, Peggy Mondo, Jan Arven

Synopsis

Roy and Johnny finish restoring their British fire engine in time to ride in the California Firefighters Parade. Driving to the parade in their old engine and in costume, they aid a heart attack victim (Stanley Adams) who insisted on driving himself to the hospital and causes an accident. While on a date, a man accidentally slips himself a drug-laced drink and passes out. Later, while en route to the parade, Johnny and Roy spot a fire in a department store, rescue shoppers, and are humiliated by their attire by the other firefighters.

"The Bash"

Episode #4.14

Production #40620

Airdate: December 28, 1974

Writer: Preston Wood

Director: Christian I. Nyby II

LACoFD Technical Advisor: Richard Neal (PM0009)

Guest cast: Adam West (Vic Webster), Karen Jensen (Monique Morris), Larry Delaney (Ted MacReady), Paul L. Smith, Marcus Smith, Morgan Jones (battalion chief), Vince Howard (police officer), Jim B. Smith (police officer), Charlene (bear)

Synopsis

After they rescue an actor (Adam West) trapped on a set with an angry bear, Roy and Johnny are invited to a Hollywood party and meet a very sexy lady (Karen Jensen). The station responds to a man who threatens to blow up his house during a standoff with police. A man (Marcus Smith) suffers trichinosis from eating undercooked bear meat.

Notes

Larry Delaney appeared only this once on *Emergency!* but later appeared in *The Rangers* and *Pine Canyon Is Burning* as Engine 78's Captain. Randy Mantooth's Land Rover appears in this episode.

"Transition"

Episode #4.15

Production #40621

Airdate: January 4, 1975

Writer: John Groves

Director: Georg Fenady

LACoFD Technical Advisor: Jerry Smith

Guest cast: Colby Chester (Gil Robinson), Elisabeth Brooks, Lora Kaye, Joyce Davis, James Chandler

Synopsis

A former high school classmate of Johnny's (Colby Chester) is assigned to Station 51 as a new paramedic trainee and finds the transition from the hospital to the field a little overwhelming. A cobra bites a man, whose roommate has a heart attack. The firemen rescue a man trapped in his kitchen and have to deal with hydrogen sulfide. The squad responds to two calls at an amusement park.

Notes

Colby Chester also appeared in the World Premier movie as firefighter Tom Wheeler, and Johnny's partner on Rescue Squad 10.

Locations

The rescues at the amusement park were filmed in Long Beach at The Pike. In one scene you can see the HMS Queen Mary ocean liner in the background. For more information on The Pike, see episode 6.13, "An Ounce of Prevention," because it was also filmed there.

"The Smoke Eater"

Episode #4.16

Production #40619

Airdate: January 11, 1975

Writer: Edwin Self

Director: Joseph Pevney

LACoFD Technical Advisor: Michael Lewis (PM0037)

Guest cast: John Anderson (Captain, Bob Robertson Station 10), Lee Harcourt Montgomery, Sid Haig, Sharon Faron, Anne Whitfield, Burt Mustin (old man with burning chair), Lin McCarthy

Synopsis

While Captain Stanley is on vacation, a senior "old school" Captain (John Anderson) fills in and doesn't think that Gage and DeSoto should be practicing medicine. Dr. Brackett uses an old-fashioned sedative on a biker (Sid Haig). Johnny and Roy treat an asthmatic boy (Lee Harcourt Montgomery)

rescued from a storm drain, which impresses the Captain. Dr. Early has an overabundance of oranges.

Notes

Burt Mustin portrayed a Fire Chief in fourteen episodes of *Leave it to Beaver.*

The nickname "smoke eater" or "leather lungs" refers to old-time firefighters who were on the job before self-contained breathing apparatus became commonplace.

Captain Robertson says he is from Station 10 in Encino Canyon, a two-man brush station. They forgot that Station 10 is where Gage worked in the World Premier movie with an engine, truck, and Rescue Squad 10.

"Kidding"

> Working title: Kid Stuff
>
> Episode #4.17
>
> Production #40605
>
> Filming began: October 31, 1974
>
> Airdate: January 18, 1975
>
> Writer: Roland Wolpert
>
> Director: Wes McAfee
>
> LACoFD Technical Advisor: William Hoke
>
> Guest cast: Paul Fix, Laurette Spang, James Ingersoll, Joyce Jameson, Norman Bartold

Synopsis

Johnny is assigned to conduct a school tour of Rampart Hospital and finds it takes more than balloons and bubble gum to satisfy inquisitive youngsters. A disturbed man (James Ingersoll) takes his wife (Laurette Spang) hostage with a knife. A woman (Joyce Jameson) gets stuck in her doggie door. A famous writer attempts suicide in his garage. An airplane overshoots the runway and crashes into a loaded school bus.

"Magic"

> Working title: Prestidigitation
>
> Episode #4.18
>
> Production #40616
>
> Final revision: November 5, 1974

Filming began: November 11, 1974

Airdate: January 25, 1975

Writer: Robert Hamner

Director: Christian I Nyby, II

LACoFD Technical Advisor: Mark Hefley (PM0079)

Guest cast: James Gregory (Dr. Brackett's father), Bernard Fox, Tony Georgio (Lorenzo the Magnificent), Dick Yarmy

Synopsis

Johnny and Roy respond to a call where a magician is locked in a trunk suspended over water. Surgeons at Rampart operate on a very important patient—Dr. Brackett's father. A man is injured when his newly built fireplace explodes. A man is trapped in bed by a live transformer that has crashed through his roof after a vehicle hits a power pole. A sheared-off gas main causes complications, while Johnny attempts to free a woman trapped in her car.

Notes

Paramedic Mark Hefley: "Working on the show was a very enjoyable experience. The cast and crew were great to work with. I remember spending a lot of time with the writers coming up with ideas or them asking me what we would do in various situations. Before too long, other firemen on-duty would sit in and relay experiences and solutions. Having the writers come to the paramedic stations helped bridge the gap with our peers by letting them contribute." Mark would work on two other episodes, 5.7 and 6.11.

"It's How You Play the Game"

Episode #4.19

Production #40609

Airdate: February 1, 1975

Writer: Jim Carlson

Director: Joseph Pevney

LACoFD Technical Advisor: Bob Hoff (PM0071)

Guest cast: Dennis Patrick (Trader Jack), Cliff Osmond, Ryan MacDonald, Maggie Sullivan, Hal Baylor (animal trainer), Scott Gourlay (Officer Scotty)

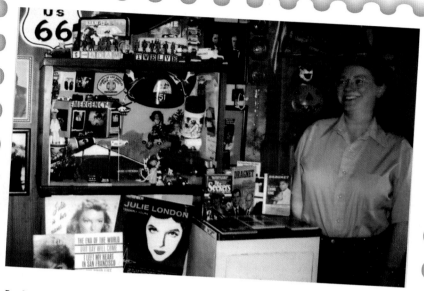

Fan Cornelia Shields stands with her *Emergency!* Shrine of collectibles.
Source: Courtesy of Cornelia Shields.

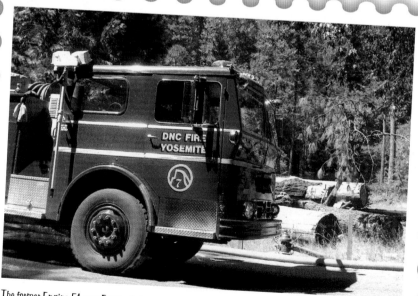

The former Engine 51, now Engine 7, in service at Yosemite National Park in California.
Source: Courtesy of David Stone.

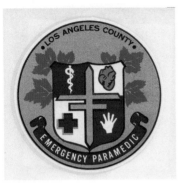

Official Los Angeles County 'Emergency Paramedic' decal.
Source: Courtesy of Los Angeles County Fire Department, Photo Unit.

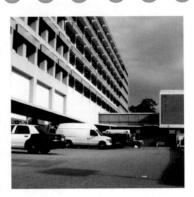

Emergency Room Entrance at Los Angeles County Harbor UCLA Medical Center.
Source: Courtesy of Harbor/UCLA Medical Center; Rozane Sutherland, photographer.

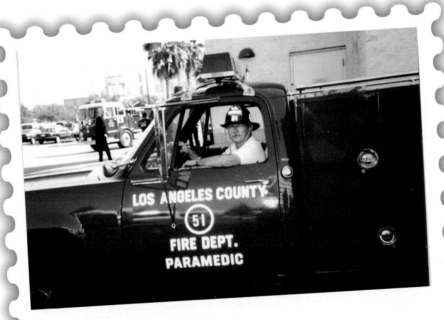

Squad 51 with Yokley in driver's seat at the 1998 Convention.
Source: Courtesy of Richard Yokley.

Synopsis

A friendly game of softball between Station 51 and Station 36 takes on a whole new meaning after Johnny wagers the entire cost of the post-game barbeque on the outcome, without the rest of the crew's knowledge. Chet becomes Station 51's only hope when their star pitcher, Captain Stanley, breaks his arm during a fire. A drunk driver becomes violent after a car accident. An auto dealer (Dennis Patrick) is trapped in a car with a tiger during a commercial shoot. A man with a slipped disk is stuck on a waterbed. A structure fire is complicated by moonshine.

Notes

This script was unusually long. The second draft was 61 pages, and the final shooting script was 81 pages.

For West coast viewers regarding the segment with the Auto dealer and a tiger, think entrepreneur "Cal Worthington." Bob Hoff filled in for Kirk Kington P0063 (who was originally assigned to do this episode) and was on the set during the infamous tarantula incident. Kirk Kington was on the original Rescue Squad 20. After attending paramedic school, he returned to his old station in Norwalk and was assigned to the new Paramedic Squad 20. Kington would work on other *Emergency!* episodes as a Technical Advisor.

Locations

The drunken driving incident was filmed on Universal's Denver Street.

"The Mouse"

Episode #4.20

Production #40626

Revised: December 26, 1974

Airdate: February 8, 1975

Writer: Edwin Self

Director: Christian I. Nyby II

LACoFD Technical Advisor: Richard Atkins

Guest cast: William Zuckert, Ronnie Schell, J. Pat O'Malley (Joe Wilson), Peter Palmer (bar patron), Lee Paul (bar patron), Barry Cahill (Pasadena Fire Captain), Harold Frizzell, Tracey D. Hurd (young girl)

Synopsis
Chet becomes obsessed with ridding the station of an uninvited guest—a mouse that Marco names Herbert. A man is trapped in a house fire with burglar bars on the window that delay the rescue. Roy and Johnny attempt to break up a bar fight. A jet plane crashes into an apartment complex in Pasadena and requires assistance from LA County. On this dangerous call, one of the LA County firemen is splashed with jet fuel, catches fire, and falls from the first-floor balcony.

Notes
In this episode, Johnny and Roy state that they are on B shift, not their usual A shift. In another error, Pasadena firefighters are visible stretching lines in the background while Captain Stanley is on the radio with dispatch, and then the first Pasadena engine arrives on scene.

The Pasadena firefighters as seen in this episode were not portrayed by Pasadena Fire Department (PFD) firefighters, according to PFD retired Captain David Leonard. Leonard further states, "To look authentic, the brand new Yellow Nomex fire gear was rented from Pasadena FD, so new that most of it was not even issued to the guys yet. This prompted Johnny's response of, "They do good work, but sure look funny. They previously had been wearing the same canvas type turnouts as LA County.""

The following is recalled by Tracey D. Hurd-Parker, the little girl in the pink robe who was at the apartment fire incident. She is seen running along the corridor of the apartment building.

> I remember clearly that when I was instructed on what to do, they didn't tell me about the fire. So if I have a horrible look on my face, it is because I was truly frightened. I do remember one of the actors carrying me around on his hip and also, after the scene, one of them took me back into the area and showed me how they can turn the fire on and off with a switch. They probably remember me running out and either crying or yelling for my mom! My mom said the Screen Actors Guild called her about the part the night before.

Notes
The Y-Not Beer bar was an actual bar that was used for exteriors.

The apartment fire was actually filmed in Pasadena at 775 Worcester Avenue (cross street, E. Orange Grove Boulevard), about a mile east of the Rose Bowl. The apartment buildings are still there.

"Back-Up"

Episode #4.21
Production #40623

Airdate: February 15, 1975

Writer: John Groves

Director: Georg Fenady

LACoFD Technical Advisor: Robert Hoff (P0071)

Guest cast: Keenan Wynn (Wild Bill Martin), Michael Conrad (football player), Patch MacKenzie (admitting nurse), Bill Conklin, Anne Schedeen (triage nurse), Brian Cutler (Tom Dwyer), Scott Gourlay (Officer Scotty)

Synopsis

Johnny gets upset by all the frivolous calls that take time away from helping people in need. Fireman Bill Wilson fills in for Chet and makes one of Chet's stew recipes for dinner. A lonely old cowboy (Keenan Wynn) fakes back pain to get a free ride to the hospital. An overdose victim is brought directly to Rampart. A retired football player "Old 87" is shocked after kicking in his TV screen and needs defibrillation. The patient's trip to the hospital is interrupted because the ambulance with Johnny and Roy in the back with the patient is involved in an accident. They finish their journey in the hosebed of the engine.

"905-Wild"

Episode #4.22

Production #40622

Filming began: December 11, 1974

Airdate: March 1, 1975

Writers: Buddy Atkinson and Dick Conway

Director: Jack Webb

Produced by: William Stark

LACoFD Technical Advisor: Lynn Seeley

LA County Animal Control Technical Advisor: William Preston

Guest cast: Mark Harmon (Dave Gordon), Albert Popwell (Les Taylor), Gary Crosby (Walt Marsh), Laura Huddleston (little girl), David Huddleston (Barney "Doc" Coolidge), Burt Mustin (Grandpa), Rose Ann Zecker (secretary)

Synopsis

The episode opens with Johnny and Roy responding into a suburban canyon area to a medical call for a "man-down, bleeding." They discover a Bengal tiger on the premises of a small store and call in Animal Control. Later, a brushfire threatens the area, and Animal Control is confronted with rescuing several animals, including an elephant. Rampart Hospital becomes a veterinary surgical center with Dr. Brackett operating on an injured goat with instructions given over the phone by Animal Control's head veterinarian (David Huddleston).

Notes

905-Wild stars Mark Harmon (*240-ROBERT, NCIS*) and Albert Popwell (*Dirty Harry*) as paramedic Animal Control Officers, and Gary Crosby (*Adam-12*) as head of the Los Angeles Bureau of Animal Control. Rose Ann Zecker (aka Rose Ann Deel) (*Sierra, Adam-12*) is the unit secretary.

This episode was produced for Jack Webb/Mark VII Productions as a development project for a possible series; the series was never developed.

SEASON 5

"The Stewardess"

Episode #5.1

Production #42805

Filming began: June 16–23, 1975

Airdate: September 13, 1975

Writer: Preston Wood

Director: Christian I. Nyby II

LACoFD Technical Advisor: Robert Forsythe (PM0034)

Guest cast: Gretchen Corbett, William Wintersole (Kirk), James Ingersoll (David Cort), John La Due (Flight Captain Dowell), Tom Williams (Mr. Penner)

Synopsis

While flying back to Los Angeles on Trans-California Airways from a paramedic convention in Sacramento, Johnny and Roy assist one of the flight crew (Gretchen Corbett) when a fellow passenger (Tom Williams) has a heart attack. Johnny later dates the stewardess. The crew battles a chemical plant fire. A man injured in a motorcycle accident is an undiagnosed epileptic.

Locations

The chemical plant fire was filmed at the Hollywood Technicolor Plant at Eleanor and Cahuenga in Hollywood. It is now the site of the UCLA Film and Television Archive, 1015 North Cahuenga Boulevard., Hollywood. Just 7 blocks south of LAFD Station 27 and the LAFD Museum.

The motorcycle accident scenes were filmed on Universal's Colonial Street and Circle Drive.

"The Old Engine Cram"

Episode #5.2

Production #42802

Filming dates: July 1–7, 1975

Airdate: September 20, 1975

Writer: Preston Wood

Director: Dennis Donnelly

LACoFD Technical Advisor: Gil Gillespie

Guest cast: Bernard Fox (Mr. Kerner), Christopher Nelson (Arnie), Smith Evans (Marilyn Dennis), Kim Hamilton (Estelle Lee Dickins), Dick Yarmy

Synopsis

Johnny and Roy think they have a buyer (Bernard Fox) for the old fire engine they restored. A fireman is injured during a training session with a dangerous chemical—sulfur trioxide. A man suffers a back injury from a motorcycle accident, and a child is diagnosed with polio. A man having a heart attack comes to the station. Johnny and Roy perform an ocean rescue of a man who has fallen off a cliff on Catalina Island, aided by the U.S. Coast Guard.

Notes

Shortly after this episode aired, a similar, real-life cliff rescue involving LA County paramedics and the Coast Guard was performed near Rancho Palos Verdes. Robert Cinedar informed *Paramedics International* magazine in 1976 that he knew of at least seven instances whereby *Emergency!* had filmed a rescue and shortly thereafter a similar incident occurred in the field.

A script written earlier by the writer was rewritten and retitled, thus airing as "The Old Engine Cram." The sulfur trioxide segment, the man having a heart attack at the station, and the child with polio that now appear in this episode all came from the writer's unfilmed script. (See "The Reading Game" in Chapter 13.)

The U.S. Coast Guard unit used in this episode was Unit 1443.

Johnny refers to the British fire engine as a 1923 Paige in this episode, even though it is the same 1934 Dennis from "The Old Engine" (episode 3.2) and "The Parade" (episode 4.13). Preston Wood wrote all three of the episodes involving the British engine; there is no explanation for the mis-identification by the writer.

Regarding Paige fire apparatus, they were an American company in Detroit, Michigan, that provided chassis for fire apparatus but not until 1928 under the Graham-Paige division. The forerunner to Graham-Paige was the Paige-Detroit Motor Car Company; they manufactured Paige-Detroit automobiles, Paige automobiles, Jewett Automobiles, and Paige trucks from 1909 through 1927, but no fire apparatus. Graham-Paige actively promoted specialty uses for their chassis, funeral cars, fire trucks, etc. They did not build the bodies themselves.

"Election"

Episode #5.3

Production #42803

Filming dates: June 6–12, 1975

Airdate: September 27, 1975

Writer: John Groves

Director: Bruce Bilson

LACoFD Technical Advisor: James Brewer

Guest cast: Maggie Malody, Hank Brandt, Jack Kutcher (Roger), Sharon Gless (Julie Robertson)

Synopsis
Roy and Johnny both run for the same seat on the Firefighters' Welfare and Benefits Committee. A sculptress (Sharon Gless) is unable to release her live model (Jack Kutcher) from her work of art. A construction worker is trapped on a crane. Dispatch reports a victim at the base of a cliff, and Johnny and Roy respond with the Coast Guard. A man gets his arm stuck in the drain of his washing machine, while his brother-in-law swallows the pull-tab from a can of beer.

Notes
Beer and sodas were manufactured with pull-tabs from 1963 to 1975, when they were replaced by safer Stay-tabs. Before that, it was commonplace for people to place the pull-tab inside their beverage after opening.

Locations

What is seen as the U.S. Coast Guard facility for Los Angeles in this episode is in fact the Air Control Tower at the Long Beach airport. See also "The Boat" (episode 6.19). Commander Sommer of the Air Station in Los Angeles states, "The sign out front had me for a bit, it appears to say Los Angeles, but a fictional sign by the property people I suspect." He says, "it looks like one of our signs, and could be, but they can do marvelous things with duct tape." He said that they work a lot with the movie and television people so they are quite familiar with what can be done.

The actual U.S. Coast Guard Air Station, Los Angeles, is located at the extreme West end of the airport complex at LAX between runways 6R and 7L at 7159 World Way West.

The construction site, a multi-story building with a man on a crane, was filmed at 233 Wilshire Boulevard in Santa Monica. However, some scenes with the "Titan Crane" were filmed on the "Laramie Parking lot" at Universal.

"Equipment"

Episode #5.4

Production #42808

Filming began: May 28, 1975

Airdate: October 4, 1975

Writer: Robert Hamilton

Director: Kevin Tighe

LACoFD Technical Advisor: Robert McCullough (PM0038)

Guest cast: Lloyd Haynes (Captain Stone), Jessica Rains, John Laurence, Hal Bokar (Station 8 firefighter), Kristine Marie Greco (nurse), Vernon Weddle (Roy's roommate)

Synopsis

Johnny pulls an overtime shift at Station 8 on their engine, where a lack of available equipment and a squad backup may have cost a heart attack victim his life. The station captain (Lloyd Haynes) becomes frustrated when the inability to transmit data on the patient results in his demise. A child falls from a swing. Back at Station 51, Chet is injured in an explosion, and Roy is injured in a fireworks warehouse fire.

Notes

Johnny sits behind the Captain in the jump seat on the engine at Station 8. Although Captain Stone was supposedly trained as a paramedic, LA County protocols at the time would have prohibited him from practicing. This rule was changed in 1976, allowing promoted paramedics to work in the field when necessary.

The call sign for Station 8 is actually KMG356 and is used as such in this episode. Although the transmitter has since been removed, it is still licensed as such by the Federal Communications Commission.

The open cab Crown seen here is a hose wagon/pumper combo. Although the Captain in this episode is African-American, LA County would not promote its first African-American Captain until 1977, two years after this episode aired. He was Hershel Clady, who was the department's first African-American Engineer in 1975.

Locations

This episode was actually filmed at Station 8, including interior shots of the kitchen that was unchanged since the TV series 'Rescue 8' filmed there 15 years earlier. To this day the station is still relatively unchanged.

"The Inspection"

Episode #5.5

Production #42807

Filming began: July 21, 1975

Airdate: October 11, 1975

Writer: Bruce Johnson

Director: Georg Fenady

LACoFD Technical Advisor: Louis Danes

Guest cast: Wolfman Jack, Jeanne Cooper (Evelyn Fennady), Warren Berlinger (Frank Fennady), Roger Bowen, Gerald Michenaud (Paul), Sam Lainer, Boot the dog

Synopsis

The station tries to prepare for the Chief Engineer's impending inspection. A woman (Jeanne Cooper) is convinced that her husband's (Warren Berlinger) heart transplant means he doesn't love her anymore. "Lucky" Collins, a parachutist, is snagged on a power pole, and KJV TV director (Wolfman Jack) attempts to direct the operation. The station attempts to free a teenager (Gerald Michenaud), whose car has overturned in the Los Angeles River.

Notes

One error is visible in this episode—the clock with the Chief Engineer's picture changes time from 2:08 P.M. to 6:45 P.M. Did it really take that long to shoot that scene, even with camera changes? Chief Houts doesn't actually appear at the station until "Above and Beyond...Nearly" (episode 5.20).

"The Indirect Method"

Episode #5.6

Production #42804

Airdate: October 18, 1975

Writer: Michael Norell

Director: Joel Oliansky

LACoFD Technical Advisor: Robert Hoff (PM0071)

Guest cast: Elayne Heilveil (Karen Overstreet), Dick Bakalyan (Dewey), Anne Loos (Mrs. Hurley), Joan Crosby, Macon McCalman, Stephen Parr, Bill Conklin

Synopsis

A female paramedic trainee (Elayne Heilveil) from a hospital in Redding, California, is training with the paramedics at Station 51. She feels the difficulty of being a woman in the fire service, but her rudeness and lack of compassion alienate her from the rest of the station. A freeway construction threatens an old couple's house. A man tries to commit suicide by handcuffing himself to a gas pipe in his home and then changes his mind. A house fire traps paramedics and a female invalid on the second floor, and the only person who can help is the trainee. Roy falls off the roof after becoming shocked by power lines. The trainee's quick response in treating Roy proves she has potential.

Notes

The LACoFD often provided paramedic field training for civilians and firefighters across the state. They would not hire their first female firefighter until 1983—Cindy Fralick, who become the subject of the 1986 TV movie *Firefighter*. Fralick later became a paramedic and was promoted to Captain.

As of 2005 LA County has only 28 females on the job, ranging from firefighter through battalion chief.

Bob Hoff, the Technical Advisor, commented, "the person portraying the female paramedic constantly had to be advised on the use of the fire and medical equipment, putting the stethoscope in her ears to get a reading, etc." Bob spent time on the set going over all the fire equipment even to the point of showing her how CPR is done. Bob said, "I thought I was being 'set-up' by the crew, as at her request, I performed chest compressions and even mouth to mouth resuscitation on her so that she could see how it was done. I really thought someone was filming this and I would end up seeing all this at a wrap party, but it was for real and she was genuinely interested." Bob went on to say, "The regulars were so familiar with what they needed to do more often than not there was not much for me to do. It was the guest actors that we constantly had to work with."

See Chapter 5 on Mike Norell's take on this episode dealing with a female on the job.

Dick Bakalyan does *not* portray the department mechanic in this episode.

Locations
The fire scene was shot on Universal's back lot for the exteriors, then on a sound stage for the interior firefighting scenes. Because the fire coming out of the propane was not good enough, Bob recalled:

> They applied rubber cement on the walls and lit that off as well. That created much more heat than anticipated, and due to the repeated takes, one of the fire stops made out of corrugated metal warped and fell into the set. That in turn shot the fire and heat up and lit off the sound stage fire sprinkler system. That alerted the studio fire department and while we made sure all the fire was turned off, (propane tanks) and were trying to cover all the cameras, evacuate people, what arrives but Engine 60—to the embarrassment of us all.

"Pressure 165"

Episode #5.7

Production #42810

Filming began: August 5, 1975

Airdate: October 25, 1975

Writer and producer: Edwin Self

Director: Georg Fenady

LACoFD Technical Advisor: Mark Hefley (PM0079)

Guest cast: Chef Mike Roy (himself), Bing Russell (David Winslow), Del Monroe (Walt), Derrel Maury, Bill Harlow, Art Balinger (Battalion Chief Conrad)

Synopsis

Roy and Johnny are airlifted to Catalina Island to assist the local doctor in treating a diver with decompression sickness by using a hyperbaric chamber. A famous TV chef (Mike Roy) is embarrassed to admit he accidentally set his kitchen on fire. Johnny, long teased by the crew about his culinary skills, tries his hand at cooking a French seafood meal, Bordure de Soles a La Normande, a fish and shellfish dish that started out as white and then turned "an interesting green color."

Notes

The Coast Guard helicopter (unit 1443) and other Catalina location shots for this episode were filmed earlier during the filming of "The Old Engine Cram" (episode 5.2) which aired earlier in the season. The Technical Advisor, Mark Hefley, advised, "The long distance exterior shots were filmed a few months before on Catalina Island prior to the actual filming of the rest of the show. I recall that part because one of the extras had to remember whether or not he had a mustache at the time."

Chef Mike Roy was in fact a famous TV chef of the time in the LA area and on the CBS Network. In addition to his radio and TV shows, he authored several cook books before his death in 1976.

Locations

Hefley also stated, "They built the mock hyperbaric chamber in a sound stage at Universal." There is a hyperbaric chamber on Catalina that is operated by the University of Southern California. It is located on the campus of the Wrigley Marine Science Center at Big Fisherman's Cove at the west end of the Island. For treatment, the chamber is compressed to pressures as great as 165 feet (hence the episode title) of seawater (fsw) by pumping in high-pressure air. The patient then breathes gas containing a high percent of oxygen (47 percent oxygen at 165 fsw, or 100 percent oxygen at 60 fsw and shallower) through a mask. On occasion, a diver in full arrest can, upon reaching a critical pressure in the chamber, regain a pulse.

"The Lighter-Than-Air Man"

Episode #5.8

Production #42801

Filming dates: The last week in July

Airdate: November 1, 1975

Writer: Claire Whitaker

Director: Wes McAfee

LACoFD Technical Advisor: John Larsen

Guest cast: James McEachin (police lieutenant), Arthur O'Connell (Ben Meduzi), Randall Carver, Sue Casey, Vince Howard, Barbara Mallory, Chuck Winters

Synopsis

Roy and Johnny are accused of hitting an elderly crossing guard (Arthur O'Connell) with the squad while en route to a rescue. The guard, a former professional acrobat known as "The Lighter-Than-Air Man" was involved in similar cons in the past. A couple hit a fire hydrant (Randall Carver and Barbara Mallory) on the way to their wedding. A camper on fire is driven up to the station with a child trapped inside. A truck hauling insecticide overturns. The station is collecting trading stamps to raise money for a barbeque.

Notes

Trading stamps were quite popular in the 1950s through the 1970s and could be exchanged for points or merchandise. These stamps could be obtained at grocery stores and gasoline stations and were often stored in special stamp books. The most popular stamps were S&H Green Stamps, Top Value, and Gold Bond.

"One of Those Days"

Episode #5.9

Production #42817

Filming began: September 23, 1975

Airdate: November 8, 1975

Writer: Preston Wood

Director: Joseph Pevney

LACoFD Technical Advisor: Gary Davis (PM0003)

Guest cast: Lara Parker, Marla Adams, Penelope Windust, Shirley Mitchell, Ross Elliott, Bill McLean (hotel manager)

Synopsis

An elderly woman's stomach problems lead to a family brawl with Johnny and Roy caught in the middle. Roy and Johnny respond to a hotel with a broken elevator, a two-car accident with no victims, and a deaf child trapped in a burning building. Meanwhile, Dr. Brackett deals with a civic-minded mother (Marla Adams) who has little time for her sick child with meningitis.

"Simple Adjustment"

Episode #5.10

Production #42812

Filming began: September 12, 1975

Airdate: November 22, 1975

Writer: Robert Hamilton

Director: Dennis Donnelly

LACoFD Technical Advisor: Gil Gillespie

Guest cast: Joan Crosby, Elisabeth Brooks (Marla Ekberg), Jane Dulo (salon owner)

Synopsis

Johnny is convinced that with a simple adjustment, he can devise a better way to log the squad's calls. They install a tape recorder into the squad's dashboard to hopefully lessen their paperwork. A beauty operator has a total personality change after an overdose of diet pills and makes a play for Johnny. A man suffers a stroke, and his daughter insists the squad transport him to a distant hospital and not to Rampart, which she considers to be a charity hospital, even though Rampart is much closer. The station responds to a fire in the engine room of a ship in a salvage yard.

Notes

The fire boat used in this episode, seen previously in "Foreign Trade" (episode 4.9), is incorrectly identified as LA County Boat 110; it is actually Long Beach Fire Department's Boat 20.

Locations

The bridge seen in the background at the ship fire incident is the Gerald Desmond Bridge, which connects the Long Beach Naval Shipyard and the container terminal docks. Long Beach Fire Station 20 houses Engine 20 and Boat 20 at the base of the bridge on the east side near where this was filmed.

"TeeVee"

Episode #5.11

Production #42813

Filming began: September 3, 1975

Airdate: November 29, 1975

Writer: John Groves

Director: Christian I. Nyby II

LACoFD Technical Advisor: Joe Cappel

Guest cast: Lin McCarthy (Clair Howells), Laurie Burton (Jane Ellis), W. T. Zacha, Heath Jobes (John Whitaker)

Synopsis

Chet and Johnny attempt to fix the station's TV but end up blowing it up instead. Johnny and Roy rescue a man from a flash fire in a sewer. An aquarium filled with exotic fish causes problems for Dr. Brackett, who is bitten by a catfish. A man (Heath Jobes) spatters glue in his eyes. An explosion of a ruptured gas line in a home results in a mudslide trapping the victim, Johnny, and Roy.

Notes

Dr. Brackett's office is room number 127, which is the real fire station number of Station 51.

"On Camera"

Episode #5.12

Production #42815

Filming began: October 2, 1975

Airdate: December 6, 1975

Writers: Rod Peterson and Claire Whitaker

Director: Christian I. Nyby II

LACoFD Technical Advisor: Lloyd Leyh

Guest cast: Peter Palmer (George Antonio), Leigh Christian (Paula Hughes), Helen Page Camp (mother), Paul Micale, Will MacIntyre Walker (Gary), Scott B. Wells (workman), Harold Frizzell (ambulance attendant), Johnny Miller (tar man)

Synopsis

TV news commentator, Paula (Leigh Christian), and her reluctant photographer (Peter Palmer) are assigned to do a documentary on Squad 51. The assortment of emergencies encountered includes a rattlesnake bite, a stuntman dangling from an I-beam, a boy who falls down a cliff, and a man (Johnny Miller) trapped under a burning truck of hot tar.

Notes

Johnny Miller, the stuntman of the vehicle accident that trapped him with spilled flaming tar, recalls:

I don't know what the tar was made of, but was [it] very hard to wash off. That gag was very dangerous, it was before fire protecting jell was invented. My lower body was wrapped in asbestos under my pants, and then liquid glue was put on my lower body plus the debris that was on me. The glue was highly flammable! Ritter fans were set up in front of me out of camera to control the fire and keep it off my back or I would have been well done. On 'Action' I was on fire, special effects turned on the fans to control the fire........HOT to say the least. Did the flames go across my back, YES! Special Effects did a great job for me and I was not burned.

The rescue! Water every where flames soaring, the boys shouting commands, 'We found the victim, need assistance.' Needless to say it was a stunt I won't forget. After all that, I was hot water logged, they strapped me to the gurney and (after filming the scene) feathered me. I was not a happy camper and I won't repeat my dialog. It took 2 hours to clean up. Was it fun? Oh yes, now just another memory in a career I love."

Locations
The stunt man scenes were filmed at the Valley Generating Station, 11801 Sheldon Street, Sun Valley, California, a steam generating facility. It is located northeast of the intersections of I-5 and the 170, between Burbank and San Fernando.

"Communications"

Episode #5.13

Production #42809

Airdate: December 13, 1975

Writer: Mark Saha

Director: Dennis Donnelly

LACoFD Technical Advisor: Bruce Mortimer

Guest cast: Cynthia Sikes (Karen Martin), Craig Hundley (Gary Welton), Ted Gehring (Tom Blasmore), Barbara George (Diane Kenner)

Synopsis
Radio communications between Squad 51 and Rampart go awry when they are outside of their district covering for another squad. The paramedics deal with an airline stewardess (Barbara George), who refuses to allow them to treat her for an overdose of sleeping pills. A teenager gets his arm caught in a pressing machine, and Dr. Brackett may have to amputate. Two kids out for a joyride end up on the roof of a house. While rescuing a man trapped under a car, Johnny and Roy inadvertently cause an explosion. Chet buys a pair of skis and starts a fire in the station while trying to refinish them.

"To Buy or Not to Buy"

Episode #5.14

Production #42806

Filming began: October 13, 1975

Airdate: December 20, 1975

Writer: Keith A. Walker

Director: Georg Fenady

LACoFD Technical Advisor: Mike Williams

Guest cast: Robert Pratt, Allan Vint, Susan Gay Powell, Fay DeWitt, Nicholas Worth (Charles), Patch MacKenzie (Martha)

Synopsis

Roy thinks about buying a house, and Johnny gives him unsolicited investment advice. Responding to a fire in an abandoned house, the station finds two children trapped inside. Two driving school students are involved in an accident. An epileptic boy is rescued from a bridge. An Indian boy breaks his arm in a minor traffic accident, and Johnny and Roy search for his lost dog.

Notes

Fay DeWitt is the cousin of actress Joyce DeWitt ('Three's Company').

Locations

The bridge used in this episode is the Colorado Boulevard (Highway 134) Bridge over Arroyo Park in Pasadena, also nicknamed the Suicide Bridge. The 1,467-foot-long and 150-foot-high concrete bridge was built in 1913 and is listed on the National Registry of Historic Places.

The Rose Bowl is just about a mile north.

"The Wedworth-Townsend Act"

Episodes #5.15 (Part 1) and #5.16 (Part 2)

Production #42898 (Part 1), #42899 (Part 2)

Airdates: December 27, 1975, January 3, 1976

Writer and director for the nonflashback sequences not confirmed; most likely R.A. Cinader

Credits from the World Premier are shown minus the writers and director

Synopsis

This is a re-airing of *Emergency!*, the World Premier, in flashback format. After returning from a run, Johnny and Roy reminisce about the start of the first paramedic program in Los Angeles and how much it has changed. The movie opens with the squad backing in to the station, and Johnny and Roy getting out of the squad and going into the station's dayroom. Engine 51 (the Ward LaFrance) is there, but there is no sign of Captain Stanley or the others.

Because this episode is aired in two parts, a "To Be Continued" is shown with the surgery to reattach arm on the girl. The second part continues from where the surgery scene begins.

Notes

In this flashback, Johnny states that he was working at Station 8 on the rescue squad. It was filmed at Station 8, but in the original airing of the movie, it was identified verbally and on the apparatus as Station 10. The same mistake would be heard in the movie *The Greatest Rescues of Emergency!*, when Johnny and Roy are promoted to captain.

"Right at Home"

Episode #5.17

Production #42821

Filming dates: October 30–November 6, 1975

Airdate: January 10, 1976

Writer: Preston Wood

Director: Georg Fenady

LACoFD Technical Advisor: Kirk Kington (PM0063)

Guest cast: Poindexter Yothers (Eddie Lapeer), Sandra Balson (Joan Hanrahan), Peggy Stewart (Martha Felt), Steven Marlo (Swede), with Alan MacLeod (Senior Pilot, LACoFD) and Larry Younkers fireman/observer in the left seat)

Synopsis

Dr. Brackett rides along with Copter 10 of the LACoFD and flies to Fire Camp 9. They respond with engine and Squad 51 to a vehicle accident. Roy agrees to take care of the child (Poindexter Yothers) of the accident victim and is appalled when the child proceeds to wreck his home and neighborhood reputation. The station responds to a residential fire at night.

Notes

In this episode we see Pacoima Air Field at 12605 Osborne Street, Pacoima, site of LACoFD Air Ops, now known as Barton Heliport, named after Chief Pilot Roland Barton (seen as a pilot in episode 1.1). On the flight line are Copters 10, 11, 14 (all Bell 204-205/UH1 Huey/Iroquois); Copter 4 (a Bell 206 JetRanger/OH58 Kiowa), later to be seen in the Kent McCord movie *Pine Canyon is Burning;* and Copter 2, which is a Bell 47G.

Copter 10 with Dr. Brackett aboard is actually flying into Fire Camp 9 located in the Angeles National Forest on Los Pinetos Mountain between Sylmar and Santa Clarita.

Dummies, not stunt doubles, were utilized for portions of the truck accident rescue, filmed on Upper Falls Lake Road at Universal.

Filmed for this episode but not utilized was the burning boat rescue with Copter 10. It was filmed at Valencia Lake in Castiac. It would be seen later in the season in "Grateful" (episode 5.21). The residential fire was used in its place.

"The Girl on the Balance Beam"

> Episode #5.18
>
> Production #42818
>
> Filming began: November 10, 1975
>
> Airdate: January 17, 1976
>
> Writer: Robert Hamilton
>
> Director: Christian I. Nyby II
>
> LACoFD Technical Advisor: Robert Lee
>
> Guest cast: Patti Cohoon (Nancy Benedict), Charles Knox Robinson (Allan Benedict), Patricia Morrow (Jennie Carter, gym coach), Brian Baker, Dorothy Schott (Sylvia, movie director), Andrea Bell, William Bryant (Captain, Engine 14), Ronnie Schell (Jasper), Robert Hackman, the Albia triplets (as the baby)

Synopsis

A former athlete (Charles Knox Robinson), who has dreams of Olympic glory, pushes his teenage daughter (Patti Cohoon) beyond her abilities. The station rescues an actress hung up on a high wire in a TV studio. Johnny and Roy free drunk driver (Ronnie Schell) trapped in his car by using the Jaws and aid an infant (baby Albia) in respiratory distress. The station responds to a train fire involving ammonium nitrate.

Notes

The 16-month-old triplets were seen only one at time as they were swapped out every 5 minutes, conforming to child labor laws, and portrayed only one character.

In the background in one scene, there is a blue background and an airplane hanging in front of it. On the tail of the plane is a "tga" sticker, which is for TransGlobal Airlines. The airline name made up for the *Airport* movies that Mickey Michaels did the set decorations for. See Chapter 5 for more on Michaels.

Locations

The segment involving gymnasts was filmed at the La Cañada High School, about 13 miles north of Los Angeles. The segment involving the girl caught in the studio rafters on a wire was filmed on a Universal soundstage.

"Involvement"

> Episode #5.19
>
> Production #42820
>
> Filming began: October 21, 1975
>
> Airdate: January 24, 1976
>
> Writer: John Groves
>
> Director: Dennis Donnelly
>
> LACoFD Technical Advisor: John Larsen
>
> Guest cast: Anne Seymour (Nurse Milly Eastman), Dawn Lyn (Jean Clark), Jean Allison (mother, Dorothy Clark), Milton Frome (salesman), Del Monroe (Steve Carson)

Synopsis

Rampart's former emergency department head nurse (Anne Seymour) tries to commit suicide. A paraplegic child (Dawn Lyn) almost drowns in a swimming pool and gives the hospital staff a tough time. The nurse and child must share a room. Johnny and Roy help a woman who fainted and find her wrapped in plastic wrap, in an effort to lose weight. A family suffers from carbon monoxide poisoning. A car becomes trapped under a liquid hydrogen truck.

"Above and Beyond...Nearly"

Episode #5.20

Production #42823

Airdate: January 31, 1976

Writer: Preston Wood

Director: Christian I. Nyby II

LACoFD Technical Advisor: Joe Bartak, Jr. (PM0073)

Guest cast: Lucille Benson (Annie), Liam Dunn (Amos), Florence Lake (Maggie), Linda Dano (Joyce), Kristin Larkin (Carol), Grant Goodeve (Larry), Hal Baylor (Frank), with LA County Fire Chief Houts (as himself) and LACoFD chopper pilot Joe Kelly and LACoFD crewmember firefighter Dave Bowers

Synopsis

Roy and Johnny receive commendations for bravery from Chief Houts for an incident they can't remember. Johnny and Roy treat a 101-year-old man who breaks his ankle while dancing. In a nighttime response, the station rescues an injured man after a 30-foot fall from a cliff. A man has an apparent heart attack in his dentist's office.

Notes

Joe Bartak:

> I did just the one episode as the Technical Advisor, talk about pressure with the 'real' Chief Engineer on the set. I was at several other filming sites where they rode with us in the squad and filmed footage of the squad going code. Funny thing about the two stars was they had to be shown how to do CPR and all the routine stuff over and over again; made for job security for us. A lot of us worked as extras at different locations when they needed real firemen. I even stood in for Randy [Mantooth] once. It was a great and fun experience. I was just telling someone the other day how that program changed EMS during my career, what an asset it was to all of us; we have come a long way since then, for the better.

Johnny Miller was the stuntman in the stokes at the cliff rescue. He states, "I was high off the ground, 250 feet, with the chopper over head; it was a heart pounder for sure."

The copters did not fly with copilots. The crewman in the left seat was a firefighter in the early days. In this particular case, Dave Bowers later became a paramedic when they went to the paramedic program at Air Operations.

Liam Dunn (Amos) appeared as a long retired Fire Department of New York firefighter in the TV pilot *The Quinns* (filmed in the winter of 1975), which aired on ABC in July 1977, a little over a year after his death.

At the end of the episode, the comment by Chief Houts while pointing to Johnny, "By the way, don't forget to get your hair cut," was an ad-lib by Houts.

Locations

The dancing 'old-timer' segment was filmed at the E'Questre Inn at 1600 Riverside Drive in Burbank, now the Riverside Inn apartment complex. It was also used in the movie, *The Wild Life,* with Chris Penn and Eric Stoltz, released in 1984. See "Insanity Epidemic" (episode 6.14).

The day and night cliff rescue scenes were filmed in Bronson Canyon, near the site of the tunnel rescue in the World Premier.

"Grateful"

Episode #5.21

Production #42819

Filming began: December 1, 1975

Airdate: February 7, 1976

Writer: Michael Norell

Director: Georg Fenady

LACoFD Technical Advisor: Gerry Smith

Guest cast: Dick Van Patten, Zina Bethune, Paul Brinegar (Grady), Ruth Buzzi, Royal Dano, Thomas Bellin, LACoFD helicopter pilot Ted Hellmers

Synopsis

After a couple (Dick Van Patten and Ruth Buzzi) is injured when a car goes through a restaurant window, they become Station 51's biggest fans and get in the way of the paramedics as they try to do their job. An elderly man (Royal Dano) tries to save his friend's life by copying a medical technique he saw on television, CPR, and ends up doing more harm than good. A child is struck in the eye by a pellet from a BB gun. Johnny and Roy respond to a boat fire via Copter 10.

Notes

The Jaws of Life® is used by Marco in this episode, and the Hurst name is clearly visible.

Michael Norell (Captain Stanley) did not recall the sequence regarding the improper use of CPR between the two old gentlemen when asked about the story line. He was asked if it came as a result of critics of the show, including Dr. Nagel, regarding medical techniques used on *Emergency!* and other medical dramas. Norell advised, "I don't remember that story line at all, sorry. If I used it, it was just a little bit of satire on my part, not the result of any complaints by critics. I don't know of anything that came as a result of responding to critics." However, by the next season, a CPR disclaimer is seen at the end of each episode. The *New England Journal of Medicine* said in 1999 that the medical TV show *ER* misrepresents CPR, giving viewers a skewed perception of its usefulness.

Performing CPR on a "live" person for television and film is difficult to make look authentic, because some liberties must be taken. This includes the use of tight shots or cutaways. The victim is often a mannequin in the tight shots showing only the torso and proper hand placement, straight elbows, and depth of compressions. In the long shots where you see both the CPR giver and the actor/victim, the "correct" procedures are not possible. Why? Compression of the chest $1^1/2$ to 2 inches (4 to 6 cm) on an adult who is indeed "alive" can cause serious damage. To compensate for the "look" of the depth, the actor giving CPR must bend his or her elbows.

Locations
The boat rescue scenes were filmed at Castaic Lake State Recreation Area, off of the I-5 at the foot of The Grapevine. The scenes were originally filmed for the episode "Right at Home" (episode 5.17).

"The Great Crash Diet"

Episode #5.22

Production #42822

Final revision: November 24, 1975

Filming began: November 19, 1975

Note: Was actually 18th episode of the season to film

Airdate: February 21, 1976

Writer: Timothy Burns

Director: Joseph Pevney

LACoFD Technical Advisor: Richard Atkins

Guest cast: Michael Mullins (Bob Jensen), Holly Irving (Sarah), Rick Podell (Frank)

Synopsis

An experiment in firefighter nutrition becomes an obsession for Chet, to the dismay of his colleagues. While conducting a fire inspection at a marine park, Roy and Johnny get splashed by Corky, a killer whale, and rescue a diver trapped in an aquarium. A birthday boy eats too much raw bread dough and gets a severe stomachache, and a pregnant woman suffers complications while her mother is being treated for a possible heart attack. Following a vehicle accident, Captain Stanley is nearly electrocuted by a downed high power line as a result of the car hitting the power pole and starting a fire.

Notes

The killer whale, Corky, as seen in this segment, along with Orky was moved to SeaWorld San Diego when Marineland of the Pacific closed. The pilot whale, Bubbles, along with several dolphins was also relocated to SeaWorld. One of this book's authors, Richard, had the opportunity to work and play with Bubbles and several of the Dolphins while working at SeaWorld.

Locations

The trapped diver segment was filmed at Marineland of the Pacific, located at 6610 Palos Verdes Drive South, Rancho Palos Verdes. Marineland closed in 1987, but some of the original structures, parking lot, and entrance gate with the stylized T-shaped wave sign are still there. Other television programs shot there were *The Beverly Hillbillies* and *Sea Hunt*. Recent movies filmed on the site include *Charlie's Angels* and *Pirates of the Caribbean,* where they constructed the Fort as Port Royal Jamaica.

"The Tycoons"

Episode #5.23

Production #42816

Airdate: February 28, 1976

Writers: Mark Massari, Robert Hamilton, and John Groves

Director: Georg Fenady

LACoFD Technical Advisor: Richard Neal (P0M009)

Guest cast: Robin Clark (Chris), Sheila James (Phyllis), Ted Gehring (Mr. Hobson, owner of Davey's Dogs), Mary Moon (Leigh), John Wyler (Roger), Vince Howard

Synopsis

Johnny gets everyone but Roy excited about buying a nearby rundown hot dog stand, Davey's Dogs, and creating Station 51 Enterprises. An over-zealous neighbor (Sheila James) extinguishes a dumpster fire prior to the arrival of Engine 51. An 18-month-old toddler is treated at Rampart with unknown respiratory problems. Dr. Brackett has trouble with a victim of a gunshot who refuses to admit that he has been shot. A 30-year-old man is injured by debris kicked up from a lawnmower, sustaining a penetrating chest wound. The station responds to a chemical plant fire. The episode ends with Roy finally agreeing to contribute toward the purchase of Davey's Dogs when Captain Stanley walks in and advises that it has burned down during the previous shift; this event leaves Chet, Roy, and Johnny in the classic monkey pose of "see no evil, hear no evil, and speak no evil."

Notes

The segment with the man injured by the lawnmower was filmed for "Election" (episode 5.3), which aired earlier in the season. The gunshot segment was filmed for "Simple Adjustment" (episode 5.10), which also aired earlier. In an unusual move, all three writers are credited for this episode. Because the segments were already filmed and unused, they were inserted into this episode.

Sheila James-Kuehl (Zelda Gilroy on *The Many Loves of Dobie Gillis*) is currently a California Democratic Senator serving the Los Angeles area. After reviewing the tape that was sent to her, she stated, "I was doing a lot of freelancing at the time and I don't recall doing this part but glad I was portraying someone that was trying to be professional, with her notebook and all, someone in control."

The hot dog stand segment and the child who has ingested the detergent (slightly modified for this episode) is the only thing that survived from the original script, which also originally included the rescue of a man in a mini-submarine and the rescue of two children trapped in an abandoned missile silo at a former Coastal Artillery site.

Locations

At one time there were sixteen Nike missile silo sites in the Los Angeles area. All deactivated by 1974, one is leased by the LACoFD, located in Malibu at 24666 W. Saddle Peak Road off Piume Road, so more than likely it would have been filmed on this site.

"The Nuisance"

Working title: The Pest

Episode #5.24

Production #42824

Written: December 1, 1975

Final revision: January 7, 1976 (yes, after it began shooting)

Filming began: January 5, 1976

Note: This was the 21st episode of the season to film

Airdate: March 6, 1976

Writer: Robert Hamilton

Director: Randolph Mantooth

LACoFD Technical Advisor: Robert McCullough (PM0038)

Guest cast: Gretchen Corbett (Nurse Mary Lynn Smith), Carole Cook (Nurse Beauxchet), James G. Richardson (Craig Brice), Jean Shawlee, Coleen Gray (Clair), Joseph Perry, Matthew "Stymie" Beard (bar owner), Marla Adams (as a bored, neurotic housewife who is a patient on a TV soap on Johnny's hospital room TV—uncredited)

Synopsis

While responding to a late night call at a local bar, Johnny becomes the victim of a hit-and-run driver, resulting in a broken leg. With Johnny in the hospital, Roy is temporarily teamed up with "the world's most perfect paramedic," Craig Brice (James G. Richardson). A man suffers from heart problems. The station responds to a fire in an abandoned warehouse where Roy, Marco, and Brice become trapped. Roy and Marco are injured, but Brice escapes unharmed. Roy and Marco are roommates in the hospital and Johnny comes by to see them in his wheelchair. Johnny tries to make a date with his physical therapist (Gretchen Corbett).

Notes

Note that Randy Mantooth directed this episode and episode 6.14.

The soap opera scenes shown on TV in Johnny's room were written by Hannah Shearer, her first writing bit for the series. She would assist in writing for several others including cowriting some of the after-series movies.

Both Randy and Marla would end up as cast members of *General Hospital,* but not at the same time—Randy as Richard Halifax (1992–1993) and Marla as Mildred Deal (1987).

Joseph Perry is Matthew Perry's *(Friends)* father.

The fire department PIO being interviewed about the firemen trapped in the collapsed building (as seen on Johnny's hospital room TV) is not Dick Friend; he was an uncredited actor portraying an unnamed PIO.

SEASON 6

During this final season, at the end of each episode, thereby shortening the story line by 30 seconds, was a CPR disclaimer. Several of the *Emergency!* actors did voiceovers over a scene from *Emergency!*, showing Johnny, Roy, and the squad, along with some of their equipment, demonstrating CPR. It began right after credits and the "hammer hitting" the Mark VII logo.

The voiceover said:

> This is (name of actor); what you are watching is a scene from *Emergency!* showing a simulation of cardiopulmonary resuscitation, better known as CPR. When respiratory or cardiac arrest occurs, and it can happen to anyone, anywhere, and at anytime, permanent brain damage begins after 4 minutes and death can occur after 6 minutes. CPR is the only method by which life can be prolonged until help can arrive. CPR is easy to learn and easy to do, but, CPR cannot be learned by watching *Emergency!* or any other television show, and done wrong it can be worse than useless. It takes about 4 hours of proper instruction to learn how to save a life. So do it now and learn to do it right. For further information about CPR training programs in your community, contact the American Heart Association, the American National Red Cross, or your local fire department.

This disclaimer may or may not have been a result of the episode called "Grateful" (episode 5.21), in which one of the actors performs CPR on his friend, "like I saw on TV." He thought his friend was having a heart attack and, in doing so, did more harm than good for him. This disclaimer was cut during later syndication and TVLand's airing. An audio of this disclaimer is all that is known to exist.

The Game

Episode #6.1

Production #44906

Filming began: August 7, 1976

Note: Episode #105 of the series; 7th episode filmed for the season, but the 1st to air

Airdate: September 25, 1976

Writer and director: Christian I. Nyby II

LACoFD Technical Advisor: Gary Davis (PM0003)

Guest cast: Larry Carroll, Jack Knight (football fan), Jack Carter (Drew McWhorter), Steve Drexel, Polly Middleton, Laurie Kennedy (Paramedic Coordinator), Jesse Wayne

Synopsis
Roy and Johnny draw duty for the big University of Southern California Trojans football game at the LA Coliseum. While there, they treat a TV announcer (Jack Carter), a fan (Jack Knight) with food lodged in his throat, an overly excited man with breathing difficulties, and an injured photographer on the sidelines. A woman accidentally pulls her husband off the roof into a tree in another incident.

Notes
This episode was to originally begin shooting on June 22, 1976, becoming the third episode of the season to be filmed (episode 101 of the series). The Technical Advisor for the episode, Gary Davis, attended the production meeting to go over the final revisions of June 16 for shooting the following week. The episode got delayed and did not begin shooting until August, becoming the seventh episode of the season to be filmed.

There was no actual game going on at the time of filming. Although filmed at the stadium, the use of stock footage of a game and extras to fill portions of the stands made it look authentic.

This is the only series episode written and directed by the same person, Christian I. Nyby II. He would write and direct two post-series *Emergency!* movies.

"Not Available"

Episode #6.2

Production #44912

Filming dates: July 13–20, 1976

Note: Episode #103 for the series; 5th episode filmed for the season

Airdate: October 2, 1976

Writer: Preston Wood

Director: Cliff Bole

LACoFD Technical Advisor: Kirk Kington (PM0063)

Guest cast: Arnold Turner, Wayne Heffley (Holt), Scott Arthur Allen (firefighter/paramedic Kirk), Bill Boyett (Engine 39 Captain), Kristen Banfield, Dorothy Love (Florence), Ivy Bethune (May), Burton Cooper (Reed)

Synopsis

Roy and Johnny are frustrated when calls for minor problems leave them not available for those who really need their help. Saddled with a rule that prevents various squads from crossing into each other's assigned territory, Gage and DeSoto nearly lose a patient due to their long travel time, which could have been more easily reached by another squad. The squad responds to a man with a possible heart attack, a woman who fainted outside a grocery store, and a man trapped in a car. Roy must rescue an escaped prisoner stranded on the side of a downtown high-rise building.

Notes

It is stated in this episode that there were thirty-one squads in service in LA County that responded to 60,000 incidents a year, although it is not known if this information is factual.

Bill Boyett as Captain of Engine 39 later appears as William Boyett in the role of Chief McConnike.

Locations

The fainting woman at the grocery store was filmed in Burbank. The car accident was also filmed in Burbank on Chandler Street near Clyborne and Burbank Boulevard.

The call to the trailer park was filmed at 11644 Hartsook Street in North Hollywood.

The building used in the rescue of the prisoner is the San Pedro Municipal Building, also known as San Pedro City Hall at 638 Beacon Street. Built in 1928, it housed the jail on the top floor (the seventh floor) and the San Pedro Fire Department on the ground floor, which opened up onto Harbor Boulevard.

The fire station part of the building began operation in 1928 as Station 36, when the building opened. Closed in 1972 when LA City annexed the area, it is now a fire museum that opened in 2003 and is run by the Los Angeles Fire Department Historical Society. The theme of the museum is Harbor Fire-Fighting and Rescue. It contains four retired Los Angeles Fire Department fire apparatus and many displays of LACoFD and harbor-related items such as a fireboat and dive display, hose fittings, various tools and equipment.

The building has recently been renovated, and today, many LA City entities as well as the Councilperson of the 15th District occupy many of the offices.

The LAFD Museum in Hollywood is located at 1355 North Cahuenga Boulevard and is the former site of LA City Station 27. This museum is run by the Los Angeles Fire Department Historical Society. The museum is open Saturdays from 10 A.M. to 4 P.M. For more information, visit its Web site at http://www.lafd.org/lafdhs.htm.

"The Unlikely Heirs"

Episode #6.3

Production #44904

Filming began: June 11, 1976

Note: Episode #100 for the series; 2nd episode filmed for the season

Airdate: October 9, 1976

Writer: Timothy Burns

Director: Georg Fenady

LACoFD Technical Advisor: Richard Atkins

Guest cast: Paul Brinegar (Max), Bennye Gatteys (Cheryl), Jim Stathis (Stuart) and Simba (the cat), with Sam Lainer and Duane Lewis (LACoFD dispatchers)

Synopsis

The station rescues a homeless man (Paul Brinegar) from a fire, only to discover the man's mattress had $80,000 in it. When the grateful victim tries to give the station a $20,000 reward, he is turned down because of department regulations. After a bride (Bennye Gatteys) faints while walking down the aisle and ends up in the hospital, Dixie and Dr. Early come to the rescue. A light plane crashes into a warehouse, causing an explosion, requiring assistance by Foam 127.

Notes

Jim Stathis would later be seen in another fire program, *Rescue 77* (episode 1.5).

"That Time of Year"

Episode #6.4

Production #44905

Final revision: June 29, 1976

Filming began: July 1, 1976

Note: Episode #102 for the series; 4th episode filmed for the season

Airdate: October 23, 1976

Writers: Mort Thaw and Edward Robak

Director: Dennis Donnelly

LACoFD Technical Advisor: Bob Lee Hancock (PM0177)

Guest cast: Ronnie Schell (Allan), Dave Pritchard (Jack), Pamela Shoop (Marcia), Meg Wyllie (Mrs Pastone), Don Fenwick (Larry), Linda Gray (Judy)

Synopsis

Roy gets more advice than he wanted while trying to plan his vacation. A fire at a nightclub causes more problems for Roy as a patron (Linda Gray) insists that her boyfriend (Don Fenwick) is still inside. Roy is seriously overcome by smoke and heat during the rescue, which threatens his vacation plans. A self-defense instructor has a very enthusiastic student, and a pair of hang-gliders crash into the side of a cliff.

Notes

Watch for Linda Gray, in the *Emergency!* movie *The Steel Inferno.* She would go on to play Sue Ellen Ewing on the long-running, prime-time 1980s soap, *Dallas.*

After the scene in which Linda Gray is talking to Mike Norell about her boyfriend still inside the burning building, the director (Dennis Donnelly) did not yell "Cut" and kept the cameras rolling. Prompted by Dennis before the scene, Linda turned to Mike and said, "What ya doing after the fire?" and just broke Mike up.

From TA Bob Lee Hancock: "I was most surprised by the amount of time it took to shoot each episode. I worked on the episode for 8 days, for about 45 minutes of actual TV time. Reading the scripts, looking for sites to shoot, and then going over the footage and cutting room stuff. I mostly enjoyed the crew and staff and how well they worked with the TAs....One thing I remember changing was the set decorators were putting donuts on plates, with knifes, forks, and napkins for each firefighter at the table. I remember telling them that was not the way a donut would've been eaten at a firehouse. You should have seen the looks I got."

"Fair Fight"

Episode #6.5

Production #44903

Written: April 27, 1976

Filming dates: June 2–9, 1976

Note: Episode #99 for the series; 1st episode filmed for the season

Airdate: October 30, 1976

Writer: Preston Wood

Director: Kevin Tighe

LACoFD Technical Advisor: Robert Hoff (PM0071)

Guest cast: Terry Kiser and Anne Schedeen (Wes and Margo Hubbard), James Ingersoll (lab guard), Jack Binder

Synopsis

Claiming that it is actually therapeutic, a husband and wife (Terry Kiser and Anne Schedeen) become embroiled in several violent arguments with tragic consequences. The station gets a new mascot (Henry), who turns out to be a real ball of fire. Johnny and Roy break into a top-secret lab during a fire. During an attempt to rescue two men trapped underground in a tunnel collapse, Johnny ends up needing to be rescued himself.

Notes

Technical Advisor Bob Hoff states that Randy Mantooth had a tough time getting through the window with his breathing apparatus on and kept hitting the frame of the window with the bottle. Although realistic, Bob insisted, the scene was cut by Cinader because it looked too unprofessional to him.

Locations

The top-secret lab incident was filmed at the Shell Oil Cracking Plant, near 190th Street and Vermont in Carson, south of the junction of the Harbor (I-110) and San Diego (I-405) Freeways.

"Rules of Order"

Episode #6.6

Production #44907

Airdate: November 6, 1976

Writer: James G. Richardson

Director: Georg Fenady

LACoFD Technical Advisor: Louis Danes

Guest cast: James G. Richardson (Firefighter/Paramedic Craig Brice), Larry Manetti (Firefighter/Paramedic Bert Dwyer), Vince Howard,

Buck Young (lineman), Ray Ballard (press agent), Bert Holland (Hoover), and Captain/Paramedic Bob Belliveau (as himself)

Synopsis
Johnny and Roy are asked to be on a paramedic advisory committee, but so is Johnny's nemesis, Craig Brice. A power pole worker (Buck Young) is injured when a car hits the pole he is working on. The station must rescue two injured mountain climbers stranded on the side of a building.

Notes
Uncredited in this episode is paramedic Bob Belliveau, who sits in on the paramedic committee, who recalls:

> I learned a great deal during "Rules of Order," especially my few lines. The real actors don't put as much effort into learning lines because they're used to it, they ad-lib, and they have teleprompters. I came to appreciate their skills at acting. I was supposedly paired up with the "Mr. Right" (Craig Brice) of the paramedics, and I was supposed to act a bit on the crude side, which probably came easy. Also, I was buddies with the dog (some of Mr. Cinader's humor), because I'm not much of a pet person.

Larry Manetti is end-credited as Firefighter/Paramedic Bert Dwyer in this episode although he is called Charlie. It was Bryan Cutler who portrayed Firefighter/Paramedic Bert Dwyer earlier in "Daisy's Pick" (episode 4.7) and "Fugitive" (episode 4.5). Manetti would portray a different character in the *Emergency!* movie, *Most Deadly Passage*. Manetti will be more recognized as Orville "Rick" Wright in *Magnum P.I.*

"The Exam"

Episode #6.7
Production #44911
Airdate: November 13, 1976
Writer: Tom Egan
Director: Richard Bennett
LACoFD Technical Advisor: Robert Lee
Guest cast: Bridget Hanley (Molly), Jodean Russo (Mrs. Cooper), Allan Lurie (Sam Cooper)

Synopsis
Johnny and Roy prepare for a recertification exam, which a number of their fellow paramedics have already failed. A fireman's widow becomes too

dependent on the station for help with all kinds of minor problems. A TV sports fan (Allan Lurie) experiences shortness of breath. A car chase stunt goes wrong on a movie set at World Studios, and a deadly fire results.

Location
The car crash ends up on the steps of Sparticus Square at Universal.

"Captain Hook"

> Episode #6.8
>
> Production #44909
>
> Airdate: November 20, 1976
>
> Writer: Susan J. Alenick
>
> Director: Christian I. Nyby, II
>
> LACoFD Technical Advisor: Ray Thompson
>
> Guest cast: Joe Maross (Captain Hookrader), Jim B. Smith (police sergeant), Chad States (Terry), Rick Podell (Mike Kendall), Vince Howard, William Bryant (Captain, Engine 45), Bert Williams (Carter), Joann Hicks (Sally Robbins)

Synopsis
Eager to celebrate the scheduled retirement of an unpopular Captain (Joe Maross), Station 51 overdoes its enthusiasm for the going-away party. Johnny and Roy take care of a woman (Joann Hicks) dressed in a polar bear costume when she is overcome by heat exhaustion. A young man is injured in a tire explosion and refuses pain medication. The station rescues two California Highway Patrol officers when their helicopter crashes. A family becomes hysterical when they think their sleeping mother has died.

"Computer Terror"

> Working title: Checkmate
>
> Episode #6.9
>
> Production #44917
>
> Filming began: September 29, 1976
>
> Note: Episode #110 for the series; 12th episode filmed for the season
>
> Airdate: December 4, 1976
>
> Writer: Bruce Shelly
>
> Director: Georg Fenady

LACoFD Technical Advisor: Robert McCullough P0038

Guest cast: Ted Gehring (Clinton), Zitto Kazann (Alvie), Russ Grieve, Walt Davis (Henry)

Synopsis
A computer mistake gives Johnny a paycheck in thousands, instead of hundreds, of dollars. A man is injured when he falls asleep in an auto salvage yard and ends up in a car crusher. An overly affectionate dog causes major problems for Roy, Johnny, and a man with a bad back. Roy takes an unexpected swim in a pool during a medical call. Johnny rescues a man trapped on a scaffold who becomes injured while hanging the building's logo.

Notes
They used the same building for climbers stuck on the side of the building in "Rules of Order" (episode 6.6) as they did for the guys stranded on the scaffold in this episode.

The pool scenes were filmed on Universal's backlot at Bristol Court, not at a faux residence but at the time a complex called the "Sacramento Arms Motor Court." The site was used for countless scenes in film and television, and it was also the site of the series *90 Bristol Court,* airing on NBC (1964–1965). Jack Klugman (*Quincy M.E., Odd Couple,* and even *Third Watch*) portrayed one of the residents in the "Harris Against the World" segment, who was a superintendent of a major Hollywood studio. If the guys left the pool area without going through the house and went through the back gate, they would end up on the Western Set.

"Welcome to Santa Rosa County"

Working titles: Loan Out; Welcome to Canyon County

Episode #6.10

Production #44916

Final revision: October 5, 1976

Filming dates: November 8–15, 1976

Note: Episode #114 for the series; 16th episode filmed for the season

Airdate: December 25, 1976

Writer: Preston Wood

Director: Christian I. Nyby II

LACoFD Technical Advisor: Richard Neal (PM0009)

Guest cast: James Jeter (Sheriff Bittner), Carla Layton, Paul Deadrick, Mike Cassidy, Bill Watson

Synopsis

Johnny and Roy take a fishing trip to Santa Rosa County, but it turns into a working vacation when they must rescue climbers (Paul Deadrick and Mike Cassidy) trapped on a cliff and help a man injured in a boat explosion.

Notes

Randy Mantooth's real Land Rover is used in this episode. Note the California State Firefighter Association sticker on the windshield. "Richard's Ambulance" arrives to transport a burn victim. It's the white over yellow (1968–1971) Chevrolet Suburban used in several episodes (with "Mayfair" logo) and the movie *The Steel Inferno*.

Locations

The cliff rescue was filmed in the San Gabriel Mountians near Kratka Ridge (Angeles Crest Highway), just past the tunnels, about 51 miles from Los Angeles. The scenes with the sheriff and Johnny and Roy discussing the paramedic program and the training of volunteers over lunch was shot at the Angeles National Forest Visitor Center in Big Pines. The lake for the fishing scenes was at Jackson Lake, near Wrightwood. Other scenes were shot at the Methodist Camp above the center of town in Wrightwood.

"Paperwork"

Episode #6.11

Production #44913

Filming began: August 20, 1976

Airdate: January 8, 1977

Note: Episode #107 for the series; 9th episode filmed for the season

Writer: John Groves

Director: Georg Fenady

LACoFD Technical Advisor: Mark Hefley (PM0079)

Guest cast: Peter Kastner (Marty), Laurie Kennedy (Nurse Patterson), Peter Brocco (professor), Michael Masters (workman), William Bronder (tree trimmer), Jeff Cotler (Mike)

Synopsis

A computer error and Rampart's new supply system create extra paperwork for all members of Station 51. A child (Jeff Cotler) falls into a storm drain and nearly drowns. A research assistant (Peter Kastner) accidentally drinks ancient Mesopotamian wine. The station responds to a warehouse fire and treats a workman (Michael Masters) suffering from burns.

"Loose Ends"

Episode #6.12

Production #44908

Airdate: January 15, 1977

Writer: Dee Murphy

Director: Dennis Donnelly

LACoFD Technical Advisor: Charles Gibson

Guest cast: Walter Mathews (Ed), Tara Talboy (Tina), William Boyett (Battalion Chief McConnike), William Bryant (Fire Captain), Vince Howard (police officer), John Zonda (police officer)

Synopsis

The squad responds to a traffic accident, and Johnny and Roy are shocked to find that Dr. Brackett is one of the patients. Dr. Brackett blames himself when the accident claims the life of the driver leaving a little girl (Tara Talboy) fatherless. Roy and Johnny treat an undercover police officer suffering from chest pains. The station responds to a fire at a rail yard involving ammonia.

Notes

Johnny is not wearing his paramedic-identified helmet at the accident scene although Roy is.

"An Ounce of Prevention"

Episode #6.13

Production #44914

Airdate: January 22, 1977

Writers: Mort Thaw and Ed Robak

Director: Christian I. Nyby II

LACoFD Technical Advisor: Unknown

Guest cast: On Ferris wheel: Peggy Webber (Helen Phillips), Richard Carlyle (Bert Phillips), Barbara Ellen Levene (Ginnie).

Other cast: Frank Farmer (Frank Bartell), Maureen Lee (Donna Bartell), Chad States, Dave Barry (Tom Jensen).

Synopsis

Several people are trapped on a Ferris wheel. A child ingests pesticides. Johnny volunteers Roy and himself to discuss fire prevention on the "Tom Jensen Show" (Dave Barry), where they become the stars of a real-life emergency on the set as a member of the production crew is injured. Jensen keeps the cameras rolling while Gage and DeSoto do their work.

Notes

The Ferris wheel rescue was filmed in Long Beach on the site of The Pike, along the area of Ocean Boulevard and Pacific Avenue. Much has changed since the mile-long Pike along Ocean Boulevard opened in the early 1900s with the first roller coaster, the Cyclone Racer, extending out over the ocean. The Pike officially closed in 1979.

Other prominent buildings seen in this episode are the New Long Beach City Hall and Library complex, the 100-year-old Clock Tower, both along Pacific Avenue, the Ocean Center Building (southwest corner of Ocean and Pine), and the building now known as the Verizon building (southwest corner of Ocean and Pacific in front of which the Ferris Wheel was erected).

Today occupying the site of The Pike are three stories of subterranean parking; above that are two, nine-story residential towers and next to that are some retail structures. They command a grand view because looking South across Shoreline Village and the Los Angeles River, one will see the Queen Mary and a Russian submarine docked across the harbor. Until recently Howard Hughes's "Spruce Goose," more correctly known as the "Hughes Flying Boat, H-4, HK-1," was also on display near the Queen Mary. The Spruce Goose, built in 1947, is now on display in Oregon at 500 NE Captain Michael King Smith Way, McMinnville, Oregon.

"The Pike at Rainbow Harbor," near the site of the original, features an oceanside corridor, open-air marketplaces, theater, antique carousel, and Ferris wheel with photos and artifacts from the historic Pike.

In actuality the closest fire station to the area is actually Long Beach Station 1, a stone's throw from The Pike, and it had paramedics at this station at time of filming. Long Beach had fifteen paramedics graduate in 1972 after attending classes at Harbor General Hospital and after 4 weeks of clinical work at St. Mary's Hospital. When the clinicals were completed, the firefighters began 8 weeks of internship ride-a-longs with three LA County paramedic squads.

"Insanity Epidemic"

Episode #6.14

Production #44901

Filming dates: August 1976

Airdate: February 5, 1977

Writer: Robert Hamilton

Director: Randolph Mantooth

LACoFD Technical Advisor: Unknown

Guest cast: Robert Pratt (gas station attendant), Bill Zuckert (Bill Nelson, gas station owner), Nancy Fox (skating instructor), Vince Howard (police officer), Harold Frizzell (ambulance attendant), Ellen Moss (Thelma), Vincent St. Cyr (Bruno), Betty Ann Carr (Lucy), Susan Alpern (Jody), Robert Shayne (Raymond Foster), Angela May (Sandy Foster), William Boyett (Chief McConnike)

Synopsis

Captain Stanley panics when he learns that McConnike (William Boyett), one of his former Captains, is the new Battalion Chief and is coming to the station for an inspection. Marco has a close call during a fire at a gas station after the irate station owner ordered the attendant to turn the power to the pumps back on, resulting in the explosion and fire. A man (Robert Shayne) is hit in the chest by a nail from a nail gun. Brawling clowns in an ice show cause problems for the crew. A car drives off an overpass and crashes into a truck filled with pesticides, trapping two teenagers (Betty Ann Carr and Susan Alpern); the Jaws are used. Chet tries to coax Henry the dog off the couch and into the dog house by getting in it himself.

Notes

In a bit of continuity, McConnike had already appeared as the Chief in a previous incident with the crew ("Loose Ends," episode 6.12). This is one of the episodes aired out of order.

The man who is injured with the nail gun (Robert Shayne) was a regular in the original black-and-white television series *Superman*, starring George Reeves; he portrayed Inspector William Henderson.

Rubber cement was used for the fire trail at the gas station fire. Mike Stoker, who was on the hose line a bit, actually singed his eyebrows and eyelashes.

Locations

The gas station fire scenes were filmed at Milan's Auto Detail, in Burbank, where gas was 58 cents a gallon for ethyl, now known as premium. Cigarettes were 47 cents a pack.

Across the street from the scenes shot at the gas station is an apartment complex called the E'Questre Inn as used in "Above and Beyond...Nearly" (5.20).

The ice rink scenes were also filmed in Burbank, at Marlindo's Bowl, just down the street from the gas station and the E'Questre Inn; both were used in the film *The Wild Life*.

Scenes where Captain Stanley and Chief McConnike get drenched by a loose hose line were filmed on Universal's New York Street.

"Breakdown"

Episode #6.15

Production #44902

Filming began: October 19, 1976

Note: Episode #112 for the series; 14th episode filmed for the season

Airdate: February 12, 1977

Writer: John Groves

Director: Georg Fenady

LACoFD Technical Advisor: Bruce Mortimer

Guest cast: Dick Bakalyan (Charley the mechanic), Brian Byers (Gerald), Joan Roberts (Jane), Jean Allison (Grace)

Synopsis

Johnny and Roy fail to heed Captain Stanley's advice not to "cross the mechanic" (Dick Bakalyan) after a series of electrical shorts plagues the squad. A back-to-nature couple (Brian Byers and Joan Roberts) discover they have a variant of anthrax. The station responds to Oceanland Park to rescue an injured man from the 320-foot sky tower.

Locations

The scene where the squad makes its final breakdown after turning the corner was just around the corner from Station 127. They just turned off East 223rd Street, making a left onto Wilmington.

The sky tower rescue scenes were shot at the old Marineland of the Pacific in Palos Verdes.

"Family Ties"

> Episode #6.16
>
> Production #44910
>
> Airdate: February 19, 1977
>
> Writers: Carole and Michael Raschella
>
> Director: Cliff Bole
>
> LACoFD Technical Advisor: Frank Mrosek
>
> Guest cast: Howard Honig (Arthur Bayes), Susan Lawrence (Susan Bayse), Jimmy Van Patten (Mark), Debbie Storm (Toni), Dirk Evans (truck driver)

Synopsis

Roy's nagging mother-in-law is scheduled for her annual visit. A car runs into the back of a truck. There's a fire at Rampart. A model rocket sets an attic on fire, trapping two teenagers (Jimmy Van Patten and Debbie Storm), and Chet is thrown into a tree by the subsequent explosion. A man gets lead poisoning from home-brewed "medicine." Dr. Brackett and Dr. Early argue over attending a convention in Acapulco.

Notes

Drs. Brackett and Early were going to Hawaii in the original script.

"Bottom Line"

> Episode #6.17
>
> Production #44915
>
> Filming began: October 28, 1976
>
> Note: Episode #113 for the series; 15th episode filmed for the season
>
> Airdate: February 26, 1977
>
> Writers: Charlene and Robert Bcalver
>
> Director: Dennis Donnelly
>
> LACoFD Technical Advisor: David Heath
>
> Guest cast: Nick Pellegrino (coach), Vince Howard, Belle Ellig, Kedric Wolfe (Duke), Johnny Timko

Synopsis

Johnny and Roy clash with Dr. Morton over his conservative approach to caring for patients, which they feel is tying them up at the hospital for too long. A phosphorus grenade injures a man. While responding to a minor call, the station rescues a drowning man. A police officer (Vince Howard) and another car are involved in a traffic accident. The officer, who sustains a head injury, pulls his gun on Johnny. A coach (Nick Pellegrino) brings in one of his kids who had been hit in the head with a baseball.

Notes
Look closely as Engine 51 pulls out of the station in one scene while on location at Station 127. The photos on the right side of the large map on the wall are actual photos of fires that 127 responded to.

"The Firehouse Five, Plus One"

Working title: Firehouse Quintet

Episode #6.18

Production #44919

Final revision: December 10, 1976

Filming began: December 7, 1976

Note: Episode #117 for the series; 19th episode filmed for the season

Airdate: March 5, 1977

Writer: Christian I. Nyby II

Director: Georg Fenady

LACOFD Technical Advisor: Ray Valasek

Guest cast: Joanne DeVarona, Howard McGillin, Harold "Happy" Harriston (referee), Herb Vigran (Lou), James Westmoreland, with the starting 5 from the LACoFD Firemen's Olympics "gold medal" team (as Station 16)

Synopsis
Station 51 makes it to the semi-finals of the fire department basketball league, but a heavy load of emergency calls the night before the game dims their hopes for a victory. The station responds to a fire in a school cafeteria. A gymnast collapses at the gym where Station 51 is practicing for the game. The station must rescue an injured man from the ceiling of a soundstage at a film studio. Station 51 plays against Station 16's B shift and wins the basketball game 42 to 40.

Notes
Harold "Happy" Harriston of the LA Lakers plays the referee in the basketball game.

LA County firefighter John Price was one of the members of the basketball team for Station 16, all of whom went uncredited. Price stated: "The filming day started early around 0600 and ended at approximately 1600 hours." Price also appeared in the World Premier as the engineer on Engine 36; his name is on his turn-out coat at the pump panel. Price actually worked at Station 36.

The first California Summer Firemen's Olympics was hosted by the San Francisco FD in 1971. Price's basketball team won the silver medal, and their volleyball team won the gold. In 1972, it was hosted by LACoFD, and most of the events were held at El Camino College. That year, the team won gold medals in basketball and volleyball. Captain Dick Hammer (season 1's first Captain) was also on the Fireman's Olympics basketball team at the time but was not in this episode as a player.

Herb Vigran also appeared in the *Emergency!* World Premier as a committee member. He appeared earlier with Robert Fuller (Dr. Brackett) and John Smith (the second Captain at Station 51) in the TV western *Laramie* in 1959.

Watch the scene where the guys had to push Chet's car down the hill to the community center. In 1976, the nation's 200th birthday, the city of Burbank, as did many communities across the nation, had a project of painting all their fire hydrants in patriotic themes. You can see one on the street corner in that scene.

Locations
Station 51 practicing and the game were filmed at the McCambridge Park Building (1515 North Glenoaks Boulevard) in Burbank.

"The Boat"

Episode #6.19

Production #44926

Written: December 10, 1974

Filming began: January 4, 1977

Note: Episode #119 for the series; 21st episode filmed for the season

Airdate: March 12, 1977

Writers: Hannah Shearer, Charlene and Bob Bcalver, John Groves, and Bruce Shelly

Director: Georg Fenady

LACoFD Technical Advisor: Jim Knight

Guest cast: Dick Bakalyan, Ted Gehring, Zitto Kazann, William Boy-ett, Howard Curtis (Technician), Michele Noval (Nurse Mary), Vince Howard

Synopsis

When Charlie the mechanic (Dick Bakalyan) stores the boat he's trying to sell at the station, the crew decides to chip in and buy it. Johnny and Roy board a Coast Guard helicopter for a rescue on Catalina Island. A bookie has a heart attack, and the station has to break into his office. A basement explosion and fire in the lab at Rampart leaves Dixie among the injured needing to be evacuated.

Notes

The lab at Rampart has typically been upstairs: "Take it up to the lab." In this episode it is in the basement. However, in "Boot" (episode 2.19), the lab was in a building outside of the main hospital, where it too suffered an explosion and fire.

Assisting on the fire at Rampart were Engines 36, 236, and 73 (which is a Ward LaFrance).

Coast Guard unit 1442 was utilized in this episode with much of the same footage from "Election" (episode 5.3): same scenes of point of depar-ture from the fictitious Air Station, same large ship in the harbor passed on the way out, same shots of the helicopter rounding a point of land, same footage inside the copter with both medics looking out the windows, and same interior shots over their shoulders.

In this episode, though, Roy leans forward and asks the pilot, "What's the story?" The pilot tells about the boat crash. In "Election," it's the same scene, but the voice of the pilot answers, "L.A. reports a victim at the base of the cliff, apparently still alive, 5 miles north of Cherry Cove," in an ap-parent voiceover. It's exactly the same footage until they arrive at the site, which also appears to be in the same area, but without the boat wreckage.

There were, however, two different crewmen. In "The Boat" he wore a different helmet and had no mustache. Neither said any lines. Both ran the winch, although in "The Boat" it was hooked up to a basket and in "Elec-tion" they used the floatation collars and the Stokes.

Cherry Cove is an actual location on Catalina Island.

John Groves wrote "Election," and he was given writer's credit in this episode for using those scenes.

The Coast Guard helicopter returns from Catalina with the patients and Johnny and Roy on board and lands at the helipad at Rampart. In ac-tuality this rarely happened, with the Coast Guard typically flying into Torrance Memorial Medical Center Hospital at 3330 Lomita Boulevard, which is about 3 miles west (as a Helicopter flies) of Harbor General.

"Isolation"

> Episode #6.20
>
> Production #44921
>
> Airdate: March 19, 1977
>
> Writer: John Groves
>
> Director: Georg Fenady
>
> LACoFD Technical Advisor: Unknown
>
> Guest cast: William Bryant (Captain, Station 86), Lyndel Stuart (Dr. Slade), Bette Ford (June Edwards), Vince Howard, Glen Sipes

Synopsis

Johnny and Roy are stranded at Station 86 when a severe rainstorm washes out the only road out of the area, leaving them the only medical help in the community. While on their own, Roy and Johnny treat people injured in an automobile accident, an elderly woman with an injured hip, a man with heart problems, and a young boy suffering from bronchitis. Rampart treats a police officer hit by lightning. LA Copter 15 transports Johnny and Roy's patients to the hospital, where a power failure complicates matters. Dr. Morton accompanies the paramedics back to Station 86, where they respond to an auto accident with multiple injuries.

Notes

The fire station used in this episode was LA County Station 65 at 4206 North Cornell Road, in the city of Agoura Hills, almost 50 miles from Station 127 (that is, *Emergency!* Station 51).

"All Night Long"

> Episode #6.21
>
> Production #44925
>
> Final revision: January 27, 1977
>
> Note: Episode #122 for the series; 24th episode filmed for the season; last episode filmed
>
> Airdate: March 26, 1977
>
> Writer: Kevin Tighe

Director: Georg Fenady

LACoFD Technical Advisors: Warren Hahne and Bob Lee Hancock (PM0177)

Guest cast: James McEachin (Julius Clarke), Carmen Zapata (Marina Martinez, injured in vehicle accident), Bill Walker (James Jefferson), Vince Howard, James Griffith, Patti Jerome, Jamie Lee Curtis* (as 17-year-old Susan Ruddy)

Synopsis

Johnny is inspired to write his own version of a TV game show but is thwarted by a series of emergency calls. Roy and Johnny treat a former jazz singer suffering from chest pains. The station responds to a nighttime multi-vehicle car accident. A daredevil must be rescued from a rope strung between buildings. Johnny has a long discussion with Henry.

Notes

*Jamie Lee Curtis (18 years old) did not appear in this episode; more than likely, she was in another one of those scenes cut due to time. The script scenes with her are scenes 23 to 46 (November 1976 draft) as a babysitter whose 4-year-old charge has taken several aspirin and become lethargic, necessitating the call for Johnny and Roy. Because this was the last episode that was filmed for the season, as well as the series, it never got a chance for a reinsert into another episode. This would have been her second appearance on television; her first was in a *Quincy* episode.

Bob Lee Hancock (PM0177) replaced Warren Hahne the last two days of shooting because of a prior commitment.

"Upward and Onward"

Episode #6.22

Production #44922

Final revision: December 13, 1976

Filming dates: December 16–23, 1976

Note: Episode #118 for the series; 20th episode filmed for the season

Airdate: April 2, 1977

Writer: Michael Norell

Director: Dennis Donnelly

LACoFD Technical Advisor: Gil Gillespie

Guest cast: Leon Ames (Alec Sudhoff), Dabbs Greer (Dr. Nippert), Tom Williams (Arnold Meyers), Tabi Cooper (Jody), William Boyett (Chief)

Synopsis

Captain Stanley worries that the Battalion Chief (William Boyett) will sabotage his attempt to pass the Chief's exam because of an incident in their past. A soap opera doctor (Leon Ames) is stricken just before he is to go on the air and is rushed to Rampart. His producer, Arnold Meyers (Tom Williams), causes problems in the hospital when he attempts to broadcast from the star's sickbed. A faulty elevator during a crucial rescue attempt of ailing Dr. Nippart (Dabbs Greer) complicates treatment.

"Hypochondri-Cap"

Episode #6.23

Production #44924

Airdate: April 16, 1977

Writer: Bruce Shelly

Director: Dennis Donnelly

LACoFD Technical Advisor: Unknown

Guest cast: William Bryant (Fire Captain), George Brenlin, Bette Ford, Vince Howard, William Boyett (Battalion Chief), Lani Gustavson (oil rig foreman), Abraham Alvarez

Synopsis

Captain Stanley is convinced he has career-ending arthritis in his hands but won't see a doctor until the crew sets up an appointment he can't refuse. A man gets his hand caught in his garage door opener. The station responds to a two-alarm fire at an oil refinery.

"Limelight"

Episode #6.24

Production #44923

Note: Episode #120 for the series; 22nd episode filmed for the season

Airdate: April 23, 1977

Writer: James G. Richardson

Director: Christian I. Nyby II

LACoFD Technical Advisor: Thomas Qualls

Guest cast: James G. Richardson (Firefighter/Paramedic, Station 16), William Bryant (Captain, Engine 16), Walter Barnes (Mike Gold), Shannon Farnon (Mrs. Robinson), Steve Shaw (Earl Robinson), Jeannie Fitzsimmons (newswoman), William Boyett (Chief), Vince Howard, Maud Strand (Erika)

Synopsis

Paramedic Craig Brice (James G. Richardson) again becomes the focus of the media's attention (newswoman Jeannie Fitzsimmons), much to Johnny's chagrin. A man (Walter Barnes) with a history of heart trouble becomes agitated when his daughter Emmie is trapped under a backhoe. An overwhelmed babysitter (Maud Strand) hyperventilates. The station responds to a hardware store fire and rescues Brice.

Conclusion

Emergency! was canceled after five and a half seasons, even though it typically beat out most of the competition, mainly *All in the Family*. The show garnered a respectable 28 ratings share, envious by today's standards. The show, however, was already sold for another twenty-two-episode season. The problem was that MCA/Universal's *The Bionic Woman*, which began airing in 1976, needed an additional year for profitable syndication, unlike today where some shows go into syndication while the first season is still airing original programming. Something had to go, and a new NBC programming executive and former head of CBS Records, Irwin Segelstien, canceled *Emergency!*. Ironically, *The Bionic Woman* lasted only the additional season (two seasons total) because when Lee Major's *Six Million Dollar Man* was canceled, so was Lindsey Wagner's *The Bionic Woman*.

During this time, Segelstein wanted to replace *Emergency!* with a series titled *Quail Lake*. The 90-minute pilot/movie aired on May 18, 1977, as *Pine Canyon Is Burning*, starring *Adam-12's* Kent McCord as a LA County Fire Captain at Station 110. The same producers, writers, and directors from *Emergency!* developed the pilot for MCA/Universal Television (writer and executive producer Robert A. Cinader, directed by Christian Nyby II, produced by Hannah Shearer and Gino Grimaldi, cinematography by Frank Thackery, with music by Lee Holdridge). The series was not developed, and NBC's vice chairman Segelstein was gone 6 months later.

Randy Mantooth and Kevin Tighe were brought back to fulfill their 7-year contract and appeared in six post-series movies. This unfortunately did not include the crew of Engine 51, although the hospital cast was brought back for two of the movies.

Episodes in Alphabetical Order

"Above and Beyond...Nearly," 5.20

"Alley Cat," 3.3

"All Night Long," 6.21

"An English Visitor," 3.4

"An Ounce of Prevention," 6.13

"Audit," (Advice) 2.21

"Back-Up," 4.21

"The Bash," 4.14

"The Boat," 6.19

"Body Language," 3.12

"Boot," (Duke) 2.19

"Bottom Line," 6.17

"Botulism," 1.2

"Breakdown," 6.15

"Brushfire," 1.4

"The Camera Bug," 4.10

"Captain Hook," 6.8

"Communications," 5.13

"Computer Error," (Checkmate) 3.14

"Computer Terror," 6.9

"Cook's Tour," 1.3

"Crash," (Torch Song) 1.11

"Daisy's Pick," (Blind Date) 4.7

"Dealer's Wild," 1.5

"Details," 4.12

"Dilemma," 1.9

"Dinner Date," 2.10

"Drivers," 2.13

"Election," 5.3

Emergency! World Premier, 0.1

"Equipment," 5.4,"

"The Exam," 6.7

"Fair Fight," 6.5

"Family Ties," 6.16

"The Firehouse Five, Plus One," (Firehouse Quintet) 6.18

"The Floor Brigade," (Big Business) 3.19

"Fools," 3.16

"Foreign Trade," (The Gasoline Crunch) 4.9

"Frequency," 3.1

"Fugitive," (Communication Gaffe) 4.5

"Fuzz Lady," 2.7

"The Game," 6.1

"The Girl on the Balance Beam," 5.18

"Gossip," 4.3

"Grateful," 5.21

"The Great Crash Diet," 5.22

"Green Thumb," (How Green Was My Thumb) 3.17

"Hang-Up," (Alpha-Beta-Gamma) 1.10

"The Hard Hours," 3.18

"Heavyweight," 3.5

"Helpful," 2.12

"Honest," 2.17

"Hypochondri-Cap," 6.23

"I'll Fix It," 4.2

"The Indirect Method," 5.6

"Inferno," 3.21

"Inheritance Tax," (Inheritance and Money), 3.9

"Insanity Epidemic," 6.14

"Insomnia," 3.8

"The Inspection," 5.5

"Inventions," 3.22

"Involvement," 5.19

EMERGENCY! *Behind the Scene*

CHAPTER 13

Unfilmed Scripts

Over the course of the series, scripts by several writers were submitted to Universal and Bob Cinader, and many were passed over. Some were commissioned initially and even made it to Universal's print shop for further review, but ultimately were never used. Some were assigned production numbers and a director and technical advisor, but never went any further. We feel fortunate to have located six scripts, which are rare finds, and we have tried to arrange them in chronological order using the best information available.

"Richter Six"

Production #35716 (scheduled for season 2)
Writer: Michael Donovan
Written: August 30, 1972

Director: Dennis Donnelly

LACoFD Technical Advisor: Firefighter/paramedic Richard Neal (PM0009)

Note: Written in flashback format

Synopsis

This story opens with Johnny and Roy talking with a group of new para-medic students. One student asks about the "hairiest" rescue Johnny and Roy had ever been on. Roy begins to talk about an earthquake they respond-ed to. In a story presented as a flashback, the squad and engine respond to quake-damaged Alameda Hospital, where they meet up with Dixie and Dr. Early, who are helping to evacuate the hospital. Roy worries about his family, not having any information on that area of the county. Johnny and Roy attempt to rescue several trapped patients and hospital workers from the wreckage. Dr. Early lowers himself down on a rope at one point to finish an interrupted appendectomy on a little girl. Johnny and Roy get as-sistance from a doctor, who has been blinded as a result of the earthquake, when their patient goes into cardiac arrest. Unbeknownst to the doctor, Drs. Brackett and Morton deliver his wife's premature baby. Chet breaks his shoulder trying to tunnel under some wreckage to find survivors.

Notes

This episode, written for airing during season 2 (fall 1972–spring 1973) may have been written as a direct result of the devastating earthquake on February 9, 1971, in the San Fernando Valley, just 50 miles north of Los Angeles. The Sylmar Earthquake registered 6.7 on the Richter scale, and 65 lives were lost; at the time, it was the third worst earthquake in California in terms of number of lives lost. The Sylmar Earthquake was also the second largest in terms of property damage loss.

This script, as written, was never filmed, although pieces of it would turn up in the rewritten "Syndrome" (episode 2.16). The technical advisor assigned to this episode would go on to work on the rewritten "Syndrome."

"Treadmill in the Moonlight"

Second revision title: My Home, My Castle

Production number: Not assigned

Writer: Preston Wood

Written: August 25, 1972 (first draft)

Director: Not assigned

LACoFD Technical Advisor: Not assigned

Synopsis

Continuing theme: Roy is upset with his wife (Betty), waiting for her to make the first move in saying "I'm sorry." Station 51 encounters a vehicle precariously balanced on a freeway support beam; the driver had been chased by the sheriff and drove through barricades indicating an unfinished freeway. A new doctor in the hospital, Dr. Varner, is taking Dexedrine, and Dixie finds him asleep in his car in the parking lot. She reads him the riot act. Johnny rescues a dog named Caesar that is stuck on the roof of a two-story house after chasing a cat. Roy and Betty finally make up. The episode ends with Station 51 rescuing two kids in a storm drain during a rainstorm, with Gage driving the squad.

Authors' Notes

Obviously, Roy's wife's name would have been changed to Joanne during further script revision.

"Hostage"

Production #37411 (scheduled for season 3)

Writer: Susan Keenan

Producer: William Stark

Director: Not assigned

LACoFD Technical Advisor: Firefighter/paramedic Jim Easley (PM0033)

Guest cast: Lillian Lehman (Nurse Carol Williams), others not assigned

Synopsis

The episode opens with a fire in a house owned by Stan Johnson where Johnny and Roy rescue unconscious firefighter Roger Demick of Engine 127. Later, the station responds to Greg's Glass and Mirror Works, where the store's owner, Greg Liggatt, tells Captain Stanley that his brother-in-law, Ralph, has become trapped under a collapsed storage rack of glass. Chet thinks he is a psychic. The firefighter from Engine 127 who was injured in the fire undergoes surgery for a heart condition and ultimately must retire from the department. While returning from the hospital, Roy and John are flagged down by a person on the sidewalk. They are then forced at gunpoint to drive to a house and treat a heroin overdose patient. They are eventually rescued by Sheriff's Department officers after Dr. Brackett solves cryptic clues to their location given over the BioPhone by Roy. Marco and Chet cook up a special meal for Roy and John of Chile Rellenos à la López and Irish Stew à la Kelly.

"The Long Weekend"

Production #37427 (scheduled for season 3)

Writer: Rick Mittleman

Written: November 14, 1973 (first draft)

Director: Not assigned

LACoFD Technical Advisor: Not assigned

Synopsis

A 3-day holiday weekend makes for a hectic time for everyone. Johnny tries to decide where to take his new girl out on a date. A young boy breaks his leg falling off his horse when it's spooked by trail bikes. Johnny and Roy team up with Fireboat 110 in Marina Del Rey to rescue a teenager from an overturned sailboat. A short man is hit in the head by a turnstile. An Englishman causes a major accident when he forgets what side of the road he's driving on. An explosion injures a man when his young daughter mistakes gasoline for lighter fluid, the house catches fire, and her grandfather suffers a heart attack.

"The Reading Course"

Production number: Not assigned

Writer: Preston Wood

Written: November 25, 1974 (first draft)

Director: Not assigned

LACoFD Technical Advisor: Not assigned

Synopsis:

In a running theme, Johnny tries to convince Roy and Dixie to take a reading course with him. A large-scale training exercise at a chemical plant involves several fire units, including Station 51, dealing with a sulfur trioxide spill (SO_3). Toxic fumes accidentally overcome the crew of Engine 51, and an explosion injures a plant worker. Back at the hospital, Dr. Morton treats a youngster with symptoms of the flu who returns a week later and is diagnosed with polio. Station 51 treats a man who walks into the station and suffers a heart attack. At a second-alarm fire in a two-story warehouse, Johnny and Roy retrieve a valuable painting.

Notes

SO_3 is real; it is formed from sulfur dioxide. When coming into contact with water, SO_3 forms sulfuric acid and reacts violently. In the first drill in the script, Engine 51 attempts to control the spill with a fog line, and the resulting reactivity, a white cloud of sulfuric acid, envelops them. They are wearing full protective gear, including their breathing apparatus, and are immediately hosed down by Engine 18.

The writer rewrote this script, and several portions of it would appear in "The Old Engine Cram" (episode 5.2).

"The High Rise"

Production #42811 (scheduled for season 5)

Writer: Preston Wood

Written: 1975

Director: Not assigned

LACoFD Technical Advisor: Not assigned

Unassigned guest cast: Nurse Carol (perhaps Lillian Lehman to be cast in her recurring role of Nurse Carol Williams), Dr. McKinley (Rampart), Captain and crew of Engine 36 and Engine and Squad 20, and other firefighters, Battalion Chiefs, police officers, and civilians as required

Synopsis
A twenty-story high-rise office building (400 Graymar Plaza) is engulfed in flames on the upper floors; Station 51 leads an initial second-alarm response. A team from Rampart Hospital, led by Dr. Brackett with Dr. Morton and Nurse McCall, sets up a triage and makeshift ER in the building's parking garage. A helicopter assists in rooftop evacuations. Gage and DeSoto extricate themselves from a disabled elevator. An explosion on the nineteenth floor isolates Johnny and Roy along with two victims, necessitating a dangerous rescue in an elevator shaft. Back at Rampart, Dr. Early takes charge of the patients transported to the ER. All the while, a jewelry heist is taking place.

Notes
There were multiple revisions to this 60-minute script that never aired, and it eventually became the basis for the 1978, 2-hour movie *The Steel Inferno*, with revisions to Wood's script by R. A. Cinader. Wood received no remuneration for the movie. He was paid for the original script and received a writer's credit in the movie.

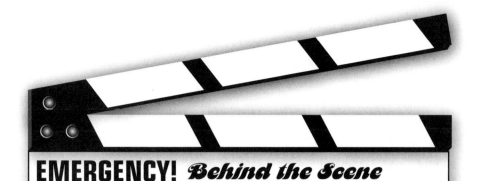

EMERGENCY! *Behind the Scene*

CHAPTER **14**

The **Emergency!** *Movies*

After the series ended on April 23, 1977, there were six made-for-TV *Emergency!* movies:

- *Survival on Charter 220*
- *The Steel Inferno*
- *What's a Nice Girl Like You Doing . . .*
- *Greatest Rescues of Emergency!*
- *Most Deadly Passage*
- *The Convention*

Each movie was essentially a 2-hour episode of *Emergency!* (runtime of 97 minutes, leaving time for commercials.) Three were filmed in Los Angeles (*Survival on Charter 220, The Steel Inferno,* and *Greatest Rescues of Emergency!*). *Most Deadly Passage* was shot in Seattle, Washington. *The Convention* and *What's a Nice Girl Like You Doing . . .* were filmed in San Francisco. The Seattle and San Francisco movies were made as pilots for a new series based on emergency medical services in different cities, but were never developed.

Recurring Actors

From the Show
Only Kevin Tighe and Randy Mantooth of the crew of A shift's Station 51 appeared in any of the movies because of their 7-year contract with the studio. When NBC decided to do the movies, the main cast members were all called back; however, contractual issues prevented the crew of Engine 51 from participating.

Deirdre Lenihan
Lenihan first appeared as a Rampart Hospital triage physician, Dr. Molly O'Brien, in the movie *Survival on Charter 220*. The 33-year-old actress would later appear as Patty McCormack's partner as San Francisco paramedic Laurie Campbell in the two San Francisco–based movies. Lenihan also appeared in five episodes of *The Waltons* as Daisy.

John DeLancie
DeLancie portrays Rampart triage physician Dr. Neil Colby in the movie *Steel Inferno*. He also portrays Dr. Dick DeRoy in both San Francisco–based *Emergency!* movies. DeLancie may be best known for his portrayal of Q on *Star Trek—The Next Generation* and on *Star Trek—Voyager*.

Patricia "Patty" McCormack
McCormack appears in "Dinner Date" (episode 2.10) as well as San Francisco Fire Department Paramedic Gail Warren in *What's a Nice Girl Like You Doing . . .* and *The Convention*. The former child actress received the Milky Way Gold Star Award as the nation's most outstanding juvenile performer of 1956 for her pig-tailed role in *The Bad Seed*. She was nominated for an Oscar as Best Actress in a Supporting Role for the same movie.

Never Filmed—*Emergency: Fire!*

While filming was underway during the third season of the show, a feature-length film with the entire cast was being planned with the working title of *Emergency: Fire!*. However, a pending writers' strike pushed NBC executives to concentrate on shooting the rest of the regular season shows before beginning a film project. When the writers' strike took place, Robert Cinader and Jim Page walked the picket lines. Several other shows never returned after that strike, and while *Emergency!* was lucky in that regard, *Emergency:*

Fire! was never produced. Marco López recalls hearing about a movie at this time, although according to Dick Friend, no details ever made it "down to our level. We were not normally included until NBC had something really concrete that we could discuss."

The film was retitled *Emergency Rescues* and was assigned production #37499. Shooting was scheduled to begin on January 8, 1974, before the season ended. However, due to the strike, "Propinquity" (episode 3.20) began filming on January 9th, utilizing a portion of the draft of *Emergency Rescues,* starting with the same location shoot and fire/rescue at the Shell Oil Cracking Plant, as well as the same director, Georg Fenady.

The Steel Inferno

Working title: The High Rise (2 hours)

Production #47101

Final revision: July 25, 1977 (still titled The High Rise)

Filming began: August 2, 1977

Airdate: Saturday, January 7, 1978

Writer: Preston Wood (revisions by Robert A. Cinader)

Director: Georg Fenady

LACoFD Technical Advisors: Battalion Chief George Harms, Captain/Paramedic Bob Belliveau (PM0001), Firefighter/Paramedic Louis Danes

Guest cast: Linda Gray (Evelyn Davis), Curtis Credel (Engine 110 Captain Mike Moore), John Furey (Station 110 Paramedic Charlie), Erik Washington (Station 110 Paramedic Dave Roberts Hall), T. Miratti (Station 110 Paramedic Bob Ryan), Anne Lockhart (Sue Adams), Brendan Boone (Davis), John DeLancie (Rampart triage physican Dr. Neil Colby), William Bryant (captain), Lyndel Stuart (triage physician Dr. Jean Wilson), William Bronder (security guard), Vince Howard (Officer Howard), Joseph Della Sorte (Sidney Clute), Robert Karnes (assistant fire chief, Battalion 7), Steven Marlo (battalion chief, Battalion 14, Philip Baker), Buck Young (battalion chief, BN 21), William Boyette (Chief McConnike)

Synopsis

A careless painter sparks an explosive fire in a high-rise building, trapping several people. Marina Del Rey Station 110 leads a three-alarm response, assisted by Squad 51. A triage team from Rampart Hospital, led by Dr. Brackett along with Dr. Colby, sets up a makeshift ER in a nearby garage. Several painters, in addition to a woman (Linda Gray) and her secretary

(Anne Lockhart), the fiancée of a paramedic at Station 110, remain trapped on the sixteenth floor. A jewelry heist is taking place during the confusion of the evacuation. A Coast Guard helicopter assists in rooftop evacuations, while back at Rampart Dr. Early and Dixie take charge of the patients transported to the ER. A paramedic from Station 110 is injured attempting a rescue, while Gage and DeSoto extricate themselves from a disabled elevator. An explosion on the twenty-first floor injures a fire captain, necessitating a dangerous rescue down an elevator shaft.

Notes

This movie was adapted from Preston Wood's original 1975 1-hour script titled "The High Rise," which was never filmed. Many scenes, story lines, and dialogue, including the address of the building (400 Graymar Plaza) from "The High Rise" script were utilized during the rewrite. Station 110 was substituted for Station 51, from the original script. Wood was not involved in the rewrite.

Locations

LA County Fire Station 110 in Marina Del Rey was used for the initial response scenes and for the final scene on the station's rear balcony. 110 is located at 4433 Admiralty Way in Marina Del Rey. Although alluded to during the series, this is the only time filming was done at this station. Boat 110 seen in the series was an 18-foot jet runabout. Engine 110, a Ward LaFrance, as shown in *Steel Inferno,* has a license plate of E996069. Although showing a different plate than the "former" E51, it is the same rig. Also seen is LA County Station 8 with the truck pulling out of the station and responding. Units seen at scene are Squad 36, Truck 8, and Squad 18. The U.S. Coast Guard Siskorsky helicopter that assisted in the movie was Unit 1442.

The building used for the high-rise fire scenes was the Oppenheimer Tower, located at 10880 Wilshire Boulevard in Westwood, California, just south of UCLA. The corridors and offices to match the building were built on a set at Universal. This location is technically within the LA city limits, and the closest responding station would have been LA City Station 37 just off Wilshire, about two blocks west of the building.

Survival on Charter 220

Working title: Charter 220 Down

Original Production #47187, #47188

Final revision: September 16, 1977

Filming began. September 20, 1977 with production number of 47111

Airdate: Saturday, 9 P.M., March 25, 1978

Writers: Christian I. Nyby II and Hannah L. Shearer (revisions by Robert A. Cinader)

Producers: Hannah L. Shearer and Gian R. Grimaldi

Director: Christian I. Nyby II

LACoFD Technical Advisors: Battalion Chief George Harms, Captain/ Paramedic Bob Belliveau (PM0001), and Firefighter/Paramedic Bob McCullough (PM0038).

Guest cast: David Ladd (Firefighter/Paramedic Pete Hansen), Jay Hammer (Charlie Stevenson), Jason Evers (Justin Manning), Barrie Youngfellow (Christine Jenkins), Marla Adams (Diana Jennings), Rebecca York (Debbie), James A. Watson, Jr., Randall Carver (Gene Wright), Jim B. Smith (Ed Crane), Jean Howell* (Emma Alden), Deirdre Lenihan (Dr. O'Brien), William Boyette (Chief McConnike), with the Compton Fire Department

Synopsis
A small plane with two people (Barrie Youngfellow and Marla Adams) and a DC-8 charter passenger jet with politicians and press corps collide. The DC-8 crashes into a subdivision in Compton just south of LA, where Johnny and Roy are already treating an injured child. The small aircraft ends up in the Los Angeles River Basin. Station 18 leads the response from Battalion 14 with assistance from the Compton City Fire Department to the plane down and resulting explosion and fire. Multiple rescues include passengers from both planes and people in the subdivision, including Johnny and Roy trapped in a collapsed home. A dog points rescue crews to an old man. Squad 51 is crushed by one of the engines from the aircraft. Station 51's off-duty C shift paramedics who live nearby assist in the rescue.

Notes
The actual Compton Fire Department appears in this movie with multiple pieces of apparatus to assist in the fire control and search and rescue of patients from the plane or trapped in the homes. All apparatus were in service, and the firefighters were on duty.

One of Compton's apparatus in the movie, a 1969 Crown 85 Pitman-Snorkel Platform, serial number F1598, original license plate number E 550322 (gold on black), appeared as Truck 411. It was in reserve as Truck 412 for about 5 years at Compton Station 3 until it was sold in 2005.

*Jean Howell previously guest starred in another LA County firefighting drama, *Rescue 8*, in an episode titled "Nine Minutes to Live."

Although the aircraft before the crash is a DC-8, it is a Boeing 707 that lies in pieces on the ground. The Ward LaFrance as Engine 60 is actually the former Engine 51.

Locations

The film was shot on a location in a redevelopment area, soon to be demolished, which contained several apartments, small businesses, and single-family homes. It covered the area between Willowbrook Avenue and South Alameda Street at East Myrrh Street in Compton. Universal agreed to clean up the area after filming, and the location is now the site of Compton's Civic Center.

The airport used for filming the establishing shots of the DC-8 at the airport, airport office, and loading of the pilots and crew was Ontario International Airport, about 50 miles east of Universal Studios.

Technical advisor Bob McCullough related a humorous story that happened while filming *220 Down*:

> Randy [Mantooth] and I were friends and neighbors on the show . . . One day he and I decided we would just see how attentive the director and the cinematographer were and we decided we would switch name badges. Of course, his said John Gage, Paramedic, and mine said Bob McCullough, Paramedic. Several more hours of filming went on and it was never noticed. Like most days, when they yelled, "It's a Wrap," we were exhausted and headed for home. We both totally forgot that we had made the switch. Randy turned his uniform into Wardrobe and went on his merry way. I am sure the wardrobe people spotted the name badge and switched it back to one of Gage's. I on the other hand went on duty at my station. No one noticed the name badge until I was leaning over a patient on a rescue. The patient looked up and me and said, "I must really be in bad shape if they sent John Gage to work on me!"

Captain Belliveau stated, "FF/PM McCullough handled this long assignment in a realistic manner. Chief Harms is a seasoned fire officer who had the experience of being on a major aircraft incident. My job was relatively easy because everybody else was good at their assignments. Coordinating with Compton Fire was a bit of problem because of difference in training, equipment, emergency operations, etc., but it all worked out."

Most Deadly Passage

Working title: Medic 1 – Seattle
Production #47112
First draft: October 17, 1977
Final revision: November 8, 1977
Filming began: November 30, 1977

Airdate: Tuesday 9 P.M., April 4, 1978

Writer: Michael Donovan

Director: Christian I. Nyby II

Technical Advisors: Seattle Fire Department

Guest cast: Jesse Vint, Anthony Herrera, George Wyner, Larry Manetti, Ted Gehring, John Kauffman (Frankie), Terence Burk, Kenneth Tobey (Ferry Captain Gordon Trigg), Cecilia Hart (Nancy Halverson), Joan Tompkins, Bill Zukert (Jason Bennet), Michael Feffer, Eric Sever (Lieutenant Mike Olsen)

Synopsis

Roy and Johnny are sent to Seattle to study the renowned "Medic One" program and the techniques used there, and they are amazed at how advanced it is compared to their own system. They are caught up in a series of near-disasters, which include a skydiver jumping off a tower; an injured man trapped on top of the Kingdome; and a fuel pumper that accidentally loaded a ferry with gasoline instead of diesel fuel, causing a ferry fire in the middle of Puget Sound.

Locations

The paramedics in this film were stationed at Seattle's Station 10, located at 301 2nd Avenue South, which is still Seattle Fire Department Headquarters, although the communications center seen in the movie has been replaced with a picnic area and an adjacent new communications facility. Fire Station 2, built in 1906, is a five-bay station located at 2334 4th Avenue.

The hospital is Seattle's Harborview Medical Center—the largest hospital in the state and home of Medic One headquarters—it is also a teaching hospital for the University of Washington. Both of these institutions contributed to the establishment of Seattle Fire Department's Medic One Program in King County by training the first firefighter/paramedics in 1970. Due to the high standards of training and education established by the Seattle training program, Seattle was called the "Best place in the world to have a heart attack," after a *60 Minutes* story in 1974. To this day, the Medic One programs throughout King County are considered models for much of the world.

Medic One headquarters are located at Harborview Medical Center, and its vehicles are self-contained paramedic ambulances.

Notes

The Duwamish fireboat has since been retired, but the Akai, the other fireboat featured in the movie, is still on duty. It's currently positioned in Lake Union so that it can be made readily available if there's a fire at one of the many marinas along the route from Puget Sound to Lake Washington.

The ferry used in the movie, the MV Klickitat, was built in 1927, and had its engines replaced and reconfigured above the car deck in 1981. It is still in service and will be until 2008 when it is scheduled for retirement.

Prior to the fire in the movie, the 256-foot-long MV Klickitat departed from Coleman Dock, where the motor home went aboard. The dock has been expanded a lot since the 1970s when there were only two slips there; now there are six. The ferry discharged its passengers after the fire at Pier 91.

The Kingdome was destroyed in a spectacular controlled demolition in 2000 to make way for Quest Seahawks Stadium.

Greatest Rescues of Emergency!

Working title: The Best of *Emergency!*

Production #47113

Final revision: March 24, 1978

Filming began: March 27, 1978

Airdate: Sunday 8 P.M., December 31, 1978

Writer: R. A. Cinader (for nonflashback sequences)

Director: R. A. Cinader

Technical Advisors: None

Guest cast: None credited

Synopsis

Flashback format. Johnny and Roy are both promoted to Captain and reminisce about their experiences as paramedics. Flashback sequences include the rescue of airplane passengers after a crash landing, a potential suicide threat from the top of a crane tower, and a girl whose toe is stuck in a faucet. The two partners remember more than thirty calls, highlighting the series' 6 years.

Notes

The script for this episode was only seventeen pages in length. Nonflashback sequences were filmed entirely on location at LA County Fire Department Headquarters.

While no guest actors were credited, Chief Bragden congratulates the dozen newly promoted Captains during the opening graduating ceremony scene. Two other firefighters promoted to Captain—Craig Brice and Robert Bellingham—appeared in several *Emergency!* episodes. James G. Richardson, who portrayed Craig Brice, was involved in another movie during the time of filming and was unavailable; this part is instead played by a tall African-American who is uncredited.

During this film, Johnny mentions he was at Station 8. This is structurally correct, but for continuity purposes wrong because the station and apparatus had been identified in the World Premier as Station 10.

What's a Nice Girl Like You Doing . . .

Working title: Code 3—San Francisco

Production #47114

First draft: January 23, 1978 (pages 1–58 only)

Final revision: February 2, 1978 (with new title and completed script)

Airdate: Tuesday 9 P.M., June 26, 1979

Writers: Hannah Shearer (story) and Michael Donovan (teleplay)

Director: Georg Fenady

Technical Advisors: San Francisco Fire Department

Cast: Paul Sylvan (Captain Pete Delaney), Patty McCormack (Paramedic Gail Warren), John DeLancie (Dr. Dick DeRoy), Deirdre Lenihan (Paramedic Laurie Campbell, PM 187), Jordon Suffin (Joe Marshal), Jon Buffington (Mike Pakula), John F. Lacues (Arlen McCoy), with Randolph Mantooth (John Gage) and Kevin Tighe (Roy DeSoto).

Guest cast: Zack Murphy, James Whitworth (Harvey Ludwig), Chesley Uxbridge (Dominick), Ed Peck, Bruce Neckels (Tony), John F. Lacues, Chris Combs, Carl Lumbly (paramedic), John Hatfield (paramedic), Tom Williams[1]

Synopsis
The story opens with a rescue of a man caught up in ship's rigging. Johnny and Roy are sent to San Francisco to study new techniques. They meet crews of the fire station and are surprised to see female paramedics. They follow along on a number of rescues, including a man stranded on support girders on the Golden Gate Bridge above Fort Dix, a boat fire on the Embarcadero, and an epileptic at a coffee shop. An ambulance transporting a heart attack victim from the Condor dance bar is involved in a fatal accident that injures five others.

---

[1] The character played by Tom Williams went through three name changes through the script revisions—from Frank Price to Frank Warren to Frank Webber.

Notes

The paramedic van (Rescue 87) is a 1976–1977 model Dodge Tradesman van cab and chassis with San Francisco Public Health Services logo.

The ship used in the high-rescue is the Balclutha, a three-masted schooner built in 1887 for trade between Europe and San Francisco that is still docked at Fisherman's Wharf and was designated a National Historic Landmark in 1985.

Locations

The film's smaller Harbor Emergency Hospital and Harbor View Clinic is a community health center in Chinatown that is still in operation at the east end of the Broadstreet Tunnel. The street going across in front is Mason Street, which is also a Cable Car route.

In the film, the San Francisco Fire Department's station alert tones and sirens are the same as those for the show's LA County Station 51.

The Condor dance bar as seen in the movie is located at 300 Columbus Avenue at Broadway in the North Beach section of the town and is currently a sports bar. This club was the site where Carol Doda made her appearance as the first topless dancer in the United States with her silicone-injected "enhancements" in June 1964. By wearing a topless bathing suit designed by Rudi Gernreich, Doda danced her way into infamy. She retired in the 1980s. Her name can be seen on the signage in the film. The Condor is actually three blocks away from Harbor Emergency, but the film arranged a 14-mile detour to have the accident. Some photos and other items from the club's past are inside.

The scene in which the Pinto cuts off the ambulance was shot at Skyline Boulevard and Zoo Road; some zoo animals appear in the distant background. However, in the film, the dispatcher directs units to John F. Kennedy Drive and Stow Lake Road, an actual intersection that is about 4 miles away.

The base referred to by the tour guide as Fort Dix (an Army base in New Jersey) is actually Fort Point, which was constructed by the U.S. Army Corps of Engineers between 1853 and 1861 to prevent entrance of a hostile fleet into San Francisco Bay. It is located underneath the south anchorage of the Golden Gate Bridge, on the northernmost part of the Presidio, and was listed as a National Historic Site in 1970.

The Convention

Production #47115

Airdate: Tuesday 9 P.M., July 3, 1979

Writer: Hannah Shearer (revisions by Robert A. Cinader)

Director: Georg Fenady

Technical Advisors: San Francisco Fire Department

Cast: Many of the same principals as the previous San Francisco–based movie:

Paul Sylvan (Captain Pete Delaney), Patty McCormack (Paramedic Gail Warren), John DeLancie (Dr. Dick DeRoy), Deirdre Lenihan (Paramedic Laurie Campbell), Bruce Neckels (Tony), Jordon Suffin (Joe Marshal), Jon Buffington (Mike Pakula), John Laurence (Arley McCoy), with Randolph Mantooth (John Gage) and Kevin Tighe (Roy DeSoto).

Guest cast: Damon Raskin (Phillip), Ray K. Goman (police officer), Sam Hoina (police officer), with the Novato Fire Protection District

Synopsis

Johnny and Roy attend another convention in San Francisco, where they meet up with the crews of Fire Station 38 and Rescue Squad 2. They assist in a number of rescues, which include a choking victim, delivering a baby while under fire from a sniper, and responding with the San Francisco Fire Department on a mutual aid response to a fire in a research laboratory in Marin County.

Notes

This film features Novato Fire Protection District's Station 4 at 319 Enfrent Drive in Northern Marin County, 27 miles North of San Francisco. One of Novato's rigs in the movie as Truck 4 was a 1968 Crown 85 Snorkel, with a Pierce body (Crown serial number F1518). Station 4 is still an active station with a paramedic engine, an ALS paramedic ambulance.

EMERGENCY! *Behind the Scene*

CHAPTER **15**

Crossovers and Spinoffs

Crossovers with *Adam-12*

Adam-12 actors Kent McCord and Martin Milner appeared in the January 15, 1972, *Emergency!* movie as their *Adam-12* characters, police officers Reed and Malloy. Their role is reprised somewhat when the *Emergency!* movie is reaired as "The Wedworth-Townsend Act" (episodes 5.15 and 5.16), shown in the middle of the fifth season. The 2-hour movie aired over a 2-week period in flashback format with Johnny and Roy commenting on how far the paramedic program has come.

Later in the first season, the crew of Station 51 is watching a TV episode of *Adam-12*, titled "Ambush" (original airdate of November 10, 1971), on their day room TV in the April 8, 1972, *Emergency!* episode "Hang-Up" (1.10). In this particular *Adam-12* episode, we see the future Dr. Morton, Ron Pinkard, as Police Officer Barrett. Marco López also appeared in "Ambush" as an LA County Sheriff but is not seen in the clips shown in the "Hang-Up" episode.

On an October 4, 1972, *Adam-12* episode titled "Lost and Found," Roy and Johnny run into Dr. Early at Rampart Hospital. Also appearing in the *Adam-12* episode are *Emergency!*'s hospital staff of Doctors Brackett and Kelly, and Nurse McCall.

Adam-12: "Lost and Found"

Episode #5.4

Airdate: October 4, 1972

Writer: Michael Donovan

Director: Dennis Donnelly

Cast: Martin Milner, Kent McCord

Special appearances: Robert Fuller, Julie London, Bobby Troop, Kevin Tighe, Randolph Mantooth, Deidre Hall (Nurse Sally Lewis)

Guest cast: Elaine Giftos (Nurse Kathy Stephens), Fred Holliday (Jay Simmons), Nancy King (Mary Simmons), Kirby Furlong (Jimmy Simmons), Chanin Hale (Irma Baker), Diane Sherry (Nurse Sheri Baker), Milton Frome (Milton Sawyer), William Boyett

Synopsis

Officers Reed and Malloy transport a boy (Kirby Furlong) in a diabetic coma to Rampart Hospital, where Dr. Brackett and Nurse McCall treat him. Dr. Early is seen briefly, with paramedics Gage and DeSoto. Malloy visits his girlfriend (Elaine Giftos), the head of a crisis center at Rampart, and they help locate a suicidal teen. When the diabetic boy runs away from the hospital, the officers lead the search.

Notes

Both the writer and director worked on several *Emergency!* episodes. William Boyett portrays his *Adam-12* character of Sergeant MacDonald and not his *Emergency!* character of Chief McConnike. Deidre Hall, who portrayed Nurse Sally Lewis in several episodes of *Emergency!* in season 2, also portrays a nurse in this episode.

Roy and John are in the episode for only about 20 seconds, which seems more like a clip from *Emergency!* that was not used and inserted into the *Adam-12* episode for a balance with the hospital staff. There was no interaction with the *Adam-12* characters, Reed and Malloy, just with Dr. Early and a young nurse that Gage was talking with.

Some *Adam-12* trivia: Jack Webb lived in Apartment 12 when a teenager in the Bunker Hill area of LA. The Los Angeles Police patrol car that worked Bunker Hill was "Car 12," which is why *Adam-12* was called *Adam-12*.

The Life You Save

Tim Donnelly narrates this educational first aid film used in schools. Produced by Filmfair in 1973, the film uses four true cases where knowledge of basic first aid saved lives, describing the first aid technique used for each situation.

NBC Starship Rescue

On September 7, 1973, Kevin Tighe and Randolph Mantooth hosted this program featuring excerpts of Saturday morning cartoon/animated programs. Among the previews were *Star Trek* and *Emergency + 4*, hence the title of the preview program. The *Emergency!* characters of Johnny and Roy and the *Star Trek* characters of Captain Kirk and others of the crew were the first adults caricatured for an animated series.

Emergency + 4

This cartoon series, also known as *Esquadrao + 4* in Portugal, debuted September 8, 1973, on NBC at 9:00 A.M. and was followed by *Star Trek*. It ran through September 4, 1976, with twenty-three "original" episodes (eleven in season 1 and twelve in season 2). In its third season, there were no original episodes; NBC would air only repeats of the first two seasons. It was produced and directed by Fred Calvert for Universal Television, Mark VII Ltd., Fred Calvert Production Companies, and NBC-TV.

The series had Johnny (who drives the squad) and Roy continuing their lifesaving roles on Squad 51 with the assistance of four kids and their pets in their own van. Tighe and Mantooth did the voiceovers for their animated characters. Instructional safety tips were interwoven into the stories, along with practical demonstrations of mouth-to-mouth resuscitation and simple medical first aid. At the end of some of the programs, Tighe and Mantooth would come out and talk to kids about certain dangerous situations and how to avoid them. Some of the life-saving tips included what to do if you see fallen power lines, what to do in case a fire breaks out in the home, how to avoid dangerous chemicals, and learning important procedures on how to save someone's life.

Even though the program was produced with the "Full Cooperation of the County of Los Angeles Fire Department" in end credits, the only identification on the squad was the 51 rondel. The words "Los Angeles Fire Department Rescue Squad" were missing as was "L.A. County" from their helmet shields. The theme song is not that from the *Emergency!* TV program, and the station only vaguely resembled its TV counterpart. It even had a fire pole to slide down from the bunk room.

GO

On September 7, 1974, NBC launched the second season of its Saturday afternoon program, airing at 12:30. *Emergency!*'s Tighe and Mantooth made a guest appearance in civilian clothes assisting in the profile of the Los Angeles County Fire Department (LACoFD) paramedics. The program, aimed at children, was hosted by Greg Morris from *Mission Impossible*. The program gave an insider's view of various occupations and activities.

The *Emergency!* stars talked about the paramedics of LA County's rescue squads. A demonstration of aid to heart attack victims and a look at firefighting and rescue gear were featured segments. Members of LACoFD were shown performing some of their various duties. GO aired from 1973 to 1976, and it was produced by Peabody Award–winning George A. Heinemann, who also produced *Ding Dong School* and *Sheri Lewis & Lamb Chop*.

Dick Friend had arranged for Tighe and Mantooth to meet with GO's production crew at LA County Station 68 in the Calabasas area of Malibu on a Saturday morning to do their filming. Dick states, "The station was fairly close to Randy's home so I picked up Kevin and we arrived at 8 A.M. as planned, but no Randy, so we joined the station crew for coffee. The film crew was anxious to get to work but still no Randy. The Captain's phone rang about 8:15. It was the Captain at Station 125, about three miles away, reporting that Randy had run into their station and wondered where we were." "They said to meet at 68's," Randy told the Captain. "But this is 125s," the Captain explained, and he pointed Randy in the right direction. Dick continues, "The Captain at 125s initially asked Randy if he was here to pull an overtime shift."

The August 9, 1973, press release with attached photo for the GO premier episode shows Mantooth and Tighe out in front of Station 68 with heavy jackets.

First Aid: Treat an Injury

A 20-minute film produced in 1975 is narrated/hosted by Kevin Tighe and was produced by Directions Unlimited Film Corp. of Beverly Hills, California. Department of Medicine, University of Southern California consulted on the project. Kevin Tighe is in plain clothes hosting what to do if a victim is burned, suffers from heat exhaustion, and other medical emergencies.

Dinah!

In the mid 1970s Randy Mantooth and Kevin Tighe made two appearances on the Dinah Shore program, *Dinah!*, to discuss the paramedic program in LA County as well as the TV show. Also appearing with them on both occasions, at the insistence of Robert Cinader, was a real LA County fire-fighter/paramedic, Robert Hoff, who was also one of the *Emergency!* technical advisors.

The hospital staff of Bobby Troop, Julie London, and Robert Fuller, along with Mantooth and Tighe, paid another visit to *Dinah!*. Johnny Miller, the assistant property master for *Emergency!*, brought along many of the medical props used on the show.

Sierra

Sierra debuted Thursday, September 12, 1974, on NBC. This 60-minute, thirteen-episode series was filmed entirely in Yosemite National Park, known as Sierra National Park for the series. Jack Morehead, Yosemite's Chief Ranger and Technical Advisor for the series, stated that no other parks were used for filming, although there were plans to go to other parks if the series was successful.

Airing against *The Waltons* at 8 P.M., this program was about park rangers and their dealings with lost hikers, enforcing park regulations, coping with visitors, and search-and-rescue incidents. *Sierra* starred:

- James G. Richardson as Ranger Tim Cassidy
- Ernest Thompson as Ranger Matt Harper
- Jack Hogan as Chief Ranger Jack Moore
- Susan Foster as Ranger Julie Beck
- Michael Warren as Ranger P. J. Lewis

John Denver wrote the words and music for *Sierra*'s theme song, which was performed by Denver's long-time friend Denny Brooks.

Kevin Tighe and Randolph Mantooth appear in a *Sierra* episode as their *Emergency* characters.

Sierra: "Urban Rangers"

Production #41315

Episode #1.5

Airdate: October 24, 1974

Writer: Michael Donovan

Director: Roger Duchovney

Technical Advisor: Yosemite Chief Ranger Jack Morehead

Cast: James G. Richardson, Ernest Thompson, Jack Hogan, Susan Foster, Michael Warren

Special appearances: Kevin Tighe and Randolph Mantooth

Story:

Johnny and Roy arrive at park headquarters (in Mantooth's Land Cruiser) to participate in a cross-training program between LACoFD and the Sierra National Park Rangers. For Johnny and Roy, this involves mountain rescue training. They participate in the attempted capture of Cruncher, the wayward bear. Johnny tries to date Julie—the only female Park Ranger assigned to the unit—but keeps getting interrupted. Roy considers a career change to become a park ranger.

Johnny and Roy go off alone on an easy day climb as part of their training and come across an injured climber; Johnny stays with the injured person, and Roy goes for help. Roy, while running to get help, trips, falls, and sustains a head injury, becoming unconscious; he is carrying his climbing helmet, not wearing it. The park rangers, noting that Roy and Johnny are more than an hour late in getting back, go searching for them and find Roy still unconscious. The rangers transport Roy to the park hospital, find Johnny and the injured climber, and rescue them as well. While visiting Roy in the hospital, Johnny, learning that Ranger Julie is now unavailable, tries to make a date with Roy's nurse.

Production

Executive producer for *Sierra* was Robert A. Cinader, and it was produced by Bruce Johnson for Mark VII Limited in association with Universal Television. Jack Morehead (for which the character Jack Moore was named) was the Chief Ranger of Yosemite National Park when Cinader approached the National Park Service about approval for the series and permission to film in National Parks; he served as the show's Technical Advisor.

The week that this particular episode aired, it was announced by NBC that *Sierra* was being canceled. It was, in fact, the first program of all the networks to have been canceled in the fall 1974 season. They would air five more already-filmed, 60-minute episodes, leaving two filmed episodes unaired.

The pilot for the series "The Rangers," that was filmed in April, aired after the series concluded on December 24, 1974 with a slightly different cast.

Ranger Butch Farabee, who was in charge of the training division in Yosemite at the time of the series, provided the security and required rangers as background extras. The "real" rangers had some initial misgivings about the series and how they were to be portrayed. Chief Ranger Morehead stated that, "Most all the Rangers supported the shooting of the series, initially skeptical, but could see the potential benefits, some were thankful that it was canceled. However, many of the Rangers worked for the series at various times during the summer, making good money during the production as extras."

Before the series began, Farabee was showing Robert Cinader the area when Farabee alertly noticed a "real" rescue situation. A hiker was trapped on a rock in the middle of the fast-moving Merced River that runs through the park. With safety rope attached, Farabee swam out in the river to perform the rescue. On the other end of the rope on land was Cinader, along with other rangers, hauling them both to safety. And true to Cinader's form, the incident was used in a *Sierra* episode titled "The Fawn," which was directed by Georg Fenady.

Dick Friend recalls that, at Robert Cinader's request, Morehead and he spent several days together, along with some of LA County's paramedics, while they were planning *Sierra*. Friend stated, "Cinader brought him down to Los Angeles and we all took one of our weekend cruises to Catalina on Bob's boat. My job was to tell him what I had learned, and in Bob's words, "see how show biz works."

Crossover Appearances

Randy's brother, Donald Mantooth, appeared in *Sierra*'s "Holiday" episode (1.6) and appeared in two *Emergency!* episodes. Hannah Shearer, later a writer and producer for *Emergency!*, was *Sierra*'s research assistant.

905-Wild

On March 1, 1975, during season 4 of *Emergency!*, a pilot titled *905-Wild* aired, the last episode of the season. The title refers to the police code for "Wild Animal Loose, Threatening." Besides the regular *Emergency!* cast, this spin-off starred Mark Harmon (*240-Robert*, *NCIS*) and Albert Popwell (*Dirty Harry*) as paramedic animal control officers and was directed by Jack Webb for Mark VII Productions with Universal Television Productions. This would be Webb's only directorial role for the series. The network never picked up the proposal.

Quail Lake

In 1977 a new NBC programming executive and former head of CBS Records, Irwin Segelstein, wanted to cancel *Emergency!* and replace it with a series titled *Quail Lake*. Some of the same producers, writers, and directors from *Emergency!* developed the pilot for MCA/Universal Television, in association with NBC, including:

- Christian L. Nyby II, director
- Robert A. Cinader, writer and producer
- Gino Grimaldi, producer
- Hannah Shearer, writer
- Frank Thackery, cinematographer

They filmed a 90-minute pilot episode, *Pine Canyon Is Burning*, but the series was not developed.

Pine Canyon Is Burning

The pilot for this series was a 90-minute episode, which aired as *Pine Canyon Is Burning* on May 18, 1977. Essentially a 78-minute movie (in a 90-minute slot), this film starred:

- Kent McCord as Captain William Stone (also in *Adam-12*)
- Megan McCord as Margaret Stone (Kent McCord's actual daughter)
- Shane Sinutko as Michael Stone
- Diana Muldaur as Sandra
- Andrew Duggan as Captain Ed Wilson
- Dick Bakalyan as Charlie (the Mechanic in two *Emergency!* episodes 6.15, and 6.19, also named Charlie)
- Brit Lind as Anne Walker (*Emergency!* episode 4.7)
- Curtis Credel as Whitey Olson
- Sandy McPeak as Pete Madison
- Larry Delaney as Captain #78 (*The Rangers* and *Emergency!* episode 4.14)

This movie also features Engine 51, the Ward, as Engine 78. Ironically, Engine 78 was the real next-in engine for that area of Pine Canyon.

Synopsis

A widowed firefighter with two children, Captain William Stone (Kent McCord), transfers to a one-man fire-and-rescue brush station in the Los Angeles foothills—Patrol Station 99 in Pine Canyon—in order to be home at night with his two children. McCord replaces veteran Captain Ed Wilson (Andrew Duggan), who is retiring from Pine Canyon station.

Locations

The opening scenes were filmed on location at LA County Station 110 at 4433 Admiralty Way, in Marina Del Rey. Station 110 is a fire station that houses two boats, a pumper, and truck.

The Patrol Station used was a real station in the Angeles National Forest that is no longer in service and is now a private residence. It was deeded to the LACoFD in 1929 and was inservice as a one-man station until 1989. The station was "old" Patrol Station 77 (also known as the Quail Lake station) at 47376 Ridge Route Road (Lake Hughes) near the intersection of Ridge Route Road and Pine Canyon Road, south of Highway 138, located East of the town of Gorman on Interstate 5 on the "Grapevine." It is a long way from Malibu where other scenes were filmed.

Equipment

The fire vehicle used in the pilot as Patrol 99 was a 1976 GMC/Emergency-1 4   4 quick attack pumper and assigned to Patrol 77 after the pilot was filmed. Later it was reassigned to Fire Station 55 on Catalina Island, vehicle shop number 49627. For some unknown reason the vehicle ID markings (GMC) were ducttaped over for the movie. After it was used in the TV show, the studio gave it to the Department. According to one source, the studio never paid for the rig. The manufacturer came after the Department for payment. After some discussion, the manufacturer took the rig back.

LACoFD Helicopter pilot Gary Lineberry, now retired, states, "I was flying the JetRanger Copter 4 at the time (registration number N4050G) and I flew Kent McCord into a set area on the back lot of Universal Studios. It was supposed to be a landing in the town of Pine Canyon. I remember it was a very steep approach into a pretty confined area, not something I would have been likely to do in the real world." Gary was a member of the Screen Actors Guild before he came to the County and did a few movies, commercials, and TV shows as a pilot. Copter 4, later reassigned as Copter 10, crashed with Gary as pilot in 1986 and he was fortunate to walk away from it. A new 206B Kiowa type JetRanger purchased in 1987, identified as Copter 10, registration number N55LA, is still in service.

Additional Appearances

Julie London and Bobby Troup

Tattletales

This CBS program was similar to *The Newlywed Game,* with three celebrity couples. The wives or husbands would go off stage with headphones, and their spouses would remain on stage. Via closed circuit TV, the sequestered spouses would be asked a question about marriage, sex, or some other embarrassing issue. On-stage spouses would try to answer the way they thought the off-stage spouses would reply. The prize money went up with each round, and the spouses changed places. After all three answered, the ones who got it right won a share of $150. After two questions, the spouses changed places for two more questions, the last being a $300 question. At the end, the couple with the most money won an extra $1000.

Julie London and Bobby Troup appeared on the show several times, in July 1974, November 1974, February 1975, and again in September 1975. In one episode, Host Bert Convy asked Julie, "How are things going on *Emergency!?*" to which Julie answers, "Everything's an emergency!" Bert replies, "Let's hope we don't have an emergency today. Let's just hope you win a lot of money."

Adam-12's Martin Milner and Kent McCord also appeared with their spouses on the program.

The Match Game

Along the same vein, Julie London was one of the panelists on the popular game show, *The Match Game,* during *Emergency!*'s fifth season from December 8–12, 1975. The host, Gene Rayburn, teased Julie, "If we have an Emergency, will you help us out?"

Rowan & Martin's Laugh-In

This show featured Julie London on September 18, 1972.

Take My Advice

The couple appeared together on this program, a panel show hosted by Kelly Lange, airing on NBC from January 5–9, 1976.

29th Annual Christmas Lane Parade

Bill Burrud hosted this parade from Huntington Park, California. The 90-minute live telecast was aired over KCOP, Channel 13, on December 4 1976, at 8 P.M. Tim Donnelly and Mike Stoker appeared.

NBC's 75th Anniversary Program

Randy Mantooth and Kevin Tighe appeared together again for this anniversary special on May 5, 2002, along with a clip from *Emergency!*, a program that was finally getting its due as one of the network's most memorable shows.

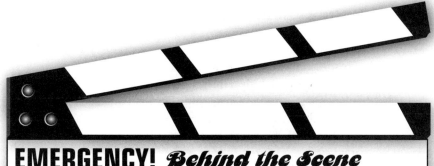

EMERGENCY! *Behind the Scene*

CHAPTER **16**

True Stories

A 12-Minute *Emergency!* Movie

Early in 1971 County Supervisor Kenneth Hahn contacted the Fire Department about wanting something that could be taken to service groups, local service clubs, city councils, and the like to show what the new paramedic program was all about. This was before *Emergency!* would do such a good job of that. The operations division approached the fire chief, who said to contact Dick Friend. Arrangements were made, and two paramedics from Squad 59, Gary Davis and Bill Ridgeway, and the County Film Unit, put a dramatized incident on film. The film was shot not far from Fire Station 36, at the home of a Harbor General emergency room nurse, who portrayed Friend's wife.

In this film, Dick Friend pretended to have a heart attack while mowing the lawn. The paramedics arrive with their engine and squad, rip off

Friend's shirt, attach patches for an electrocardiogram, and start an IV. "Ridgeway whispered to me that he was going to stick me and was it okay. Sure, I said, anything for the film. This was in the days all IVs came in pretty hefty bottles, not plastic bags." Davis said that his partner on the Squad, Bill Ridgeway, was the best IV man that ever lived. "Often while at 59s we would be called over to the hospital to start a line as the staff in the ED could not get a vein."

In the middle of the shoot, Friend recalls, the paramedics were required to respond to a call, and they left him there with the IV in his arm. "Ridgeway told me he didn't want to pull out the needle," Friend said, "because they'd have to just redo it when they came back. They shut off the flow, a fireman handed me the bottle, and they yanked out the leads from the patches, and took off. I sat on a low brick wall holding my IV bottle awaiting their return. Needless to say, the onlookers were amused. They returned, the movie [was] completed, and it turned out well, about 12 minutes long, although I never won an Oscar."

Dr. Mike Criley said he showed it dozens of times to doctors in training and always said what a remarkable job the paramedics did. "I have seen Dick die, go through at least a dozen heart attacks, and the paramedics always brought him back!" Several years later, a nurse told Friend that she saw the film while in training at Huntington Memorial Hospital. Friend went on to state, "So I got to star in my own production, just another day at the good old LACoFD."

Kicked Out of Long Beach

Universal Studios was expelled from Long Beach after they caused fire damage to a neighboring house while filming "Problem" (episode 2.1). The following account by Dick Friend, Engineer Mike Stoker, and LA County Firefighters Alan Barbee and Ray Ribar is of the night *Emergency!* was "kicked-out" of Long Beach. Dick calls it "Singed eyebrows, cracked windows, WOW!"

In this episode, a fire traps a young boy in a two-story house. Roy DeSoto wades through the smoke, finds the boy hiding under a bed, and hands him over to John Gage before all three exit the building. The house used for the shoot was located on Ocean Boulevard in Long Beach and was going to be demolished soon. Long Beach police blocked off the street during the filming. The production crew fitted the windows with propane gas jets so that flames would shoot outward, and special effects crews lathered highly flammable rubber cement on the walls to create instant flames. A tarp kept out the sunlight to make it appear like night inside the bedroom.

The cameraman, Frank Thackery, was to shoot the scene through the window using a heavy, 35-mm camera. However, the heat of the day caused the rubber cement to vaporize faster than expected, and when the flames ignited, a fireball blew Frank off his ladder. Friend recalls, "The tarp kept him from falling but he slid, face down, on the ladder with the camera banging him all the way down." Thackery's eyebrows were singed, but thankfully neither he, nor the camera, was seriously injured.

The final shoot took place around midnight. Friend had ordered a reserve pumper and crew, and they laid an inch and a half hoseline up to the second floor as a protector line. Friend and his partner, Captain Joe Day, assumed control of the inside protector line to prevent the heat of the propane fire from igniting the interior of the dwelling. They placed a ladder from the second-story bedroom up to the attic crawl hole, where Friend held the hose line and nozzle. When the director called "Cut," they would extinguish the flames.

After a long day, the actors were tired, so Cinader proposed that stunt doubles be used to avoid any possible injuries. LA County Firefighters Alan Barbee and Ray Ribar were up to the task. Ribar said that their job was simply to "drive up to the structure, bail out of the squad, and move a hose line into the burning building," but they never got that far.

The director, Chris Nyby Sr., wanted a large fire and kept asking special effects for more flames, until, as Friend recalls, the entire house started to quiver from the force of the propane. "Steam was starting to build up as the heat dried the wood structure," says Friend. "It was getting hotter and hotter." The director ordered more fire. Friend recalls that the flames were "roaring 20 feet out the front of the house" when they finally heard the sirens of approaching engine and squad, one of the few times the squad's sirens were used.

Mike Stoker recalls sitting in the engine some distance away with the squad, ready to respond. "I knew there was trouble," he said, when he could see the lights and the fire from that far away. "We were told to come in. There was this 'mark' we were supposed to hit, get out, pull hose, etc. Well, I hit the mark but the fire was so hot we could not get out," he said, and "after about the third take the Long Beach officials shut us down." The heat of the blaze cracked windows and singed the lawn at a neighboring home. "We had peeled the paint off of a neighboring house and ignited the drapes," said Stoker. Instead of holding the hoseline assisting Engine 51 and posing as Johnny and Roy, Alan Barbee and Ray Ribar went into the neighboring building, stripped burning drapes from the windows, and soaked them in the bathtub. Ray Ribar recalls, "The shoot was closed down, and we got booted out of the city."

By 2 A.M., the Long Beach fire inspector on site ordered the *Emergency!* cast and crew out of the city. As a punitive measure, they were prohibited from shooting inside the city for a full year.

To complete the episode, they converted a house on Universal's backlot to look like the house in Long Beach so they could shoot the close-ups of Johnny and Roy. The studio paid to repair all the damage.

Engine 51 to the Rescue

Once, in the middle of filming on Universal's backlot, someone spotted smoke from a brush fire at the studio's east perimeter. Universal's Engine 60 (the Crown) responded and passed the filming crew. However, "seeing the engine pass them was too much for the crew of Engine and Squad 51," said Dick Friend, "so Engine 51 (the Ward LaFrance) with Engineer Mike Stoker at the wheel, and its full studio crew, plus a couple of TV crewmen, and Squad 51 with as many as could crowd onto the small truck, set off for the fire. It looked like a scene from an early silent movie; never had fire apparatus been so fully manned. When they arrived, Engine 60 just about had the fire out, but a line was pulled off Engine 51 to assist. An engine from LA City also arrived on scene (as the fire was in the City) and marveled at the great response from the County and along with 'Engineer Stoker' even had Kevin Tighe and Randolph Mantooth on board." The rest of the cast remained on the set, waiting for their return to resume shooting.

Johnny Wrecks a Fire Truck

In "The Parade" (episode 4.13), Johnny "finally" gets to drive a fire apparatus, if only briefly. It's the old antique British engine that Johnny and Roy purchased to restore and drive in parades. The crew was filming him driving the engine from the back of the station (127) when he crashed into a concrete wall along the east side of the station (not in the script). He hit his head on the steering wheel. The technical advisor for the episode, Gil Gillespie, tended to Mantooth's cut. Randy and Gil were loaded into Dick Friend's car, and they drove to Harbor General (Rampart) emergency room to get stitches. Initially, they were ignored by the ER staff, who assumed they were filming a scene there, as they frequently did.

The next day, for Mantooth's birthday, September 19th, they celebrated with a cake, decorated with the words, "Happy Birthday Crash Mantooth," at Station 127. He cut the cake, which was sitting on the tailboard of Engine 51, for the cast, crew, and firefighters of the station.

Revisions were made to the script to explain the bandage on Johnny's forehead. The crash scene was cut from the episode, and Roy drove the engine to the parade. At the convention in 1998, Randy Mantooth indicated that the scar is still visible.

Randy Assists at a Fire

Joe Bartak (PM0073), a technical advisor, remembers fighting a structure fire in Topanga, when Randy Mantooth unexpectedly arrived on the scene.

> Station 69 had two rigs at that time, one staffed and the other used by call firemen (volunteers). During this fire I was at the door alone with no BA [breathing apparatus] and an inch and a half line knocking down the fire in this shed/garage when someone behind me was trying to push me into this smoky shed for no reason. I turned around to give him a piece of my mind (and a little boot), thinking it was one of the volunteers; it was Randy. He was across the canyon visiting some friends when he spotted the flames and decided to help. I laugh today at how excited he was to be on a real incident and trying to get me killed for no reason. Bartak stated, "He turned out to be a real friend to the LA County FD. I have seen him at several events and always wondered if he remembered the shed fire."

Doing Wheelies with Wheelchairs

Firefighter/paramedic Mark Hefley recalls having a wheelchair race with Randy Mantooth:

> Using one of the many wheelchairs used in the show, we would sit in them, pop them back on the large wheels. While balanced, he and I would have slalom races all around the soundstage. Then it somehow progressed into a "who can knock the other over first" contest. We were having a good time until Bob Cinader, the Executive Producer, came on the set. We both got our butts chewed and no more wheelchair races after that.

Bob Fuller's Fear of Spiders

Bob Fuller, the actor who portrayed Dr. Kelly Brackett, was terrified of spiders. Firefighter/paramedic Mike Lewis recalls using a rubber spider to taunt him:

> During one day of shooting one of the episodes I was working on, Ward Bond from the old *Wagon Train* series that Bob Fuller was also on stopped by to visit the set. Bob Fuller and him were in Fuller's dressing trailer on the set and the door was open as they talked. There was a small coffee table between them. I walked by the door and threw a rubber spider in there and it landed on the table between them. Bob Fuller could scream like a lady and did so as he jumped over the table and Ward Bond caught him in mid-air.

Another time, Lewis held the rubber spider on a string down from the rafters while Fuller was talking to Julie London. "Fuller cleared the desk in one jump and out came the scream." At a studio Christmas party, Lewis wore a spider ring and tricked Fuller into shaking hands. When Fuller saw Lewis approaching years later at the convention, Lewis recalls, "The first thing Fuller said was, 'No spiders allowed!'"

Actor and stuntman Scott Gourlay (Officer Scotty) played a spider trick on Fuller while they were shooting "It's How You Play the Game" (episode 4.19). The script called for Scotty to bring a paper bag to Fuller with a jar of grain alcohol inside. However, instead, he replaced the alcohol with a live tarantula. Fuller dropped the jar, and both he and the tarantula fled. Fuller refused to return to the set until the tarantula was caught.

Dr. Fuller Makes a House Call[1]

While at home one evening, Fuller received a call from his neighbor, actress Jackie Joseph, the wife of Ken Berry from *Mayberry RFD*. She told him that she had a metal wire stuck in her finger. Fuller drove over and cleanly removed the wire.

"Did you learn to do this on *Emergency!*?" she asked.

"Not really," he replied, "but that will be $65.00 for the house call after 6 P.M."

Forgotten Lines

As with any television program, lines were often forgotten or botched, but Tim Donnelly relates one worth mentioning. There was a bathroom scene in which Mike Stoker had difficulty with his lines. "Marco and I wrote his lines on a piece of paper and put it in the wash basin," Tim said, "Well, it was great to see him look in and crack up. I think after that it still took him about ten takes to get it. Mike had a great sense of humor."

Missed Basketball Shot

Tim Donnelly stated that one of his favorite episodes was the basketball one, "The Firehouse Five, Plus One" (episode 6.18). "I was the great shooter who lost it," he says. The Laker's Happy Harriston played the referee, and Georg Fenady directed. Donnelly was supposed to perform an odd shot with two hands up over the back, which later became popular with the players. "I kept telling Fenady to let me take a shot at it from a long distance, maybe 20 feet," said Donnelly, and to film it with Tim in the shot, but, says Donnelly, "He did not trust me to make it so—Cut! It took Harriston about 10 to 15 shots off camera to make it for the camera—Edit!"

---

[1] *Emergency Product News*, 8, no. 2 (April 1976).

EMERGENCY! *Behind the Scene*

CHAPTER **17**

Cross-Country Tour with the Ward LaFrance

When NBC acquired the Ward LaFrance that became Engine 51, they arranged for LA County Public Information Officer Dick Friend, LA County Engineer Mike Stoker, Captain Mike Stearns (PM0011), and Firefighter/Paramedic Ed McFall (PM0039) to fly to New York to pick it up. On April 15, 1973, these men began their 26-day, 4000-mile journey to Los Angeles Universal Studios. Along the way, they met with firefighters and fans all across the country and explained this new concept of providing emergency medical support in the field before being transported to the hospital. The Ward made its first appearance on the program in the third season in the episode, "The Old Engine."

The material in this chapter is adapted from an unpublished document by Dick Friend. We are grateful to Dick in allowing us to use his material.

Spring Vacation

Emergency! had completed its second season, and it was time for "spring vacation" in 1973. In the TV industry, they call it a "hiatus"—several months when no filming is done. It's vacation time for the actors. To date Engine 51 had been an actual in-service Crown Firecoach. Problem was, there were only several actually in service to use when filming was done all over a very large county, and the Los Angeles County Fire Department had placed 46 new Ward LaFrance "triple combination" fire engines in service.

Ward executives desperately wanted to show off their new product, and what better chance than every Saturday night on *Emergency!*. During contacts with Executive Producer Robert A. Cinader and the Fire Department, Ward agreed to loan to Universal Studios "a copy" of the engines used by the department. It was being assembled in Elmira, New York.

Cinader proposed a cross-county trip, stopping at cities along the way and working with local fire departments to help explain and promote the new paramedic concept. One problem—the actors were on vacation and unavailable. Who was to make the trip? Cinader spoke with Fire Chief Richard Houts, and it was decided a four-man crew was needed. The chief directed that I assemble the crew and make all arrangements.

Engineer Mike Stoker was a natural and now was back at his "real" job, driving a fire engine at a real fire station. Mike would be the only recognizable member of our crew. I selected Mike Stearns, one of the early paramedics. He had just been promoted to Fire Captain and worked at Station 36, not far from Station 127, which was Station 51 in the series. He had been a technical advisor on several shows.

Firefighter/Paramedic Ed McFall of Station 9 rounded out the crew. NBC gave me a list of cities that the network considered important to visit. We would start our adventure in New York City and finish at Universal Studios in Los Angeles. The Fire Chief wrote to every department along our route asking if they would be interested in having us meet with them and if they would have room. Most could house Engine 51, but not all had extra living space for the four of us. I contacted hotels or motels in those cities. It was spring, so weather should be good for the many thousands of miles.

NBC gave each of us $50 a day in cash for our expenses and covered any cost of hiring overtime personnel to fill in at our jobs. Planning was hectic, with stopover changes almost daily from NBC. Time was short. We loaded our uniforms and turn-out coats, paramedic equipment including the biocom radio, electrocardiogram (EKG) monitor, the trauma and drug boxes, and IV bottles in large wardrobe cases loaned by the studio, and they were sent air express to New York.

New York City

Stoker left a day early and went to Elmira, where he drove the engine to New York City. We flew back and were met at the airport by an NBC publicity man and Stoker in a big limo. WOW! The PR man took us to dinner; we ate, had a few drinks (we were not in our uniforms!), and we wondered what the heck we were doing. We had no credit card to use for fuel; our engine had New York license plates; and we had no registration papers. But we did have a 3-by-8-foot metal placard attached to each side of the engine, which shouted "Emergency! on NBC Saturday nights. A Cross Country Tour . . .", and on our doors was written "Los Angeles County Fire Department" and "51."

On Sunday morning, we had breakfast in our hotel, went to a nearby New York hospital where Engine 51 had spent the night in a garage, and headed for the New York Fire Department (FDNY) "Super Pumper" Station in the Bronx. We were wearing our "grungy" clothes because we had a major cleaning job to do on Engine 51. A station lieutenant met us and gave us a tour of their special "Super Pumper," which had the capability to pump thousands of gallons of water every minute. It was like a fireboat on wheels. The rest of the station crew was not interested in Engine 51—they stayed in their recreation room watching TV.

We found some buckets and cleaning material and started washing. A Deputy Chief backed in and didn't come over to see who we were. It turns out I had made a horrible error in protocol. I addressed the letter to the FDNY to its Fire Chief; it should have gone to the Fire Commissioner! To most in that fire station, we just didn't exist. Our plan had called for us to keep the engine at that station but I said we would leave, but for where? And, we had checked out of our hotel when we left in the morning because we thought they were extremely rude to us in the restaurant at breakfast. Now, we were homeless in New York City!

A New York Department of Hospitals ambulance arrived at the station and we met a young medical doctor who was to be our "victim" during a live demo on the street near Times Square Monday morning. He suggested a hotel that was near the hospital where we had kept the engine the night before.

Monday morning came and we were about to do our first public "show" at Rockefeller Center. A police officer had closed the street for a block, and we were parked at the curb at 8 A.M. with the ambulance next to us. The president of Ward LaFrance appeared, and we had an informal presentation of the keys to Engine 51. (It didn't really use any but it was a great gesture.) I jumped up into the hose bed (empty of hose) and announced to the people walking by that we were about to demonstrate a new life-saving concept now underway in Los Angeles County. Some people stopped. As I spoke, our doctor "patient" (a young doctor from New York's Department of Hospitals) grabbed his chest, let out a gasp, and did an Oscar-winning death drop to the concrete. I narrated each and every action. Stearns and McFall dashed around carrying their equipment, followed by Stoker. They did the entire number, starting an IV, even transmitting an EKG strip and talking to Rampart Hospital. (Our radio didn't really work. We faked all the conversations.) The "dying" patient already was making a remarkable recovery as he was loaded onto the ambulance gurney.

Many people chatted with us, but the policeman asked us to leave so he could reopen the street. More TV crews arrived, and we hurriedly repeated our demo. The cop was very understanding and gracious.

Next stop was Angel Island, home of the FDNY Training Academy. At a traffic signal, a policeman pulled next to us and seeing a fire engine from far away shouted: "Are you guys lost?" We were running on diesel fumes and almost coasted into the Academy grounds. We were refueled there, courtesy of the Assistant Chief in charge. We attended three meetings with medical personnel and city officials. It was Monday evening rush hour on New York highways when we finished, and we were headed for Baltimore. One of the training lieutenants needed a ride home, and it was on our way. He was our guide. We delivered him to his door. Engine 51 was parked in his front yard, where it attracted a crowd of kids and grownups.

Next Stop: Baltimore

We arrived after dark and, by following my precise directions, got lost. While parked looking at our map, a car pulled alongside occupied by two members of the local fire buff club. They escorted us to "6 Engine," a station that had been in service for more than 100 years. This was a real test of Stoker's driving. They pulled their engine out and Stoker backed Engine 51 in, with about three inches to spare on each side of the mirrors!

It was about 10 P.M. One of the firemen's wives had baked a big cake with a welcome message in the frosting, and we sat on the tailboard of our engine actually inside their kitchen! We spent a peaceful night at the dorm upstairs.

An Assistant Chief met us the next day and escorted us downtown to a restaurant, where we spent several hours with officials from the local city/county fire departments, medical providers, and TV writers for the city's two daily newspapers. All seemed very impressed with the paramedic/fire department concept. We "delivered" the writers back to their newspapers on Engine 51, and they loved it.

Baltimore Fire Chief Thomas Burke gave us a plaque commemorating our visit. Our department's art staff had made certificates that we gave to every department where we stayed or stopped, all signed by our Chief.

Our Nation's Capital Is Next

We drove to DC the next day and stayed at a very large fire station in the midst of Washington's impressive government buildings. Firemen worked a 4-10 shift (instead of 24) so they actually never went to bed, although there were many beds in their dorm. A couple of men did catch a few winks, while fully dressed, we noticed. An alarm at 4 A.M. sent them all away. When we got up, a cook had prepared breakfast for us, and the crews were returning.

They had been at a fire at The Smithsonian! I don't think anyone ever considers what a disaster a major fire in that place would be. The blaze was confined to a large electrical control room. (*Little did Dick know then that he and Mike Stoker would be back in Washington, DC, even at the Smithsonian, 27 years later still extolling the virtues of Emergency!.*)

We put on demos at the department's training center for district fire and medical personnel. A recruit class was in session, and they marched them over to observe. The department used military rank, and it looked more like the Marine Corps than the fire department, especially the way the instructors yelled at the newcomers. When we needed a "victim" to be a heart attack victim for our demo, we got one promptly! The instructor told him if we wanted him to die, "damn it, die." We spared him, however.

When we were leaving, the local fire buffs presented us with a complete AAA Trip-Tix map routing. They had earlier borrowed my notebook filled with pages of maps and directions, and the AAA had assembled one easy-to-read cross-country map for us.

We headed straight for the Capitol and drove Engine 51 almost to the Capitol steps. You certainly couldn't even get close now, and the area was somewhat restricted then. We jumped off the rig just as a Capitol cop arrived to chase us away. First, though, he took our cameras and snapped pictures of us posing with the Capitol behind.

Philadelphia and Actor Sid Caesar

We were in a large downtown station and spent the evening cleaning our gear and apparatus. As usual, it was about midnight before we went to bed because everyone wanted to talk about our trip and working with *Emergency!* Shortly before noon, we went to the NBC Studio across from Independence Square and were met by a pretty young woman who was one of their TV anchors for the noon news. We put her in the jump seat with the camera crew hanging on. Engine 51 circled the Square and stopped in front of NBC.

A large makeshift stage had been erected on the steps. We unloaded our paramedic gear. The Philly Fire Department's snorkel was parked alongside and lifted the basket to the roof and lowered actor Sid Caesar to the stage, where we talked about *Emergency!* and our trip. It was a live broadcast.

While the show was on, some fire department mechanics climbed under Engine 51, got in it, and drove away. A Fire Captain motioned "not to worry," but we did. When the telecast ended, he told us they had noticed oil on the apparatus floor where we had parked, and their mechanics had taken it to their shops to check it out. They replaced an oil seal and we got the truck back in several hours.

That afternoon, Fire Chief Joseph Rizzo came to the station and presented each of us with a personal Philadelphia Fire Department membership card. He seemed pleased with the certificate we gave him, expressing our thanks.

On Our Way to Pittsburgh . . . After a Slight Detour

We had a 5-hour drive to Pittsburgh and were slated to stay at the Grant Hotel downtown with a fire station adjacent for Engine 51. Prior to leaving Philadelphia, NBC changed our route. I called NBC in New York every day to receive any schedule updates. We were to spend the night in a city about 30 minutes from Pittsburgh; arrangements had been made for us to store the engine at one of the town's two fire stations (all volunteer), and they had made sleeping arrangements in a large motel.

We found the station and quite a crowd of their volunteers and others had assembled. There was no brass band, but we felt quite honored and pleased with the nice reception. An Assistant Chief "volunteered" his wife to do our laundry, but we declined. (We did regular laundry duty at laundromats along the route.)

The chief delivered us to a large downtown motel and invited us to spend that Friday night drinking beer with the "vollies." He left and we checked in. We were in uniform but the clerk wanted to know exactly who was "to sleep with whom." We frankly didn't care as long as there were two beds in each room. I paired up with Stearns and Stoker and Ed took the other. I used my credit card to pay. (We kept a running tab and we shared the expenses when we got home.)

A large billboard outside advertised there was a popular singing group appearing in their lounge. No way. They hadn't been there in weeks. The heated swimming pool was empty. As we made our way down a long corridor, two ladies wearing very short, tight skirts and high heels and lots of makeup passed us. One muttered loud enough for us to hear: "They let anyone in here now." They were looking mostly at Ed, who was Black.

Stoker and McFall hit their room and we ours. I asked Mike if he had heard the comment and he had. In two minutes, I announced "we are out of here," and we got Stoker and McFall and headed for the office with our travel bags. A young attractive woman was now in the office and she immediately recognized Mike Stoker. I told her there had been a mistake and we had to leave and please tear up the credit card bill. She did. We asked where she would stay if she were downtown, and she named the Grant Hotel. She telephoned them and they had plenty of rooms.

I called NBC and said Stoker would need transportation next morning from the hotel to the town where we kept our engine, but we were leaving now. We stuffed into a taxi and drove to the Grant. They even opened the steam room for us. I called the assistant chief and told him we had a change in plans and could not join them for their Friday night get-together.

At 6 A.M., an NBC limo driver joined us for breakfast and took Mike to get Engine 51. We spent the entire day at Pittsburgh's fire training academy putting on demos for fire officers and EMS officials from numerous cities and towns. Fire Chief Thomas J. Kennelly personally greeted us at the training center, even though it was a Saturday. We kept Engine 51 in one of their stations that night. We later discovered that the Pittsburgh Fire Department had not been notified that we were not staying with them Friday night.

Another "Really B-I-G Show"

It was off to the races—horse races that is—after our day of demos. We arrived at a large racetrack several miles out of town during the third race. We were led onto the track, and after the race was completed, we responded with a red light/siren around the track and stopped in front of the grandstands. The place was packed. We had brought with us a very popular local noontime radio and TV personality. A small stage had been set up. We lined up at the side of Engine 51, and he did a short interview with each of us. We were used to this now and had it "down pat." I usually would start off with a general description of our mission, talking about paramedics in the fire service. I'd then hand it off to another, but usually never in the same order. We decided this would keep us alert because you didn't know when you'd be next. One might even hand it back to you, so stay tuned.

Stearns and McFall would go more into detail about the role of the paramedic and the training required. Stoker would talk about being in *Emergency!* and driving a fire engine all across the country. We got a great reception from the large audience.

We drove the engine off the track and were ushered up into the owner's box, where we had a great dinner. We stuffed our badges into our pockets so we could "legally" enjoy a cool beer (or two). Stoker did not drink.

Ed won about $100 betting on the horses! The owner joined us and said that each Saturday night they have some kind of visiting "entertainment," including paratroopers or fireworks. He said we had drawn the biggest applause of the season. We took this with a grain of salt and another beer.

Next morning was Easter Sunday. As we departed the Pittsburgh station, their alarms went off (just like in *Emergency!*) and the dispatch center announced: "Thanks to the L.A. County Fire Department for sharing your time with us. Have a safe trip and God's speed."

We Make It to the Cincinnati Fire Department—Almost

This was one of our rare 8-hour days on the road. We were on an interstate and it was a warm day. We rotated seats, except for Stoker who always drove. Every day one of us was "Captain" and read all the maps and charts. The other two were nestled into the jump seats. It was fun waving back to people who passed on the freeway, saw Engine 51, and waved frantically. Probably to keep us awake, Stoker swung off the freeway into a very small town. We became instantly awake and waved at curious residents who stared as we drove up and down their streets, in an LA County fire engine.

On the freeway, we saw a car stopped on the other side with steam pouring from under the open hood. A couple of men were staring at the engine. Stoker came to a halt, and Ed and I ran across eight lanes. Luckily there was no fire because we had no hose, no water, not even a fire extinguisher. As we walked up, they said they had blown a water hose. "What are you doing here from LA?" they asked. We told them we had been sent to a car fire, even though "it was a bit out of our district." They appreciated our concern.

About 30 minutes later, we came across an empty car parked on the shoulder and soon after saw a young man walking, a long way from any town it appeared. We asked him if he wanted a ride to the nearest gas station. He was an *Emergency!* fan. Now he was actually riding in Engine 51. We let him out at a gas station and were told they could get him a ride back to his car with a can of gas.

We desperately needed fuel. Many of the gas stations were closed for Easter. We found one station, but they had no diesel; we were told to take the next off-ramp and follow it for a mile or so. There was this very small town: a gas station with two pumps and a small shed, a post office, a small store, and a little café. At the gas station sat an older man in his coveralls. He just stared as we pulled up and climbed off. "My God," he said. "That fire truck is so big." He was a member of the local volunteer fire department. We offered him a ride, but he said he couldn't leave.

While pumping our fuel, a teenaged girl ran over from the café. She had recognized Stoker. She was quite flustered but got out that the woman in the café invited us in for some homemade ice cream. There were about three or four people eating, and they had their noses pressed to the glass watching us. We had great ice cream and the girl followed us out. As we started to pull away, she looked at Stoker and said: "I was raised in this town. Seeing you from *Emergency!* is the happiest day of my life. Thanks for stopping here." We all darn near cried.

It was a long drive, and it was getting dark as we approached the Cincinnati suburbs—and we were again low on fuel. We stopped at a fire station but it was empty—all volunteer. The fuel gauge was bobbing on "E." We were heading down a slight incline with very heavy traffic in both directions, and the engine conked out. Mike did a remarkable job of steering clear of other cars, and we made it to the curb . . . not knowing where we were.

There was a boarded and dark brick building on our right. I saw a phone booth across the street and with trip "Bible" in hand headed over and put in a call to the Cincinnati Fire Department (CFD) headquarters. At that exact moment, the front doors on the boarded building opened, and it was a fire station! Four men came out and I ran back. They were confused and a bit leery of us. Was this some kind of trick? Their station had been blasted at and shot at because of the area. Were we on some kind of "Trojan Horse" and going to steal their fire truck? I held my book open to the letter from the CFD chief. They invited us in.

They had diesel and Mike rolled the rig back into the station so we could fill up. Shortly, a CFD rescue squad appeared and escorted us to the headquarters. When we pulled up, there stood Mickey Michaels, the set designer for *Emergency!* and a great friend of our department. I had called Universal earlier stating we were nearly out of IV bottles for our demos. He jumped on the next flight out of LA and personally brought us several cases. He rode with us for most of the way home.

We made several TV appearances with the CFD on Monday. On Tuesday, we headed for Indianapolis. After the usual greetings, we changed into our civvies and for the first time, each went our own way getting haircuts and hitting a store for extra underwear or socks.

We were back at the station to have dinner with the crew. They were sitting on a loading platform at the rear of the station having a "refreshment," or two. They got an alarm and headed for their apparatus—an engine, ladder truck, and rescue vehicle. Engine 51 was boxed in, so we grabbed our turnouts and jumped onto the nearest unit. I was in the cab of the truck company. We had only gone several blocks when the first-arriving company turned us back, but we kept going. They wanted us to get off and wander around with our LA County Fire Departments turn-outs just to baffle the onlookers.

The next day, we drove onto a large entry at City Hall and parked next to its rescue truck. It was a lot of standing and talking with those who passed by. We also visited a grammar school and chatted with the kids who tried to identify all of the paramedic gear that we held and they had seen on the TV program. These were not our favorite kind of "work" days.

St. Louis: Where's the Beef?

Our itinerary directed us to go to the famous Gateway Arch along the Mississippi. We were later than expected, but a Park Ranger was waiting and took us up in a tram to see the city. The river had flooded, and some of the river cruise boats were almost on the pier.

We pulled Engine 51 into the mechanical shops of the St. Louis, Missouri, Fire Department and took our personal luggage next door to their headquarters station. Our itinerary called for a dinner courtesy of NBC at the local studio, and we were to meet the Fire Chief. The department took us over and we were greeted by NBC people and escorted into a nice conference room, with a well-stocked bar. We were in uniform and do not drink in uniform in public. We also were all going back to the station to meet with families and friends of the firemen and talk about *Emergency!*. We had a coke. "Dinner" looked very pretty, but it was nothing but tiny little hors d'oeuvres. The Fire Chief arrived and seemed none too happy. As we all chatted, he loosened up and seemed to enjoy our company.

We soon departed for the fire station, accompanied by the Chief. He introduced us in glowing terms to the forty or fifty gathered there. He stayed almost an hour as we talked and took pictures with those present. The Chief's driver said he had not been on "the floor" for many months, and he hadn't seen the Chief enjoying himself this much in a long time.

Next day, we drove out into the suburbs to a brand new shopping mall, where we parked and displayed our paramedic gear. Practically no one came to visit. It was getting very cold and windy. About noon, a fire truck pulled up with two volunteers from a nearby town. They had seen the engine and pulled in, surprised to see Engine 51! They went to a nearby fast food place and brought us back lunch and hot drinks. At about 1 P.M., I made a phone call to NBC and said we were leaving. The volunteers led us back to the proper freeway.

Another Challenge for Stoker: Driving *In* a Mall

We checked into Kansas City, Missouri, main station and walked a half block to our hotel. The crew had invited us to dinner at 6 P.M. sharp, "not wearing your uniforms!" Stoker had laundry call, so he took our clothes to the corner laundromat. The phone rang and it was a local TV station. They were doing a documentary on new emergency medical programs and were sending a crew to the fire station to meet us. The three of us assembled what part of our uniforms weren't at the wash and headed back. We used a new Kansas City fireman as a victim and used another to fill in for Stoker. It went well and was aired that night.

We headed back to the hotel to shed our uniforms, and we were at the station on time. They led us down the street into a little tavern. As we entered, shouts and cheers went up, and they had made a big banner welcoming us. Most were off-duty firemen, families, and friends. A good time was had by all.

Next day we were led to a brand new enclosed shopping mall. Stoker carefully guided Engine 51 around large open ponds and planters, and we set up shop, with the paramedic gear and Ed and Mike on the tailboard and Stoker and I in front. Many people stopped and asked about this new paramedic concept. We signed a lot of autographs. Early on, we decided to make a circle around 51, as on the engine, and sign "For Johnny and Roy . . . " and our name. We laughed that weeks later people wouldn't remember who the heck we were anyway.

Look Out Kansas: Here We Come

The Fire Chief from the other Kansas City, in Kansas, met us at the shopping center with a couple of motorcycle officers, and the Chief's car leading went red light/siren over rush hour traffic to the Indian Springs Shopping Center in his state. We spent several hours and visited with a lot of people.

We had a full travel day and stopped in a motel in Hays, Kansas. The Fire Chief had written that they had no room in their station for the engine. It was a single-bay station within City Hall. As we checked in, the clerk told us that many people were aware of our arrival; he suggested we park the engine behind, or we would have nothing but visitors. However, laundry called and we headed downtown and parked Engine 51 outside the laundry. Soon after we had the washers running, a young man told us he was a fireman, and the Chief asked if we would drive to the station and leave the engine. They were parking their truck outside. He asked if it was okay to invite people to come over and take pictures.

When done with our laundry, we drove to City Hall and left Engine 51 and he took us back to our hotel. We invited him to join us for dinner at the local VFW hall that the chief had recommended. The chief had an injured foot and couldn't join us. The same fireman picked us up at the motel the next day to retrieve the engine.

Quite a Welcome in Denver

It was evening rush hour as we approached Denver's newest fire station on Ogden Street, just out of the downtown area. As we stopped, crewmembers rushed over carrying CO_2 fire extinguishers—it was then we noticed that smoke was coming from under the right front wheel well. A small air blower had shorted out. They blasted it with CO_2. We pulled into the station, and in minutes one of their mechanics arrived and installed a new part. Denver Fire Department had identical Ward LaFrance engines.

It snowed most of the night, a real sight for us from LaLa Land. Denver Fire Chief Merle Wise greeted us early and escorted us to another station across town. He had assembled people from city and county governments as well as many suburban Fire Chiefs from as far away as Vail. We met and gave demonstrations most of the day. That night, we went on a live TV interview program with the Chief and held meetings until about 10 P.M.

The Eisenhower Memorial Tunnel through the Rockies was closed for major repairs. The roads were icy, and we had no chains. Chief Wise arranged for the State Highway Department to meet us at the entrance and escort us through a maze of construction equipment. Once there, we were on our own, and the road had not been completely cleared of ice. We had all climbed into the front seat (all four of us) because it was very cold. As we started down, however, I opted to be in a jump seat. I explained that if we slid off the road, I could jump free but they would all crash and die in the wreckage of Engine 51. Thanks to Stoker, we made it safely.

While having a quick lunch in Vail, their Fire Chief, who had attended one of the meetings the day before, sent his volunteers over and took Engine 51 back to the station, where they steamed off the ice under our truck.

It was about 4 P.M. when we arrived in sunny Grand Junction, Colorado. We stayed at a motel and kept our engine across the street in their No. 2 fire station. At the invitation of the Chief, we drove to the headquarters station in early evening and spoke with dozens and dozens of firemen and families and friends. We finally realized we hadn't eaten dinner and headed to a nearby McDonald's. Several dozen cars followed us, and we continued visiting while we munched on our Big Macs at the engine.

Utah: Engine 51 Gives Out

Salt Lake City was uneventful for us, at least at first. The department had no planned activities for us but graciously housed us in a beautiful new station. The next day we were en route to Las Vegas. Just outside of Provo, the engine threw a section of drive shaft, and we clunked to a halt on the interstate. I had brought my portable radio and we had tried it many times, but only once got a reply from a department in Ohio that used the same frequency. We were about a mile from a small farm town we could see across the fields. Stoker and I hoofed it over there and stopped in a gas station. I asked a young man washing down the station if I could make a collect phone call, and he deferred to his boss who said no—and we were in uniform, too.

We could see "something" going on several blocks away and found a wrecking crew demolishing a small building with lots of spectators, including a state trooper. He took us to his tiny office and I called the Ward factory. It was Saturday. We were told to sit tight at the engine, and the trooper took us back. In several hours, a tow rig from Provo arrived and hooked up poor Engine 51. We arrived at a transmission repair shop just before noon, closing time. The Salt Lake City Fire Department had arranged for them to stay open.

We walked down the street and had lunch, and when we returned, the mechanics and their kids were all over Engine 51 taking pictures. Not only had they installed a new part, but they had painted it! Because of this delay, we were forced to stop over in St. George for the night. The weather was miserable.

Arrival in Las Vegas (At the Wrong Place!)

Our travel time was about 5 hours, but the weather was great all day. As we pulled off the freeway, there was Las Vegas Fire Station #1. We pulled in the rear, where a fireman was washing some fire prevention cars. He greeted us and called his Captain. We said we were there to spend the night and would do some stuff on TV the next day. He offered us one of their red cars to take our travel bags and us to our hotel on the Strip. (NBC had made these hotel arrangements for us.) I opted to call the NBC public relations person and she soon arrived and transported us.

Stoker and I were in one room and Stearns and McFall were in others; they were expecting their wives. While putting on our poolside attire, the Clark County Fire Department called and asked why we were not at "their" fire station where we were supposed to be. I had no answer but to confess we didn't know the difference and the crew at the Las Vegas Fire Department station acted as if they expected us. NBC treated us all to a great dinner and show in one of the hotels that night.

We were parked outside a shopping center next day, with the Clark County rescue squad nearby. As usual, Stearns and McFall were showing off the paramedic equipment at the rear of the engine, and Stoker and I were stationed up front. This guy came up holding a camera. He had cut-off shorts, no shirt, a very shaggy beard, and somewhat long hair. He took my picture and as he lowered the camera, I saw that it was Randolph

Mantooth! None of the others recognized him. He had been hiking and camping with his brother for several weeks and had seen a TV promotion that morning about our visit.

I told him to climb in the cab and he started moving switches up and down. I called to Stoker and said, "This guy is messing around in there. Please ask him to leave." Polite Stoker calmly asked him to stop, and Randy kept playing around. Stoker raised his voice and ordered the guy out. With that, Randy leaped out right onto Stoker, who recognized him a split second before they collided. We all roared with laughter.

The NBC public relations lady met us for lunch, and I went into a small radio studio in the mall and did a live interview. She then took me to a TV studio a mile away, and I met a local personality who was to interview me. I had no equipment to show, no anything. We still had 15 minutes until "show time" and I phoned the Clark County fire dispatcher. Yes, their rescue squad was still with Engine 51. I asked them to escort the engine to the studio as rapidly as possible. A member of the stage crew set up three more chairs. The TV host was not present.

Shortly afterward, I heard sirens and the stage man opened the back door. As Engine 51 pulled up, I said to unload all the paramedic gear and take the seats on the stage. Naturally, they complied. Seconds before we went on the air, the host came in, looked around, and was quite confused. I introduced his new guests, backed out of the set, and watched the entire interview from the control room. It went well!

Engine 51 Is Back in Its Own District

Our trip back to Los Angeles County seemed very long. We were finishing a 26-day journey unlike any other. As we crossed the San Bernardino/Los Angeles County borders, I used the radio: "LA Engine 51. We're back in our district." The dispatcher, without missing a beat, acknowledged: "Welcome home Engine 51." Shortly, we were asked to notify dispatch when we were about 15 minutes from headquarters. On arrival, Fire Chief Houts and the entire top headquarters staff were there to welcome us.

The next day, we drove to Universal Studios, where Chief Houts, Kevin Tighe, Bob Fuller, Julie London, Bobby Troop, and some studio and Ward LaFrance executives met us. Our trip was over after nearly 4000 miles!

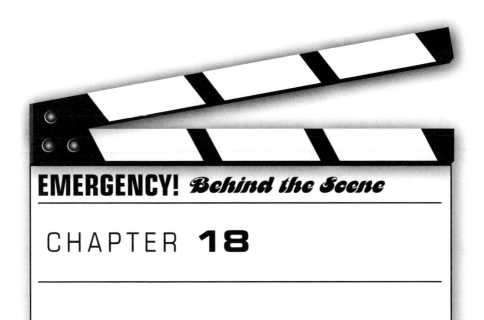

EMERGENCY! *Behind the Scene*

CHAPTER **18**

Collectibles

Although the show ran its last call in 1977, *Emergency!* collectibles are still hot. Prices continue to soar on collectibles from the 1970s and today, although none of the cast members have benefited from royalties of collectible sales. Even after 30 years, authorized products are still being released in the name of and the likeness of *Emergency!*. The list in this chapter is not all-inclusive, although it does include some that never made it into the stores.

Board Game

Milton Bradley made three versions of its *Emergency!* board game:

- Standard 11-by-17-inch version
- French language 11-by-17-inch version made by Somerville Industries for Milton Bradley in Canada
- Smaller 11-by-14-inch version, with different photo insets

Drawing Slates

At least three Johnny Gage *Emergency!* slates were licensed in 1977 by Universal City Studios. It featured Johnny on the front with a handi-talkie and the squad. On the back, it had a photo of Johnny and Roy from the last season of the program, along with directions on how to use the slate. There were two graphic versions, one with Johnny holding a radio with the writing stylus on the front and one without the radio and the stylus holder on the back. A third version, a new TV Magic Slate, offered later wrote in Magicolor© and depicted John on the front with a handi-talkie and the squad. These items all selling for 59¢ were produced by the Samuel Lowe Company of Kenosha, Wisconsin.

Lunchboxes

Produced by Aladdin Industries of Nashville, Tennessee, these steel lunchboxes came in three versions: two rectangular styles [flat panels on each side and bias-relief (embossed) panels] and one domed. Johnny and Roy are depicted along with their 51 Squad, and the name *"Emergency!"*. Roy and Johnny's helmet shields read "LA County," although the squad reads "LUEDIEI" County Fire Department, not Los Angeles.

The *Emergency!* lunchbox graphics were designed by Elmer Lehnhardt, art director for Aladdin Industries. He designed other popular lunchboxes depicting the *Beverly Hillbillies, Bonanza, Land of the Giants*, and many other television shows. He began his artistic career under the instruction of Haddon Sunbloom, the creator of the Coca-Cola™ Santa Claus.

Firefighter Sets

In 1975 Placo Toys issued an *Emergency!* Firefighter Set for children ages 3 to 5. Included in this set was a red *Emergency!* helmet (which also sold separately in yellow, black, and gold) along with a bullhorn, firefighter badge, and air tank with mask. They also released an *Emergency!* fire helmet and bullhorn set in 1975, which did not include the air tank.

Records

In 1976, a 33$\frac{1}{3}$ LP record album, 12-inch vinyl, was released with three episodes not seen on the television program. It featured cast photos on the album cover, although none of the voices are from the actual cast and no writers' credits are given. It was produced by Wonderland, a product of A.A. Records, Inc., with the Wonderland Players, and Tom Cipolla and

Bob Goemann. Included in the album is an order form for iron-on transfers for *Beretta, Bionic Woman, Donnie and Marie,* or *Elton John.*

Sheet Music

Emergency!'s theme composer, Nelson Riddle, released sheet music as a piano solo with a photo of the cast on the cover.

Publications

Comic Books and Magazines

In 1976 and 1977, Charlton Publications issued four comic books and four of the larger magazines about the exploits of Station 51. The comics cost the fan 30 cents for each issue, and the magazine size cost $1.00. The stories in these Charlton publications were stories written for Charlton and not stories seen on the television program. The Charlton Comics contained one complete story with only Johnny and Roy and the Rampart staff written in, while the crew of Engine 51 included different characters from the series. The magazine contained three to four complete stories in each issue along with cast photos and information from the TV program.

In 1979, World Distributors Ltd. in Manchester, England, issued an *Emergency! Annual,* ironically after the series was canceled. This comic was authorized by "*Emergency!* Productions" and included close-ups of the stars of the program. This rare British annual usually sells for around $100.00 (U.S. dollars) on the secondary market.

Novel

Chris Stratton wrote a novel, titled *Emergency!*, based on the TV characters in 1972; it was published by Popular Library. Stratton also published an *Adam-12* novel the same year.

Crosswords

The January 2004 issue of *TV Guide Crosswords,* a monthly publication, featured a "Lifesavers—TV Heroes to the Rescue" edition. The "New Puzzle" section featured a Johnny and Roy photo and full-page article about firefighting and paramedic programs that have aired since *Emergency!*. In the puzzle, several of the questions related to *Emergency!*, and the program was featured in the "Bonus Jumble."

It is said you can gauge how popular a program is by how often it shows up in *TV Guide*'s Crossword.

| *TV Guide* crosswords puzzles with an *Emergency!* tie-in: |

June 17, 1972	42 down	*Emergency!* starr Bobby _____.	Ans:. Troop
Oct. 19, 1974	39 down	*Emergency!'s* Roy __Soto.	Ans: De
Nov. 2, 1974	6 down	Mantooth role on *Emergency!*	Ans: Gage
Dec. 21, 1974	14 across	Randolph Mantooth series	Ans: *Emergency!*
Mar. 6, 1976	1 across	fireman Kelly	Ans: Chet
Mar. 6, 1976	48 across	*Emergency!* actor	Ans: Donnelly
Nov. 11, 1978	4 across	Emergency treatment	Ans: IV

| From seven different *Summer TV Crosswords'* puzzles during the run of *Emergency!*: |

4 across	*Emergency!* nurse Dixie	Ans: McCall
21 down	Roy DeSoto on *Emergency!*	Ans: Paramedic
3 down	*Emergency!* actor Randolph	Ans: Mantooth
25 across	*Emergency!* emergency	Ans: Fire
40 down	*Emergency!'s* Dr. Joe	Ans: Early

Released in January 2006 by Penny Press, the Word Seek book, *Remember the 70's* includes *Emergency!* as one of the answers in the "On the Tube: The 1970's" puzzle.

Television Guides

TV Guide

There are four U.S. *TV Guide* covers with cast members on the cover and related articles:

- Julie London, June 17, 1972
- Robert Fuller, August 18, 1973
- Randy Mantooth and Kevin Tighe, August 3, 1974
- Randy Mantooth and Kevin Tighe with the hospital cast, August 16, 1975

Other articles appeared in *TV Guide* on April 7, 1972 (as part of a Cleveland Armory review); July 29, 1972 (as a three-page review by New York Fire Department firefighter and author Dennis Smith); March 24, 1973, April 8, 1973, October 20, 1973, November 17, 1973, and August 9, 1975. The February 11, 1978, issue featured a two-page photo spread showing a jet crashed into a housing development for the movie *Survival on Charter 220*.

TV Week

This rare regional television guide published for the *Sunday News* in Lancaster, Pennsylvania, features a drawing of the five principal cast members on the cover. Issued for the week of September 19, 1976, the two-page article, with several photos, discusses the new TV program *Emergency One!* starring Bobby Troop. It premiered for the first time in syndication on WLYH-TV that week, joining the evening lineup on ABC.

Tele*Guia

The June 7–13, 1973, version of this foreign television guide, printed in Mexico by Editorial Television, featured Robert Fuller as Dr. Brackett from *Emergencia* on the cover, although it had no article about the program. A similar photo appeared on the U.S. *TV Guide* for August 1973. The August 21–27, 1975 issue of *Tele*Guia* featured Johnny and Roy in the squad on the cover, with a related article. Fuller appeared as Dr. Brackett on another cover in 1977.

TV Guia

Argentina's *TV Guia* for the week of August 8, 1978, featured a two-page article with photos, including one from *Survival on Charter 220.*

Under Cover

This monthly Argentinean TV news magazine included a four-page article in the issue for April 2000 with photos about *Emergencia.*

TV TIMES

A Canadian supplement to the *Montreal Gazette* for the week of January 29/February 4, 1972, featured a two-page article and photo of Julie London in her nurse uniform.

Trading Cards

The Topps Bubble Gum Company released a limited number of *Emergency!* bubble gum cards in 1972. Within the Topps set there were 27 *Adam-12* cards and 27 *Emergency!* cards. Due to poor sales in the test market area, sales were discontinued. Current price on an uncut sheet at time of printing was over $4,500.

Toys

Movie

In 1978 after the series conclusion, the Ideal Toy Corporation, in its only venture into the TV program, released an *Emergency!* "Pocket Flix" movie.

The film strip had to be inserted into a hand-held projector (sold separately) that, when held to the viewer's eye and wound by hand, allowed the movie to be viewed.

Action Sets

In 1975, Fleetwood Toys "TV Super Stars" line included TV programs such as *CHiPs*, *Adam-12*, and *S.W.A.T.* In the *Emergency!* line, Fleetwood Toys Inc. in New York issued several types of plastic action accessory kits, survival kits, and medical kits. Fleetwood also issued a seven-piece "Paramedic Kit" and a five-piece "Utility" pouch. The "Rescue Squad with Firehouse" set contained a plastic helicopter, sedan automobile, and pumper, all on a blister card with *Emergency!* photos. Strangely enough, there was no squad in the set.

The air rescue set included a helicopter with the livery of "Los Angeles County (51) Fire Dept" and five plastic firefighters; it was authorized by Emergency Productions and licensed by Universal City Studios Inc. The blister-pac card has a photo of Johnny and Roy taken from the opening credits scene of the tanker exploding behind them.

In 1981 Imperial released two City Fire Department "Emergency Team" sets, with five vehicles including the squad and engine, helicopter, Chevy Blazer, and sedan with "FD" within the gold shield on the sides of the vehicles. The box art on these two sets featured a drawing of a firefighter with a helmet shield depicting LA County Station 36.

In England, the same set was released by Trafalgar Toys (imported from Hong Kong) with the same City Fire Department and gold shield tampos (similar to a decal) on the vehicles and same box graphics, except instead of the LA County Station 36 shield there was a British firefighter.

Lights

Fleetwood released a plastic "Rescue Light" in 1975. It came with a battery and three colored lenses (amber, blue, and red). The emblem on the light was that as seen in the closing credits of *Emergency!*, the round medical emblem. Roy DeSoto appeared alone on the card stock.

Action Figures

At least three different boxed sets of the eight-inch-tall, fully jointed action figures of Johnny and Roy were released by the L.J.N. Company. One of which, released in 1973, was in their "Super Stars" series that has them wearing the blue station wear with several cast photos on the box. In the other set, the Johnny and Roy figures are wearing brown jackets, depicting their turn-out jackets, and were released exclusively through Montgomery Ward and in the JC Penney catalog (Catalog Item Number x 924-4682A) in 1978. There were no cast photos on the generic brown box. Another brown box (item 6195C) set has the Johnny and Roy figures in blue uniform with a few accessories, an ax, ladder, extinguisher, and breathing apparatus tank with mask.

The action figures in blue uniform were also released in 1973 on blister cards with seven photos from the show with an L.J.N. item stock number of 6102 and original price of $2.29. The top of the packaging was either red or black toped on the blister card. Also released in the 'Super Stars' line was an action accessory kit containing items that would fit the action figures such as a ladder, helmet with the LA County front shield, ax, radio, extinguisher, flashlight, boots, first aid kit, and Breathing Apparatus tank with mask, L.J.N. item number 6131.

Trucks

The L.J.N. Toys Ltd. Company of New York released a squad (emergency rescue truck, 70 mm, model 2000) and a Ward LaFrance Engine (emergency fire truck, 73 mm, model 2000) both 1:64 scale, in 1975. The engine has a removable dark gray ladder located on top of the engine. They both have red paint jobs, with no tampos indicating department or station number. These were distributed individually in the "Road*Stars" series with original cast photos on the blister cards and were authorized by Universal Television as *Emergency!* toys. Although the squad was a new casting, it was based on a Chevrolet 1 ton.

These two vehicles were later released in a "Road*Stars" boxed set that included vehicles from *The Rookies* (ABC 1972–1976) and *S.W.A.T.* (ABC 1975–1976).

L.J.N. was a Japanese toy company that started as a subsidiary of the Matsushita Electric Industrial Company in Japan, the makers of Panasonic products. Ironically, L.J.N. Toys Ltd. division was purchased by MCA/Universal in 1986, and MCA sold the company in 1988 to Acclaim Entertainment, a video game company.

Later the same models were issued under the Imperial (Squad - model 8284, engine - model 8211), Laramie (engine - model 8222), and JaRu (engine - model 8222) toy company names, with the engine having a white ladder and different running boards. The Laramie issue included fire extinguishers on the sides. Imperial Toys of Los Angeles issued the squad and engine using the same casting from L.J.N. Toys and using the tampo of a gold shield and FD within the logo.

L.J.N. also released in 1973 a vinyl fire station/Rampart Hospital "Emergency Action set." It was designed to accommodate the squad and the action figures. The station folds out and converts to the inside of Fire Station 51 and Rampart Emergency. The advertising description is as follows: "It is a ©1973 Emergency Productions. It features two floors of adventure for your Emergency figures; John and Roy! They sleep in bunks on the top floor and slide down the pole to their headquarters. They can enter the Emergency Room elevator from two directions and go upstairs for emergency treatment. The play set folds into a carrying case. It closes with a sturdy lock and comes packaged in a corrugated sleeve."

Dinky Toy

The front of the display box is advertised as *From The TV Series "Emergency"* and depicts two LA County firefighters. *Emergency!* Productions authorized a die-cast version of the squad by the Dinky Toys (division of British toymaker Meccano Ltd.). This Dinky #267, Paramedic Truck, is approximately 1:40 scale, 119 mm in length. It has a paper label livery of "Emergency (51) Rescue Squad" affixed to the doors. Included were Johnny and Roy plastic figures, removable yellow air bottles, and a "lapel badge." This badge is not a badge as known in the United States (a metal emblem worn over the left breast on the uniform). This is a yellow plastic badge (patch),[1] about 2 inches round, embossed with the logo as seen in closing credits of the show. The number on the firefighter's helmets on this box design as well as two other pre-production boxes was not "51"; however, the helmets were numbered for Station "8."

The Paramedic Truck was introduced in England in 1979 and was one of the very last pieces of fire apparatus released by Dinky. It was in production for that year only as the Binns Road factory of Dinky Toys, based in Liverpool England, closed down in 1979. The model was, however, available for a few years to clear unsold stock. The back of the box depicts other Dinky models available at the time, two British fire apparatus and an ambulance, in front of a burning building in a scene not related to the TV program.

The Paramedic Truck had also been intended for use in a gift set, first announced in the 1978 Trade catalog and intended for release that year. The set was allocated as item number 302 "Emergency Gift Set." In the 1978 Trade catalog the set is shown with what is clearly a handmade mock-up box, and shows a prepro resin Paramedic Truck with blue emergency lights and silver air bottles, accompanied by a red Plymouth Fire Chief sedan. The sedan is a re-liveried version of the Dinky #244 Police car. The front of the box reads, "The 'Emergency'™ Gift Pack 302. The Emergency series is one of TV's most exciting programmes. This gift set features the new Paramedic Truck and flame red Plymouth Fire Chief's car plus two figures of Gage and DeSoto, © 1977 Emergency Productions."

By the time the 1978 Dinky retail *Die-Cast Toy Catalogue #14* was released (the last catalog Dinky published and cost 5 pence or about 8 or 9

---

[1] Many of the LA County Stations have patches that are not department issue or authorized to be worn on station wear, and Station 127 is not alone. The center of the patch shows "Light Force 127" with the station engines and underneath, "Home of The Show," "KMG 365." While there are several of these prized patches for many of the stations, it does not appear, at this writing, that there is one for FS51 located at Universal Studios.

cents U.S.), the Fire Chief car had been replaced with Dinky's #288 Cadillac Superior Ambulance, complete with a patient on a stretcher. The Cadillac had started its life in 1967 as model #267 with a flashing red roof light. It was retooled and issued a new stock number in 1971 as Dinky #288, bottom stamped, "Superior Rescuer on a Cadillac Chassis," with a white-over-red paint scheme and without the flashing light on the roof. For this set, it was repainted with a white-over-yellow paint scheme. The retail catalog has a prototype of this model together with the resin prototype of the Paramedic Truck in a proper pre-production box with the livery of "Los Angeles County (51) Fire Department Rescue Squad."

The Emergency Squad #302 set was still shown in the 1979 trade catalog in the same form, but it was not put into production and released due to the factory closing. Interestingly, in this last publication, the note by the item shows that while the Paramedic Truck was licensed from the makers of *Emergency!,* the ambulance was "not licensed." Perhaps it was included because it looked similar to the Cadillac used during the first season of the show. That vehicle was a Cadillac Miller-Meteor with the Mayfair livery.

At least one prototype for this ambulance with the white-over-yellow paint scheme is known to exist, and it changed hands in 2006 for almost $200.00 U.S. This one would have been used for the catalog photography and also for showing to buyers at trade fairs. The last trade fair that Dinky attended was in 1980 at the British Toy and Hobby Fair at Earls Court in London. In 2004, four complete, finished, but unfolded boxes for the #302 set turned up in an auction lot, showing how close to production the set reached. These were identical to that shown in the 1978 retail toy catalogue and the 1979 trade catalogues.

On the base of the box and the rear, cut-out buildings were printed. Text on the box reads, "As flames rage through the top floors of a luxury hotel, guests – finding their escape route cut off to the blaze – rush to their windows. But they are too high up to jump! You're in command of the Emergency Squad. You send officers DeSoto and Gage into action. While fire services tackle the blaze, DeSoto and Gage clear the people from the burning building and rush them by ambulance to the nearest hospital. On the spot treatment is given to badly burned survivors using equipment carried in the Paramedic Truck."

Grouped by theme in the 1978 toy catalog #14 but not sold as a set, as illustrated on page 30, were three vehicles, one of which was the resin Paramedic Truck (now with red emergency lights and yellow air bottles) identified as *From The TV Series "Emergency!"* with the livery of "Los Angeles County (51) Fire Dept. Rescue Squad." It has the Paramedic Truck, along with the #288 white-over-red Cadillac Superior ambulance, and the previously released #274 Ford Transit Ambulance (129 mm in length), both with a patient on a stretcher.

When the Dinky Toy factory closed down, John Gay, a specialist model dealer in Kent, England, purchased several hundred "blank" models and leftover labels. Gay re-liveried the models with various logos and sold them. He did this with at least three of the vehicles in the Dinky line that were already painted red, on which he applied the original paper labels as seen on the pre-production resin Paramedic Truck of "Los Angeles County (51) Fire Dept. Rescue Squad." The three vehicles are included in various die-cast model books with photos, descriptions, and livery as noted earlier. The vehicles he used were the previously released Dinky #410 and #412, both Bedford CF vans, approximately 1:50 scale, first introduced as a Royal Mail vehicle and a yellow AA Service van (a roadside assistance vehicle) respectively; and #385 as a Royal Mail Truck, 1:36 scale, now all with the LA County logo.

Universal

In 1977 the Universal Associated Co. Ltd. of Hong Kong released a very realistic die-cast Dodge Rescue Truck (101 mm, 1:48 scale), in its "Champ of the Road" series. This was before Universal acquired Kidco as its American distributor and several years before it acquired Matchbox. The blister card has a likeness of Johnny in fire gear with "LA County 51" on the helmet. Another in the emergency vehicle series is the "Chevy Nirvana Paramedic Van" ambulance (99 mm) with the same likeness of Johnny on the card stock. The squad and fire truck have an "Emergency Rescue" sticker on the doors, with no other labeling. Also in the series are a Merryweather Marquis Fire Tender and a police car, all with the same catalogue number of 805. The vehicles are bottom stamped "Universal Product 1977" and were released exclusively through Kmart stores at $1.49 each. The company, Universal Associated Co. Ltd, was not associated with Universal Studios or Television. Universal Associated was in business from 1976 to 1978, when Kidco bought them out. Kidco dissolved in 1982.

Hot Wheels

Another "concept paramedic vehicle" was released by Hot Wheels/Mattel as a red "Emergency Squad" marked "50" in the "Flying Colors" series, bottom stamped 1974, released in 1975. It has also been released as the "Ranger Rig" and "Rescue Ranger." It closely resembled the vehicle on *Emergency!* but was not authorized by Universal Television as such at the time. The Emergency Squad continues to be issued with different card stock, graphics, and stock numbers. To date, there are more than 40 variations of paint schemes and logos to this casting. This includes three versions of the Forest Service Ranger truck Unit 71 as the "Ranger Rig," Hot Wheels number 7666 released in 1975. In 1998 it appeared for the first time with "51" with "Fire Dept.," "EMERGENCY," and "51" on the sides.

In 1977 the "Fire-Eater" pumper by Hot Wheels/Mattel was released marked "51." The Fire-Eater was also used in a McDonald's promotion without a blister card. This pumper was designed after an American LaFrance engine, not the Ward LaFrance that was on the show. Several variations of engine color and tampos are seen with the newest Fire-Eater released in 2003, with flames along the side of the engine.

Road Tough

In 2002 the Road Tough company in China released a pack of fourteen different police, fire, and emergency medical services vehicles. One of the vehicles is a squad that closely copies the 1974 Hot Wheels "Road Ranger" version, with slight variations. The "Squad A10," as it is identified, is bottom stamped "Made in China" with an ID number but no date. Yat Ming Industrial Factory Ltd. of Hong Kong also issued it as a single in the "Track Stars, Create-a-World" series with a few non-fire-related road signs. There are forty-three vehicles in this series.

This vehicle casting is virtually identical to the Hot Wheels and, in some cases, is even better. On closer inspection, there are several differences. The cab is diecast metal, but the utility body is plastic; the TwinSonic light bar is clear red plastic; and the underside showing the drive train is different than on the Matchbox vehicle. The utility body is the same, but inside the bed of the body there is a hose reel and the O_2 bottles are at the rear and not along the side as with the Hot Wheels. The words "FIRE DEPT." appear on the side of the utility body of the A10 Squad, and the door logo, a firefighter's shoulder patch design, has a black fire helmet with crossed ladder and ax under the words "Fire Department."

Paramedic Club

Members in the short-lived Johnny and Roy's "Jr. Paramedic Club" received a cast photo poster, a map of the LA area depicting various areas of importance regarding *Emergency!*, sixty thumbnail-size cast photos, a membership application to "The *Emergency!* Gang," and a vinyl record—a $33^1/3$ RPM record by Evatone with a message from Randy and Kevin, "A very special record for *Emergency!* Junior Paramedic club members only." Membership cost $3.00.

According to Dick Friend, membership was originally $5.00, but the price was lowered after Kevin Tighe and Randy Mantooth stormed out of a meeting of NBC Studio Executives, insisting that membership should be free. Club membership information was released only in Cincinnati as a test market.

Puzzles

Several different jigsaw puzzles were produced. Two box sets were made in England by the Pentos Company for Whitman Publishing. One scene is an LA County helicopter lowering a firefighter down to a ship that has gone aground on the rocks during a storm. The other puzzle features the squad and Ward LaFrance at the scene of a high-rise fire. They were licensed by Universal City Studios Inc. and have 224 pieces each.

A nine-piece frame-tray puzzle features a color illustration of the main cast along with the "Los Angeles County Emergency Paramedic" shield, manufactured by Lowe and copyrighted by Emergency Productions.

Three canned, 200-piece 11-by-17-inch jigsaw puzzles with different fire/rescue scenes with the words *Casse-Tete* (French for *jigsaw puzzle*) were manufactured in the United States by American Publishing Corp. A 49-piece boxed set from the same company, released in 1976, featured the "Hook and Ladder" scene that was in one of the canned puzzles. All puzzles featured photos of the cast on the outside of the can and box. Although the puzzle scenes were not from *Emergency!,* the completed puzzles were inset with actual cast photos. The American Publishing Corp. also produced a frame-tray puzzle. For ages 2 to 6, it was released in 1976 featuring a scene from one of the earlier-released can puzzles but without any cast photos.

In 2004 the Spilsbury home catalog company of Madison, Wisconsin, offered a 1000-piece puzzle titled "Television History Jigsaw Puzzle." This 24-by-30-inch puzzle includes Roy and Johnny in uniform with their helmets. In 2006, abc distributing, LLC® released the same puzzle for $6.95.

Coloring Books

Several coloring books were authorized, including one depicting Johnny and Roy on the cover with their squad, titled "*Emergency!* Coloring Book, Authorized Edition." They were copyrighted by Emergency Productions from Universal City Studios, 1977. The cover and drawings were by Pollard Studios, printed by Samuel Lowe Company. Another by the same company in the same year featured the hospital staff along with Johnny and Roy, and another with just Johnny and the squad on the cover.

Belt Buckle

Produced by the County of Los Angeles Fire Museum Association (CLAFMA) in 1979, this $2^3/8$-by-$3^1/4$-inch brass-plated buckle has an elongated Maltese cross as its border with the words "Los Angeles County" within a circle. Also within the circle is depicted a high-eagle leather helmet (LACo in lower rocker panel) above an old hand pumper. The reason for including this belt buckle is the fact that to the left of these firefighting symbols of old is a smaller Maltese cross with "51" within its center, playing on the recently canceled show. Issued as a fund-raiser for the newly organized Fire Museum, it is unknown how many of these belt buckles were made and sold, although they are back-stamped with an issue number. According to CLAFMA president, Joe Woyjeck, the molds are still in the Museum Association's possession.

Other Miscellaneous Items

- Walkie-talkies
- GAF ViewMasters, printed in English and French

Related Collectibles

In 1973 Little Golden Book (number 402) was released with the title of *The Bravest of All*. On the cover is depicted an old retired firefighter in a 1920s era, open-cab Seagrave fire engine. The helmet he is wearing depicts that of LA County Station 36.

In a generic blister card by "HK," the word "Emergency" (no "!") emblazoned over a burning plane, the (former) L.J.N. squad is now listed as an ambulance (model 8212). It was issued painted white, including the light bar, with a red cross on the back. Others in the single-issue sets, painted red, are an engine (the WLF) and a chief's sedan, a helicopter (painted white with a red cross on the side), and a motorcycle (black and white). The "squad" was released by the same company, "HK," in a camouflage version, Model 6224, and called a "rescue." It has an all-clear light bar on the roof. Others in the set were the chief's car, now called a "saloon car," a helicopter, a tank, and a jeep that looks more like a Land Rover—all camouflage paint jobs without any tampos.

Emergency! + 4 Collectibles

Emergency! + 4 collectibles include:
- Activity books.
- "Press-out and play" activity box produced in 1975 by © Emergency Productions.
- 60-page coloring book by Artcraft.
- Two different Halloween costumes issued by Collegeville in 1975 in their Tiny Tot costume series, including helmet that read "L.A. County" with "51" on the lower panel.

- Rescue truck by Fleetwood Toys Inc., 1975 (patterned after the squad, included four plastic firemen and had round "51" paper stickers on each door and "Squad 51—Rescue Truck" on the rear).
- Action photographer mini-camera, 1979 by Fleetwood Toys—used 127 film (16 photos), on an *Emergency! + 4* blister-pack card.
- Video series—an episode of the cartoon was packaged along with animated episodes of *The Jackson 5ive* (ABC 1971–1973) and *The Osmonds* (ABC 1972). The *Emergency + 4* episode is "S.O.S. Help Us," from season 2.

1998 *Emergency!* Convention Collectibles

Several items were made for the convention, including T-shirts, program books, two styles of patches, and magnets. All quickly sold out. A 3.5-hour video shows the Awards Ceremony, Q&A with the Cast and Crew, scenes of the Private Luncheon, tour of Los Angeles County Fire Department (LACoFD) Headquarters, tour of Station 127, and some other general footage of the convention, including shots in areas of the dealer's room, trivia contest, outdoor shots, etc. The video was later remastered onto DVD and is available from *emergencyfans.com*.

30-Year Anniversary Collectibles

In recognition of the LACoFD's 75th anniversary and the 30th anniversary of paramedics in Los Angeles, Code 3 Collectibles released a die-cast version of the Crown Firecoach on January 1, 2000. LACoFD authorized a Limited Edition of 5000 Crown Firecoach fire trucks in the "Classics Series," 1:64 scale ($34.95). It is identified as "Engine 60," which was one of the actual engines used in the series. Code 3 issued the same Crown with different city locations, including LA City and Honolulu, later in the year.

The next month, Hot Wheels (Mattel) also released a LaCoFD–approved (now authorized) Squad 51 in a Special Edition. It was issued in February 2000 with 1974 era Squad logos, 1:64 scale ($19.95). Ironically, they used the previous casting originally known as the "Emergency Squad" and "Rescue Ranger" for this release, still bottom dated 1974.

Matchbox (Mattel) was to issue an *Emergency!* Squad in Set 4 of their "Star Cars" series in 1999/2000. Each car in sets 1 and 2 sits on top of a decorated collector's box and is mounted on a blister card containing a cast photo or still from the TV series the vehicle represents. The back of each card lists trivia questions relating to that particular show. Each car is labeled as a Special Edition retailing at $4.99. Only a few of the 1:64 scale pre-production models were produced with the livery of "Los Angeles County (10)

Fire Dept. Rescue Squad" on the doors and with the tampo of "*Emergency!*" on the hood. Unknown is why they chose the number "10," or if they were going to change it to "51" when it was released. Even though a Star Car Premiere Collection blister card with a photo of the squad was made, this vehicle was actually packaged on a generic Premiere Collection card with a police car on the front and the box inserted upside down.

The squad would have been issue number 24 in the Star Cars series (Set 4, Issue 6). None of the cars in sets 3 or 4 were ever released because the line was dropped before these went into production because of the slow sales of sets 1 and 2. The model is officially called the "Rescue Truck" and was first issued in 1998. It was released as a "Bear Patrol Forest Service" in green, a "Lifeguard" vehicle in yellow, and a "Beach Patrol" in orange. These three releases all have working lights and sirens, which the pre-production "*Emergency!* Squad" does not have. Worldwide, there are only six known of these vehicles. Other vehicles in Set 4 (that were not released) along with the *Emergency!* truck were the *CHiPs* police motorcycle, *Charlie's Angels* Chevy Van, *Welcome Back Kotter* School Bus, *Brady Bunch* '55 Chevy, and the *American Graffiti* '57 T-Bird.

In April 2001, Code 3 Collectibles released in its "Code 3 Classic Series" its previously issued Crown now as *Emergency!*'s "Engine 51" (10,008 units) along with "Squad 51" (20,004 units), and a replica of "Station 51" (12.5 inches long by 16 inches wide by 4.5 inches high), all 1:64 scale. A year later Code 3 issued the long-awaited 1973 Ward LaFrance as "Engine 51" (15,000 units) in July 2002 to round out the "*Emergency!* Set." The initial photo of the Ward on the Code 3 site concerned collectors because the engine sported a full light bar and not the distinctive "Gumball" rotator. Code 3 advised that it was a pre-production photo mock-up, and it was soon corrected on the website. The photo resembled the engine as it is now in Yosemite National Park as Engine 7. There is even a "talking" squad, a plush toy, also by Code 3, that emits siren sounds and dispatch tones with Johnny Gage acknowledging when pressing on the squad's hood.

Project 51 Collectibles

To help defray the cost of refurbishing Squad 51 and the national tour expenses, several items were commissioned specifically for Project 51. They include an 18-by-24-inch poster with the likeness of Johnny and Roy, the squad, helmet, and LA County paramedic patch; a white, Project 51 T-shirt, with the Project 51 emblem on left front chest, a fireman badge, and the engine and squad on the back in full color, with "On the Road to D.C." below; and a replica MSA Topguard helmet with paramedic front shield and paramedic sticker on the sides as worn in final season of *Emergency!*. The helmet was also available with firefighter front shield with a 3-inch gold sticker, and the number 51 in black, placed on the side of the helmet.

Also handed out was the squad, on heavy stock cardboard with full graphics that could be punched out and assembled. The cardboard squad was about 8 inches long. A navy blue baseball cap was sold with the lettering "Los Angeles County" in white arced across the top front with "51" below in red and "Fire Dept." (in white) below the number. Another style ball cap had the words "Project" arced over the gold and a red "51" roundel. A dark blue (cobalt) coffee mug was offered with the County of Los Angeles Firefighter badge with Squad 51 and the Ward fire engine from the TV series on one side and a "51" in gold and surrounded by red (like the squad and engine roundels) on the other, with the signatures of Kevin Tighe and Randolph Mantooth as part of the mug as well. Around the mug itself is "Project 51" in gold, and on the bottom all the way around the mug is the date "May 16, 2000" and "Road to D.C." in gold.

Along the way to Washington, D.C., several members of the cast autographed photos and other *Emergency!* memorabilia items for the hundreds of people that lined up at each stop to see the famous squad.

Videos and DVDs

Authorized VHS-format videos of many of the episodes once only available from Columbia House or Jems Communications are now available only on the secondary market.

Between 1995 and 1996, Jems released four VHS volumes of six episodes each. They did not include the World Premier movie, but the season 5, two-part flashback version titled "The Wedworth-Townsend Act" (episodes 5.15 and 5.16). There were six episodes from season 1, five episodes from season 2, four episodes from season 3, two episodes from season 4, three episodes from season 5, and two episodes from season 6. Also included were two post-series movies.

In 1998 Columbia House released a total of nineteen VHS tapes, containing one tape of the 2-hour World Premier and eighteen tapes of two episodes each. They would include the same episodes from the Jems Communications release plus an additional twelve. They included various episodes from every season and excluded the post-series movies: six episodes from season 1, seven episodes from season 2, thirteen episodes from season 3, seven episodes from season 4, only one episode from season 5, and two episodes from season 6.

Announced by Universal annually since August 2002 was the much-anticipated release of the World Premier and first season, eleven episodes, on DVD. It would not be until August 2005 that Universal would finally release the two-DVD set of the World Premier and eleven 60-minute episodes (first season). The DVD contains the original first-season opening credits. However, they mistitled the World Premier as the Wedsworth-Townsend Act. Not only was the Senator's name misspelled, but the original TV Movie was titled simply, *Emergency!*. The Wedworth-Townsend Act aired as a two-parter in season 5 in a flashback format with Johnny and Roy discussing how the paramedic program began. There are other graphic errors on the DVD box too numerous to mention.

February 2006 saw the release of season 2 with better graphics. The depiction of the Crown and the squad leaving Station 51 below the cast photo was similar to the season 1 set. Season 3 was released February 13, 2007. These are the only *authorized* DVDs of *Emergency!* that have been released, and none of the releases contained any "extras."

The DVDs were made available in several markets across the United States (region 1 format only), including sets from CLAFMA. Although slightly more expensive from the Museum than from other retail outlets, the added incentive was that they were autographed by Randy Mantooth. Along with Randy Mantooth's autograph on the season 1 DVD box cover was a Fire Museum trading card with a photo of the squad in front of Station 127. The card was not available separately at the online store. The Museum also had Mantooth autograph the seasons 2 and 3 sets.

Cast Member Items

Rare collectibles include those items made exclusively for the cast or crew. The following includes a few notable items.

Mark VII Tray

A glass tray was given out by Jack Webb for Christmas 1972 in recognition of the programs that Mark VII Productions had on the air at the time during the 1971/1972 season. This included *Adam-12, Emergency!, Hec Ramsey, O'Hara, U.S. Treasury,* and *The D.A.* This glass tray, which is roughly the shape of a large piece of pie, measures 7 inches by 7 inches at its widest and tallest points. The glass is smokey gray in color with "Mark VII" in black lettering with the five television programs and the date "1971–1972" lettered in gold.

Mugs

There are at least two versions of mugs. The LACoFD Benefit and Welfare fund sold a simple cream-colored ceramic mug with brown speckles and a raised Maltese cross affixed (ceramic) with "51" in the center. The other is an official Mark VII Production Company mug. It is a light cream mug with the Paramedic logo in gold, as seen in end credits with the word *Emergency!* in red over the logo and "Mark VII Ltd." in gold letters on the other side.

Belt Buckles

In 1976 and 1977, numbered brass belt buckles were ordered and sold by the LACoFD Benefit and Welfare Association. Number 1 was presented to Robert Cinader, and numbers 2 and 3 were presented to Randy Mantooth and Kevin Tighe, respectively. The hexagon-shaped buckles were solid brass, approximately 2 inches tall by $2^1/4$ inches wide and lettered "SQUAD" over "51" within the circle. On the lower portion of the buckle were two crossed trumpets. According to Dick Friend, not many were made (although he had number 36 and number 497 has recently surfaced). Many firefighters involved with the show were not even aware that the buckles existed.

Baseball Game Specialty Items

The following items were especially made for the *Adam-12* vs. *Emergency!* baseball game, shortly after the arrival of the Ward LaFrance. The ballgame took place at Elysian Park (835 Academy Road) just north of Dodger Stadium.

- Jackets—red jackets with "Emergency" in black arced over "51" in a circle, also in black.
- T-Shirts—white T-shirts with the "51" logo on the front, about 4 inches round, colored (as is on the side of the squad and engine), with the word "Emergency" arced across the top of the roundel in black; also made in kid sizes.
- Ball caps—yellow cap with the letter "E" on it in red.
- Shorts—probably not official because only one member is wearing them; red shorts with "EMERGENCY" across the back.
- Banner—placed on the side of the fence around the ballfield, says "BURN THE BACON—All Bacon shrinks when it hits The Fire."

Basketball Tank Top

Made for "The Firehouse Five, Plus One" (episode 6.18) for the basketball scene were tank top shirts with "51" in a circle. The opposing team from Station 16 wore yellow tank tops with L.A.Co.F.D. and "16" within a circle silk-screened in black.

Antenna Flag

This item was given out at an end-of-season wrap party as a table centerpiece decoration, but for which season is unknown. It is a 7-inch-long by $5^1/4$-inch-high red flag with $^1/2$-inch gold fringe on three sides. In the center is the 5.5-inch diameter, gold "51" roundel, like what appears on the doors of the squad and engine (51 within a circle). It is double seamed on one edge, without the fringe, which could have been used to slip over a vehicle antenna, or in this case a miniature flag base with staff. It was made by Universal Studio's seamstress Gina Casey.

Where to Find *Emergency!* Collectibles

Photos of many of the collectible items discussed in this chapter may be found online, at fan sites like *emergencyfans.com*. Others are on display at the Los Angeles Fire Department Historical Society and Museum in Hollywood at "old" LA City Fire Station 27 located at 1355 North Cahuenga Blvd, (two blocks south of Sunset). http://www.lafdhs.com/

Many other items have been found in collector magazines such as *The Toy Shop* and on Internet auctions. For the past several years, new and *unauthorized Emergency!* collectibles (that are not NBC/Universal authorized) have entered the market. Consisting of mugs, magnets, shirts, mouse mats or mouse pads, mini-badges, and many other items, most are emblazoned with photos of one or more members of the cast or photos of the squad or engines. There is nothing wrong with new collectible items being made by private individuals and sold for the pure enjoyment of this or any other television program or movie, just as as it is made known that these items are "new."

EMERGENCY! *Behind the Scene*

CHAPTER **19**

The Convention

From October 9–11, 1998, in Burbank, California, a special *Emergency!* convention took place. "*EMERGENCY!* 98, The Boys Are Back in Town" drew virtually the entire cast, many of the crew, and special appearances by Squad 51 and Engine 60. Close to 1000 fans from seven countries attended, which was much greater than the convention organizers had anticipated. The Burbank Airport Hilton and Convention Center was overwhelmed with enthusiastic *Emergency!* fans.

The convention was sponsored by Jems Communications, Straight Streams Magazine, Laedral Medical Corporation, the International Association of Fire Fighters, and many others without whose help the convention would not have been possible.

Attendance

Those in attendance included:

- Cast members
  - Tim Donnelly, who played Chet Kelly
  - Robert Fuller, who played Dr. Brackett
  - Marco López, who played a firefighter using his own name
  - Randy Mantooth, who played Johnny Gage
  - Ron Pinkard, who played Dr. Grey and Dr. Morton
  - Mike Stoker, who played a firefighter using his own name
  - Kevin Tighe, who played Roy DeSoto
  - Bobby Troup, who played Dr. Early
- Guest stars
  - Randall Carver
  - Patti Cohoon
  - James McEachin
  - Tom Williams
- Crew
  - Laurann Cordero, female costumer
  - Dennis Donnelly, director
  - Georg Fenady, director
  - Harold Frizzell, stuntman/double
  - Gino Grimaldi, producer
  - Mickey Michaels, set decorator
  - Johnny Miller, stuntman
  - Ed Self, producer
  - Hannah Shearer, producer
  - Cynnie Troup, script supervisor
- Los Angeles County Fire Department (LACoFD)
  - Dick Friend, Public Information Officer
  - Jim Page, technical consultant and writer
  - P. Michael Freeman, Fire Chief
  - Daryl Osby, Chief
- LA County Explorers

- Staff of the County of Los Angeles Fire Museum
- Technical Advisors
  - Bob Belliveau
  - Jim Brewer
  - Mike Lewis
  - Michael Stearns
  - Bob McCullough
  - Bruce Mortimer
  - Mike Williams
- Honored Guests
  - Jean Cinader, wife of the late Bob Cinader
  - Laurette Lanier, wife of the late Sam Lanier, dispatcher
- Convention organizers
  - Cynthia Hawkins, convention co-chair
  - Rozane Sutherland, convention co-chair
  - Laura Aguiar, production coordinator
  - Carol Barta, facilities/programming coordinator
  - Lisa Damiani, merchandise designer
  - Maribel Rios, international coordinator
  - Tangee Taylor, merchandise coordinator
  - Erika Bartlett, program designer

Program

Friday night consisted of registration and a welcome reception with music from the 1970s, snack bar, photography sessions, trivia, and other games. Special merchandise was for sale, including T-shirts, magnets, and limited edition patches; all quickly sold out. Several of the cast and crew members who were staying at the hotel came down for the fun and mingled with the guests.

Saturday included vendor displays; fire-and-rescue vehicle displays (including Squad 51 and Engine 60); question-and-answer sessions with the cast and crew[1]; autograph sessions; auction of memorabilia; and viewings of *Emergency!* episodes, bloopers, and music video. It also included an

---

[1] Fans waited for the cast to enter the stage for the Q&A session and burst into excited applause when the *Emergency!* theme music started playing loudly and the cast surprised the audience, rushing in from the back door, high-fiving the audience as they made their way to the stage.

awards ceremony, where the members of the engine, squad, and hospital staff of Rampart each received a special plaque presented by Jim Page and LA County Fire Chief P. Michael Freeman. When Randy Mantooth received his Honorary LA County Firefighter plaque, he stated, "We had no idea the show would have this kind of impact," and Kevin Tighe agreed, "It was an honor for us to do what you [firefighters and paramedics] do on a day-to-day basis. Playing a Paramedic to serving now as a hospice volunteer, helping others is my link to EMS."

Huge gift baskets (large wicker laundry baskets) were presented with items sent in from fans in fire departments and civilian life from all over the world, including:

- Jems video of *The Best of Emergency!*.
- Convention T-shirt and program guide.
- A memory book made up of comments and stories from fans about the show and its stars.

Coauthor Richard Yokley had the distinct honor of presenting Bobby Troop (Dr. Joe Early) with his presentation basket at the awards ceremony on Saturday. Bobby Troop had such a great wit and sense of humor! He didn't think anyone would remember him or care that he was there, but he was wrong. I am so glad that I had a chance to talk with him, even though only briefly.

An auction of *Emergency!* memorabilia, including donations from the cast, followed the presentation. The autograph session, that was scheduled for only 2 hours lasted for well over 4, and the cast happily gave their signatures again and again, without complaint, until the last fan came through the line.

On Sunday, the convention went on tour to LACoFD Headquarters and TV's Station 51 (Station 127). At the headquarters, fans toured the museum, dispatch, and training facilities with Marco López, Tim Donnelly,[2] Dick Friend, and Mickey Michaels. Demonstrations included a helicopter water drop, rappelling, and response to a real car explosion. Equipment was on display, and attendees were invited to try on gear. Afterward, fans traveled to Station 127, and firefighters put nameplates on what would have been Johnny's and Roy's lockers, although they were reversed. Despite hoards of people wandering around the station, the firefighters were very accommodating.

---

[2] Years later, Tim Donnelly said that the "most important piece of memorabilia" he had from *Emergency!* was the honorary LACoFD plaque he received at the convention. At the convention, Tim was also seen collecting signatures from everyone on his *Emergency!* lunchbox.

Some of Convention Co-Chair Rozane Sutherland's favorite memories:

- Seeing the faces of the cast and crew when some of them saw each other for the first time in over 20 years.
- Tim and his lunchbox.
- Bobby's eyes as he would tease me, asking me every time I went up to him, "Have I told you what blue eyes you have?"
- The way the fans reacted when the tones went off at the start of the cast Q&A session. I think everyone was expecting the doors behind the stage to open and the cast to come in from there. But nope, we had them in the back with the back doors opening and making their entrance! Ha ha!
- Seeing the cast just walking around the hotel and lobby and the reaction of the fans seeing them, how they could just walk up and talk to them.

Stuntman Johnny Miller had this to say about the *Emergency!* Convention: "Memories of the good times and hard work can never be taken away from those who were fortunate to have them. Thanks for the memory and the opportunity to revisit cast and crew of a great time of my life!"

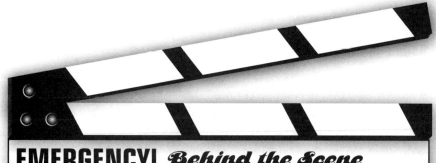

EMERGENCY! *Behind the Scene*

CHAPTER **20**

Project 51: On the Road to DC and The Smithsonian

Project 51 was established as a nonprofit corporation founded to promote public awareness of the history and success of emergency medical services (EMS) and the role that *Emergency!* played in its development. In 2000, Project 51 sponsored a national tour that featured Randy Mantooth, a fully restored Squad 51, and original medical equipment and clothing from the show. The tour included a visit to Washington, D.C.'s National Mall and an induction ceremony of *Emergency!* memorabilia at the Smithsonian Museum of American History.

Funding

No corporate sponsors were obtained for Project 51's tour. Funding was by payroll deductions of the LA County firefighters to the Museum Association, donations from *Emergency!* fans, and sale of Project 51 items.

Squad Restoration

In preparation for its national tour and appearance, Squad 51 underwent a 6-month, $30,000 restoration (**Photo 20-1**). The squad was literally taken apart down to its axles and put back together. In addition to a new engine, transmission, brake work, new suspension components, and much more, the vehicle received new paint—spec color Dupont 674 Fire Engine Red. This color is the current color for the County apparatus and is also what was used in the 1970s when the squad rolled off the line and what Universal used when painting the utility body.

The lettering design on the doors and rear of the squad were restored to 1972 Fire Department specifications. The Museum Association obtained from the Department of Motor Vehicles the original TV license plate numbering from the series for the squad, E999007.

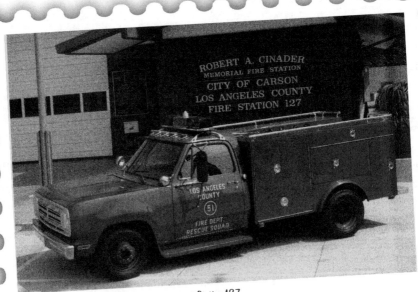

PHOTO 20-1   Refurbished Squad 51 in front of Station 127.
Source: Courtesy of Joe Woyjeck, County of Los Angeles Fire Museum Association.

History of the Tour

The Project 51 tour unofficially began on October 17, 1999 in Irvine, California. One year earlier, Cynthia Hawkins, a fan of *Emergency!*, developed the idea. She contacted the Smithsonian Institution about the possibility of accepting equipment from the TV program into their archives to celebrate the 30th anniversary of America's EMS program. Cynthia was also a Co-Chair of the highly successful *Emergency!* reunion convention held in Burbank California in 1998.

Irvine's Orange County Fire Department sponsored a Fire and Safety Expo on October 17, 1999. More than 2000 attendees came to get their first look at the refurbished squad, several of the *Emergency!* stars were on hand to sign autographs, and Project 51 items were sold.

Every member of the Project 51 board, save for one, participated in the cross-country journey; the journey was to originally include more than thirteen cities in its itinerary, but that proved to be a scheduling nightmare and the journey was trimmed back to six cities. It took ten to twelve people at each stop to remove the merchandise from the bright red trailer. The squad had to be cleaned and polished at each stop and mirrors reattached, because it would not fit in the trailer with the mirrors on.

Fundraising Events

Prior to the national tour, Project 51 members along with the squad attended various functions promoting the tour. They consisted of a one-day event at the LA County Medical Association Conference, a sales-autograph-signing event in the Los Angeles Civic Center, and another at the Universal Studios Courtyard on April 27, 2000, the official send-off.

Other Project 51 functions included attendance at the National EMS Today Conference & Exposition in Orlando, Florida, held on March 25 and 26, 2000, at the Orlando Convention Center. Project 51 had an exhibit and merchandise for sale; Randy Mantooth was available for autographs and to have his picture taken with fans. Jim Page also attended.

The squad also appeared at the International Association of Fire Chiefs Rescue-Med Conference in Las Vegas, Nevada, on April 16 and 17, 2000, at the Orleans Hotel. Randy Mantooth and Marco López were there to sign autographs.

Press kits were sent to the fire departments in the cities where they were scheduled to participate in various activities. Radio and TV station interviews were set up. A Project 51 website was established so that fans all across the country could track their progress and see photos taken at each of the events.

Schedule

May 3: The National Fire and Emergency Services Dinner held at the Washington Hilton and Towers attended by Randy Mantooth. Project 51 merchandise was available, and Mantooth signed autographs for the fans before the dinner. Mantooth was given an award for his and Kevin Tighe's contribution to the development of the nationwide EMS system.

May 4: In Baltimore, Mantooth and others participated in the Preakness Parade press conference and later flew to Chicago, where they met up with other members of the entourage for the next day's events (**Photo 20-2** and **Photo 20-3**).

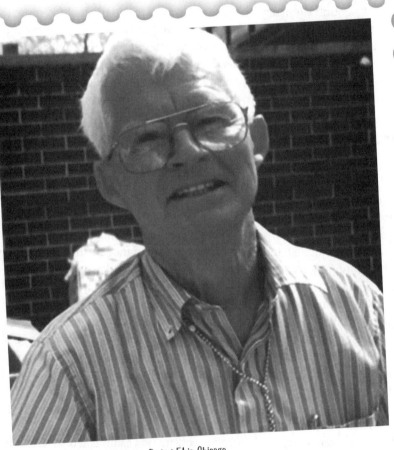

PHOTO 20-2   Dick Friend during Project 51 in Chicago.
Source: Courtesy of Connie Duncan.

May 5: A 30-minute radio interview at a downtown Chicago nightspot called the Blue Agave Restaurant on West Maple Street. The next day they all went to the Chicago Fire Department's training center (on the site of the infamous O'Leary barn) for their first real "show," which included sales of Project 51 items and an autograph signing session. Food was available and was prepared by some Chicago Fire Department retirees in the training center kitchen. Well over 1000 people waited in line for hours, some from as far away as Canada. Six hours later, Mantooth and others were still signing autographs.

May 6: Day off for preparation and planning, printing more press packets, and touring New York City.

May 7: Visited New York's Long Beach Fire Department on Staten Island, where they again set up shop inside their large Fire Headquarters station. Live TV interviews were given, and the volunteer firefighters grilled hamburgers and hot dogs for the many visitors.

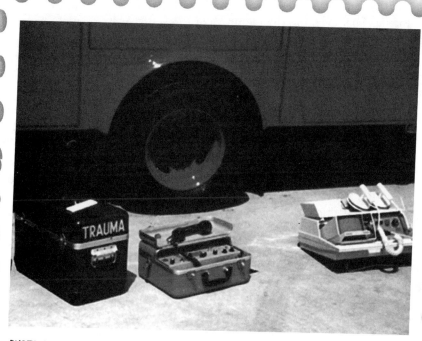

PHOTO 20-3   Gear by squad during Project 51 event in Chicago, including trauma box, BioPhone 3502, Datascope MD2 defribrillator, and the HT-220 portable radio.
Source: Courtesy of Connie Duncan.

May 11: Baltimore: Randy Mantooth went to Camden Yards, home of the Baltimore Orioles, where he was to throw out the first pitch that evening for Firefighter/Paramedic Night. Everybody else was escorted into the owner's suite. Before the game, the large Jumbotron screen lit up with the opening scenes and sounds of *Emergency!*. Just as the squad was pulling out of Station 51, Mantooth drove Squad 51 out onto the warning track. He ended up at the pitcher's mound, where he threw out the ceremonial first pitch. Several live TV interviews were performed during the game, with a telephone interview later that evening on a radio station.

May 12–13: Baltimore's Preakness Parade with Mantooth as Grand Marshal; he stood in the back of the squad waving to the large crowd. Everyone else got aboard various old fire apparatus right behind the squad. Interviews followed the parade.

May 14: In Washington, D.C., "*Emergency!* Fest" activities were sponsored by the Hyattsville Fire Department and *Firehouse Magazine*. Several hundred tickets to the luncheon (at $35.00 a plate) were sold for people to dine with the *Emergency!* stars Randy Mantooth, Ron Pinkard, Marco López, Mike Stoker, and Tim Donnelly. There was a Q&A session, and clips from the TV program were shown. Kevin Tighe, who was unable to make the trip, sent his greeting via tape from London, where he was filming a movie. That evening, the members of Project 51 were treated to a special tour of the White House normally off-limits to visitors. Escorted by the Deputy Assistant to the President, they toured the West Wing and were able to see the only portion of the original White House that was still visible.

May 15: Visited the Hyattsville (Maryland) Fire Department Headquarters *Emergency!*Fest. Food was prepared for the visitors and tables set up for autographs and selling of the Project 51 merchandise. More than 2000 people came. Again, Randy Mantooth, Ron Pinkard, Marco López, Tim Donnelly, and Mike Stoker were on hand to sign autographs for the fans. In the evening, the International Association of Fire Fighters sponsored a reception and dinner.

May 16: Induction of *Emergency!* artifacts into the Smithsonian Museum of American History.

The Smithsonian Institution

The Project 51 tour concluded with a private ceremony held in the Presidential Suite of the Smithsonian's Museum of American History on May 16, 2000. At this ceremony, the museum displayed several donations of key props used in the series, including Johnny's and Roy station uniforms (without LA County badges), fire gear, and helmets, Mike Stoker's turnouts, medical equipment, radios, and original scripts that the museum had recently acquired.

These items had been officially approved by Dr. Ramunas Kondratas, curator and chair, and Jane Rogers, collections manager, for the Fire-and-Rescue collections and were displayed at an October 16, 1999, reception held at the Gene Autry Museum (Museum of the American West) in Los Angeles, to celebrate the LA County Fire Department's (LACoFD) 75th anniversary. When asked about the possibility of the squad being put on display at the Smithsonian, Rogers replied that the Smithsonian just didn't have enough room.

At the induction ceremony, speakers included Dr. Spencer Crew, director of the Smithsonian's National Museum of American History; Dr. Ramunas Kondratas, curator and chair; Chief P. Michael Freeman, LACoFD; Dr. Michael Criley, cardiologist responsible for developing paramedic training in Los Angeles; and Dr. Eugene Nagel, cardiologist responsible for developing paramedic training in Miami.

Randy Mantooth also spoke about his involvement in the show, "I am not so sure I like the word 'museum' used in close conjunction to my name, but what an honor for all of us who have participated in developing and building a concept that has saved countless lives. I am only a spokesman: it is those in the stations and in the field and hospitals that deserve the honors."

Sitting in the audience, Dick Friend and Mike Stoker realized it had been 27 years since they were here, then on the new Engine 51, and now on a virtually new Squad 51. Both now realized they had contributed to the development of the nation's EMS system.

The items accepted into the Smithsonian's Division of Cultural History in the National Museum of American History, Behring Center, included:

- BioPhone
- Oxygen unit with carrying case
- Two defibrillators
- Defibrillator monitor
- Two trauma boxes, complete with supplies
- A splint box
- Three firefighter helmets (including Randolph Mantooth's and Kevin Tighe's)
- Uniform shirts
- Turn-out gear and boots worn by Randolph Mantooth and Mike Stoker
- An original script from the show

None of the items are currently on display; so don't go looking for them. And none of the docents or guides will know anything about the *Emergency!* items if you ask them about it. Dick Friend advises, "We were told that the materials would be divided into several Smithsonian sections and not be 'shown' for a year or so."

According to Jane Rogers, Museum Specialist, "The objects have gone to two different divisions in the museum. The paramedic equipment, which was actual equipment used by the Los Angeles County Fire Department in the 1970s, was sent to our Medical Sciences division. These include a Biophone, oxygen unit with carrying case, two defibrillators, a defibrillator monitor, two trauma boxes, complete with supplies, and a splint box. The other items went to the Entertainment Collections because they were used in the television show and were not used for actual firefighting although they were authentic items used in LA County at the time."

In late 2004 Jane Rogers said, "Unfortunately these objects have never been on display and are currently in our storage areas. Due to the federal budget constraints, a fire exhibit is not in our current plans although perhaps we can include some of the objects in a smaller case sometime in the future."

Those in attendance at this event included:

- Project 51 Board of Directors
  - Jim Page, executive director and LACoFD Battalion Chief, retired, technical consultant to *Emergency!*
  - Dan Dingillo, president and assistant chief LACoFD
  - Gino Grimaldi, vice president and *Emergency!* producer
  - Hannah Shearer, secretary and *Emergency!* producer
  - Steve Martin, treasurer and LACoFD Captain
  - Randy Mantooth, Johnny Gage on *Emergency!*
  - Ed Self, *Emergency!* producer
  - Jean Cinader, widow of executive producer, Robert A. Cinader
  - Dick Friend, LACoFD Public Information Officer, and advisor to *Emergency!*
  - J. Michael Criley, who created LACoFD's paramedic training curriculum
  - Eugene Nagel, who created Miami Fire Department's program
- LACoFD
  - P. Michael Freeman, Fire Chief
  - Franklin Pratt, medical director
  - Rudy Castro, photographer
  - Paul Schneider, Paul Oyler, Ron Ripley, and Gil Garcia, who helped restore Squad 51

- Ron Stewart, writer of LA County's first paramedic training manuals
- Jordan Pearl, County of Los Angeles Fire Museum Association
- Frank Harris and Pam Graham, drivers of the 75-foot transport trailer
- *Emergency!* cast members
  - Mike Stoker, engineer
  - Marco López, firefighter
  - Tim Donnelly, firefighter
  - Ron Pinkard, Rampart doctor
- Cynthia Hawkins, honorary chairperson who first contacted the Smithsonian about accepting equipment from *Emergency!* into the National Archives

The ceremony concluded, and everyone went out onto the front steps of the museum to have their photo taken with the Squad. It later returned to the LA County Fire Museum on board its 75 transport.

Concluding Ceremony

The American College of Emergency Physicians launched national Emergency Medical Services Week at a ceremony with Project 51 members at the national mall in Washington, D.C. Representatives of the United States Fire Administration and DC Fire Department were present, along with Jim Page and Randy Mantooth. They spoke about the history and importance of EMS and how *Emergency!* helped spread these life-saving services across the nation.

After the tour, Project 51 disbanded, and all the funds it collected were distributed to nonprofit groups such as burn centers, fire prevention projects, and museums.

EMERGENCY! *Behind the Scene*

CHAPTER **21**

Life After Emergency!

The Apparatus

Engine 51[1]

The Ward LaFrance Engine 51 is spending its retirement at Yosemite National Park **(Photo 21-1)**. Until 1987, it sat relatively idle on Universal's backlot as a reserve rig (Engine 260), but it was then pressed back into service for the Yosemite Concessions Service (YCS) at Yosemite National Park in California. At the time, the Concessions Service at the Park was operated by MCA, who also owned Universal Studios. The Park was looking for an engine to replace its 1937 Seagrave, and MCA approached LA County Fire Chief John England. He arranged for the Ward to be transferred to the National Park. Now 35 years old, the engine is still a first-line pumper at

---

[1] Additional information may be found in James O. Page, *The Paramedics, An Illustrated History of Paramedics in their First Decade in the USA* (Morristown, NJ: Backdraft Publications, 1979).

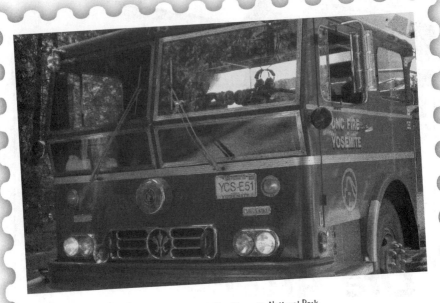

PHOTO 21-1   The former Engine 51 (now Engine 7) at Yosemite National Park.
Source: Courtesy of David Stone.

the Park and is staffed by a paid on-call crew of ten firefighters who work for the Park.

Originally on a $1.00 a year lease agreement, MCA sold the engine to YCS in 1993 for $5,500. A few minor modifications have been made to the engine. Engine 7, as it is now known, is running with license plate number YCS E51. The engine was originally owned and operated upon arrival to the park by Yosemite Park & Curry Company and is now owned and operated by Delaware North Parks & Resorts at Yosemite Inc. (DNC). The engine generally stays in a firehouse at 9006 Village Drive, across the street from the Village Store, and it goes on only about twelve responses a year, according to David Stone, Manager of Security, Fire, and Life Safety in Yosemite. In Yosemite, The National Park Service (NPS) is the primary agency for fire response. Part of the park's contractual obligation with NPS is to maintain a structural fire response crew of ten paid on-call firefighters and one Type 1 structural engine. He says that this engine still attracts lots of attention. "During good weather, the engine is usually parked on the apron in front of the firehouse. The firehouse receives a steady stream of visitors from around the world to take a picture of, or with, the engine. As a result of the related patch trading that takes place, we have nearly 1,000 fire patches from around the world."

History in Yosemite

The engine was in service with Los Angeles County Fire Department (LACoFD) at Station 60 at Universal Studios. At some point its name changed from Engine 60 to Engine 260 around 1983. Its last maintenance with the LACoFD was March 31, 1987, and it was leased to Yosemite Park and Curry Co. on April 24, 1987. According to the vehicle title, ownership transferred on June 29, 1993, and DNC acquired the engine later that year. According to David Stone, the engine arrived from Universal Studios completely stripped of its ladders and equipment and had 27,432 miles on it. As of December 31, 2003, it had 34,600.

"When the engine arrived in Yosemite," Stone relates, "the firehouse had to be raised 4 inches to accommodate the engine. The engine has less than 1-inch clearance on top, and 3 to 6 inches on each side to the mirrors on each door. The 500-gallon water tank was replaced in 1995 by Hi-Tech in Oakdale, California. The old tank had begun to leak, and upon removal we discovered a significant (1- to 2-inch-thick) growth of what were obviously ocean barnacles in the tank. Apparently Yosemite's very high quality fresh water did not agree with them, as they were all dead."

Only minor modifications have been made to the engine, as needed, including adjustments to the hose bed, seating, and installation of a light bar. NPS is sensitive to the engine's historical nature but understands that operational concerns take priority. In April 1999, the cab upholstery was replaced, although efforts were made to match the original material as closely as possible, and the heat-embossed design was duplicated by hand stitching. In May 1999, two external mast-floodlight assemblies were added to aid night responses; Stone insists that installation was completed in a manner to make restoration simple **(Photo 21-2)**.

A more major overhaul was completed in 2000 to upgrade the equipment to meet new standards. "Historically, some type of mechanical impairment or outright failure of the vehicle occurred during 5 percent to 10 percent of our attempts to use it, including at least once annually during an actual alarm response," says Stone. "Most of these failures were attributed directly or indirectly to lack of regular detailed preventative maintenance and routine replacement of aging seals, hoses/lines, etc. These issues were successfully addressed with the help of the DNC garage staff and an outside contractor." Modifications included repairing the diesel engine head, replacing hoses and fittings, cleaning the fuel system, installing a diesel exhaust filtration system, replacing tires, repairing the electrical system, installing floodlights, replacing batteries, rewiring spotlights, installing an

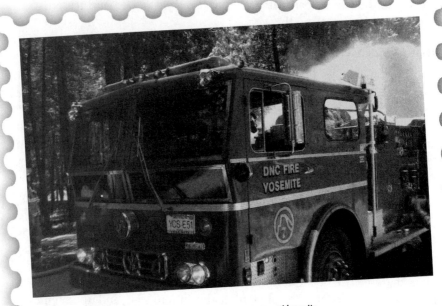

PHOTO 21-2   The former Engine 51 during a training evolution at Yosemite.
Source: Courtesy of David Stone.

electrical distribution block, resealing the water tank, reconfiguring the hose bed, and installing new crew seats. The rear taillights were not replaced with LED-style lights for historical preservation. Stone said, "For fans and friends of Engine 51, rest assured it is in good hands and treated well by firefighters who care for it and take honor in responding to calls with it. The contract with NPS currently expires in 2011. At the end of the engine's service life, every intent is to reunite it with Squad 51."

"With the arrival of the Ward, YP&C.'s old Engine 7, a 1937 Seagrave pumper, was sent to the LACoFD Museum, to be used as a display or parade engine," according to Stone.

Squad 51

On February 18, 2002, Randolph Mantooth co-hosted an event with Jim Page at the Petersen Automotive Museum in Los Angeles, honoring the first 40 paramedics from the Los Angeles area **(Photo 21-3)**. The group included firefighter/paramedics from Los Angeles City and County Fire Departments, McCormick Ambulance Company, and the Inglewood Fire Department who were taught at Harbor General and at Daniel Freeman Hospital. The ceremony was co-sponsored by the County of Los Angeles Fire Museum Association (CLAFMA) and the Peterson Automotive Museum; more than 250 invitees attended the ceremony. The squad was inducted into its collection on a 1-year viewing contract in its "Cars of Hollywood" exhibit. Part of the ceremony included having the special guests, the firefighter/paramedics, sign a specially prepared backboard that travels with the squad. Several of these early paramedics are still on the job, but with the mandatory retirement age of 60, most will be retiring within the next few years.

In February 2003 the squad was taken to the Hall of Flame Museum in Scottsdale, Arizona, where it remained until May 2004, where even more people were able to view the famous television vehicle. LACoFD Captain

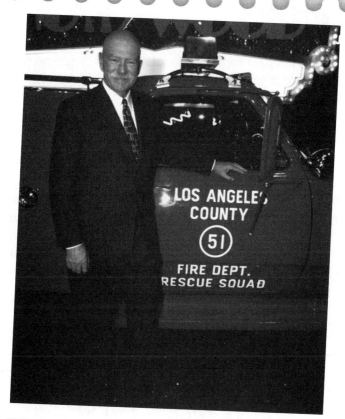

PHOTO 21-3 Jim Page in front of squad at the Peterson Automotive Museum.
Source: Courtesy of County of Los Angeles Fire Museum Association Collection.

Joe Woyjeck, CLAFMA President, indicated that the Association would like the squad to be on a roving exhibit where people can get up close to this famous vehicle. Plans are underway for other exhibit venues.

More work still needs to be done on the squad, according to Paul Schneider, museum director and a LACoFD Captain, to get it totally back into 1972 condition. Detail work, such as the installation of Dodge nameplates and other chrome work, needs to be accomplished.

There are plans to refurbish the storage compartments with some of the original medical gear and tools used on the program; an original trauma box was recently located. On a recent visit, this author was shown the original "Body Guard" turn-out coats as worn by Gage, DeSoto, and Mike Stoker that will eventually be placed in the squad. Over the course of the series, more than one set of gear was used on the program, which accounts for turn-out coats worn by DeSoto and Stoker, now also at the Smithsonian.

Television Appearances

McCloud

Scenes from Station 10 in the 1972 *Emergency!* World Premier were later used in NBC's *McCloud* episode titled "Fire" (6.03), which aired November 16, 1975. The New York Fire Department (FDNY) responds to a high-rise apartment building that has been torched by an arsonist, and where McCloud and his girlfriend have become trapped [McCloud's girlfriend, Chris Coughlin, is played by Diana Muldaur (*Star Trek:TNG*, Dr. Kate Puaski, *Pine Canyon Is Burning*). Later, McCloud poses as a businessman to crack the arson ring.

The editing on the apparatus responding segment was a real mismatch. The opening scenes are from a FDNY station with a Mack CF; the firefighters gear up and approach the engine but then a cut is made to LA County Truck 10, the Crown Firecoach. There are varied scenes from the apparatus startup at Station 10 as depicted in the *Emergency!* World Premier. There are close-ups of the LACoFD apparatus leaving, and then the scene changes to the fire ground showing a building well involved with a Mack CF arriving.

Hardy Boys

Footage from the *Emergency!* movie *The Steel Inferno,* showing the squad and engine, appears in a *Hardy Boys/Nancy Drew* episode ("Arson and Old Lace," 2.21, airdate April 1, 1978), complete with background "radio chatter" from the movie. Also appearing is Colby Chester (*Emergency!* and *The Rangers*) and Vince Howard (*Emergency!*), as a police lieutenant. Pernell Roberts (*Bonanza*) portrays the Fire Chief. Janet Julian (Janet Louise Johnson) portrays Nancy Drew.

The Steel Inferno

Engine 51, the Ward LaFrance, in its final act as an engine on *Emergency!*, portrayed a different engine company. In the *Emergency!* movie *The Steel Inferno*, airing January 7, 1978, the Ward was numbered Engine 110.

Escort

When Robert Fuller received his Hollywood "Walk of Fame" star in 1975, he reportedly was driven to the ceremony in Squad 51.

ChiPs

The squad and engine made a guest appearance on *CHiPs*, in the episode "Mait Team" (2.15) airing January 13, 1979. The engine and Squad 51 are shown pulling out of Station 51 and responding to a motor vehicle accident.

The China Syndrome

The Ward appears in this 1979 film; it approaches the freeway on-ramp just before Jack Lemmon peels out in his BMW. The engine is shown coming toward the intersection (toward the camera) as Lemmon is approaching. Engine 51 is shown as Lemmon peels out as he sees the traffic stopped to let the engine through. He turns right and passes the engine and races toward the freeway. There's no fireman in the No. 4 seat (where Chet sits in Engine 51).

Fire: Countdown to Disaster

This 1984 National Fire Protection Association training film opens with Engine 51 arriving at the scene of a fire in front of the Hammond Chemical Co. In the 1-minute clip, the engine arrives and the crew enters the building to save an individual.

Hunter

"Fire Man," an episode of NBC's *Hunter* (1984–1991), aired May 4, 1985, and contained shots of the engine and squad from inside Station 51, leaving as well as responding. They also used the responding scene from Station 8 from the *Emergency!* World Premier.

The Great Los Angeles Earthquake

This 1990 made-for-television movie includes stock footage of Squad 51 and Engine 51 responding from the station. Scenes from the Earthquake ride at Universal Studios Theme Park were also utilized.

Blood Work

The squad does not appear in this 2002 Clint Eastwood film, but its license plate does—affixed to an LA Police Department vehicle. Plate E999007 has also been seen in various other projects filmed in Vancouver.

Miscellaneous Appearances

The film rental company Hollywood Fire Authority owns a former LA County Ward LaFrance, so recent television spotting may include *Desperate Housewives,* McDonald's commercials, *24, Alias, Cold Case,* and the TV movie *Combustion.* It is often numbered as Engine 56 and, in homage to *Emergency!,* background firefighters often appear with "51" on their helmets.

While the *Emergency!* World Premier was being filmed, the actor Michael Gregory read for the role of one of the regular cast (he does not recall the particular role). He said that unfortunately he didn't get the part and never worked on the show: "My longest running job was as 'Dr. Rick Webber,' cardiovascular surgeon and resident heartthrob, on *General Hospital*" (1976–1978). Gregory's coincidental role was that of a Fire Chief in the 2004 movie, *Combustion* (airing as *Silent Killer* on Lifetime) starring Michael Gross (*Family Ties*), Gabrielle Carteris (*BH 90210*), and Joe Lando (*Dr. Quinn-Medicine Woman*). The coincidence is that Gregory worked with Hollywood Fire Authority's Ward LaFrance engine, as he would have had he worked on *Emergency!.*

Good Morning America

On the long-running ABC program of July 9, 1986, a reunion of sorts was held to include Kevin Tighe, Randy Mantooth, Bobby Troup, and Robert Fuller. GMA host Joan Lunden showed clips from various shows, and they all discussed pranks and the serious side of the program. Robert Fuller stated, "A lot (of time) was put into it, Joan. We had technical advisors on the set, paramedics everyday. Every time we did an operation we had a doctor, Dr. James Lewis from Harbor General Hospital. So we knew what we were doing, and the truth of the matter is that most of our series and our scenes were used as training films throughout the country and South America, Mexico as training films for the paramedics."

Bobby Troup, in discussing the paramedic program stated, "Of all the television shows in the United States, I think *Emergency!* did the most public service, because when we started, nobody had ever heard of the paramedic program and there were only three in the country. By the time we finished, six or seven years later, there were thousands of them all over. It was a common word."

Michael Norell

Some 11 years after Captain Stanley appeared on *Emergency!*, he made a special appearance in the 1987 made-for-TV movie *Pals*, starring George C. Scott, Don Ameche, and Sylvia Sydney for which he wrote the screenplay. In one key scene, an actress is leaving behind her motor home and, grabbing a beloved photograph, declares, "I ain't leavin' without my autographed picture of Captain Hank Stanley of *Emergency!*." During rehearsal, Norell recalls, the actress, Miss Sydney, in his words a "very salty old lady," demanded, "Who the hell is Captain Hank Stanley?" Norell explained that, "It was sort of a private joke, that it was a very obscure character I'd played on TV and that my four fans would get a kick out of it, and she said, 'Aw, that's cute.' And so she played it as written."

Randy Mantooth

Before Randy became a paramedic, he portrayed a hospital intern. Randy's first role on television was in Dennis Weaver's *McCloud* (1970–1977) series, in the episode titled "The Man From Taos," which aired September 16, 1970. This was the first episode of the *McCloud* series.

In 1986, Mantooth gave the closing remarks at the County of Los Angeles Paramedic Training Institute's one-hundredth class. Eleven fire departments were represented, graduating thirty-three firefighter/paramedics, eleven of which were from the LACoFD. One member of that class, Joe Woyjeck, currently a paramedic/captain for LACoFD, worked hard on producing the program for the graduation of Class #200 on March 29, 2007, and in which Randy Mantooth spoke again.

In 1991, Mantooth appeared on *MacGyver,* "The Prometheus Syndrome," airing on October 7, 1991, as an LA City Fire Department Fire Inspector. Mantooth's character is killed off early on in the episode as a result of a bomb explosion set off by a psychopathic arsonist for revenge against firefighters. MacGyver uses a firefighter's badge to get out of one of his infamous jams. "Old" LA City Station 27 in Hollywood, now a Fire Museum, was used for exteriors.

In an October 1997 episode of *Diagnosis Murder* (1993–2001), titled "Malibu Fire," Mantooth portrays Bill Tremont, mayor and volunteer firefighter of a small community near Malibu threatened by fire. In the episode, there is an LA County GMC 4-door rescue unit with a large "51" on the side and "Rescue 51" on the rear, although it is not *the* squad. Robert Fuller and Jennifer Tighe (daughter of Kevin Tighe) also appear in this episode, which was directed by Christian I. Nyby II. The cinematographer was *Emergency!*'s Frank Thackery.

In 2001, Mantooth appeared on the Learning Channel's *The Secret World of Paramedics*. He was interviewed for the 60-minute program that featured clips from *Emergency!* and scenes of a "Project 51" event taken at Universal Studios' new Station 51. Paramedics from across the country told stories and anecdotes about their profession. Airdate for the program was January 8, 2001. On this program, Mantooth revealed that at first he was more impressed by the size of his paycheck than the contribution the show was making to emergency medicine, but that soon changed, and now he is blown away by the number of people who tell him they became paramedics because of Johnny Gage.

In 2005 Randy Mantooth was named the honorary chairman for CLAFMA.

USAR-I

In 1999, Randy Mantooth began work on a TV pilot titled *USAR-1* (Urban Search and Rescue), based on a real USAR team of LACoFD. If this show is picked up, Kevin Tighe will have a semi-recurring role, which will be the first time the two co-stars will have worked together since *Emergency!* However, Mantooth insists that the two actors will not be reprising their *Emergency!* characters. "Anyone expecting *USAR-1* to pick up where *Emergency!* left off will be disappointed," he said.

After receiving approval from LA County Fire Chief P. Michael Freeman, Mantooth and the program's Emmy-winning producer, Hayma Washington (co-executive producer for *The Amazing Race*), did several ride-alongs with LA County's USAR 103 to learn more about USAR and the role they play in fire service. *USAR-1* promises to be similar to the *Emergency!* series in its realistic and dramatic portrayal of LACoFD operations. The show would draw its story lines and technical advisors from real USAR stories and personnel, and it hopes to use actual footage of LACoFD responses.

According to Mantooth, the main characters would include a captain, engineer, and two firefighter specialists on a 28-ton USAR rig along with a three-man Air Ops team consisting of a pilot and two firefighter/paramedics. "They are trying to outfit *USAR-1* with Sikorsky (UH-60) Black Hawk helicopters," said Mantooth, who hopes to be one of the executive producers and an occasional director. "We are going to try to be as responsible with USAR-1 as Bob Cinader was with *Emergency!*."

In 1999, *USAR-1* was unsuccessfully pitched to CBS and three other networks in 2001. Mantooth and Washington pitched it again to several networks in 2004, and again at CBS in 2006, but it has not yet been picked up.

Hollywood Squares

On Hollywood Squares, Randy appeared as a square on "TV Doctors Week," February 9 through 13, 2004. Photos from *Emergency!* were shown.

Fire Serpent

In February 2007, Randy Mantooth played a 40-year-veteran wildland fire-fighter in the TV movie *Fire Serpent*. His character, who believes that the fire is alive, mentions having worked for LACoFD, among other places.

Randy's Namesake Appearances

The first few episodes of the firefighting/paramedic drama *Third Watch* on NBC shows a firehouse Dalmatian named Mantooth. When Randy Mantooth met up with John Wells, *Third Watch* producer, Wells told him that their field research showed an overwhelming number of fire stations had dogs named Mantooth.[2] "In a September 8, 1999 interview Randy commented, "We've named our Labrador Retriever in *USAR-1*, John Wells."

In the TV series, *The Pretender* (NBC 1996–2000), Jarod (Michael T. Weiss) often took on the name of someone associated with his new profession. In the 1996 episode "Under the Reds" (1.16), he plays paramedic Jarod Mantooth.

Although not yet selected, Randy Mantooth continues to be nominated each year since 2001 for a Hollywood "Walk of Fame" star.

In the book *Mr. Monk Goes to the Firehouse* (2006) by Lee Goldberg, based on the *Monk* TV series, the Captain's name in the San Francisco firehouse is "Captain Mantooth." The book was adapted for one of the episodes of the TV series and aired July 28, 2006, as "Mr. Monk Can't See a Thing" (episode 5.4). Although the Fire Captain's name is not used on the show, there is still an *Emergency!* connection—when the engine gets toned out to respond to a fire, Station 51's two-tone horn and claxon are heard.

Kevin Tighe

Tighe appeared in a cameo as LA City Battalion Chief Kieran Ryan in the 1-hour pilot episode for *The 119,* produced for CBS and Paramount Television in 1997. This show was filmed utilizing the new LA City Fire Station 112, at 444 S. Harbor Blvd., Berth 86, Ports O'Call for exterior and interior shots. The helmets and uniforms sporting the station number "119" are the same helmets and uniforms used for Randy Mantooth's and Robert Fuller's appearances in the *Diagnosis Murder* episode "Malibu Fire" filmed a few months later.

In May 16, 2004, Tighe appeared on *Law & Order: CI* as Dr. Lindguard and, in what was perhaps an inside joke, said that he had been in the medical profession for more than 30 years. The *TV Guide* listing for the episode stated: "Guest starring Kevin Tighe (*Emergency!*)."

Tighe has appeared on *Lost* as Lock's evil father in several episodes from 2005 through 2007.

Kevin has been very active for several years in hospice care and support for terminally ill patients and their families.

---

[2] According to A&E Network's monthly *Biography* magazine.

Marco López

Marco López lives near Las Vegas and appears in commercials, still cooks, and at one time owned and ran a catering business called Marco's Catering.

López advises that all the recipes named on the show were scripted and not real (such as Roy's Beef Whatever, Roy's Eggs Lupin, Chet's Eggs Rasputin, Capt's Clam Chowder, Butterscotch Bean Dip, and Johnny's Green Stew) and that all the food specialties that he personally made were not used on the show, even though they were popular at cast parties. López even published a small cookbook, which includes his favorite chili recipe, published here with his permission.

    1 large onion, coarsely chopped
    1 medium green pepper, chopped
    1 large celery stalk, chopped
    1 large clove garlic, minced
    3 tablespoons oil
    4 pounds ground beef chuck
    $1^1/_2$ teaspoons minced jalapeno chilies
    $^1/_2$ cup chili powder
    1 tablespoon ground cumin
    1 teaspoon garlic salt
    1 teaspoon onion salt
    1 teaspoon liquid red pepper seasoning
    2 bay leaves, crumbled
    2 teaspoons salt
    $^1/_4$ teaspoon freshly ground black pepper
    $^2/_3$ cup beer
    1 (16 oz) can stewed tomatoes
    1 (8 oz) can tomato sauce
    1 (6 oz) can tomato paste
    2 tablespoons honey
    $1^1/_2$ cups water (about)

Stir fry onion, green pepper, celery, and garlic in oil in large dutch oven pan or kettle for 8 minutes or until tender and golden brown. Add beef and cook until crumbly. Add jalapeno chili, chili powder, cumin, garlic salt, onion salt, red pepper, seasoning, bay leaves, salt, pepper, beer, tomatoes, tomato sauce and paste, honey, and enough water to barely cover ingredients. Cook over low heat, uncovered, stirring often, for at least 3 hours or until chili is thick and flavors are well blended. Adjust seasoning to taste if necessary (10–12 servings).

Marco has an unpublished cookbook containing more than 30 recipes (and still growing) that he prepared for the cast and crew of *Dragnet* and

Emergency!. The book is available for purchase (contact coauthor Rozane Sutherland through Erika and Rozane's Emergencyfans.com website for more details). The book also includes some photos of him on the set of *Emergency!*.

The *Emergency!* cast also had fun by throwing the best parties around, López said. There were about 15 other television series getting made at the same location, and "everybody used to invade our parties." López also used to enjoy cooking for the company on the set kitchen. This was the biggest similarity between the real López, who has been to culinary school, and his character.

Robert Fuller

Years after playing Dr. Brackett, Fuller got a role in the 1990 parody of *The Exorcist,* titled *Repossessed,* in which he portrayed Dr. Hackett. He also had a voiceover as a doctor in *Seinfeld* episode 8.13, "The Comeback." Fuller also appeared as a retired ranger in an episode of *Walker, Texas Ranger*, which aired January 15, 2000. The actress who plays his wife was Marla Adams, who also appeared in *Emergency!*. In this episode, "Dr. Brackett" is paged over the public address system in a hospital scene.

Jim Page

Twenty years after the show debuted, Page had the idea that videotapes of the 1970s show *Emergency!* could be repackaged and sold. He knew many people in emergency medical services had been inspired by the show as youngsters and knew how popular the show still was among this group. When he approached his bosses at *JEMS (Journal of Emergency Medical Services),* they were unimpressed and thought the idea was too risky. Page replied, "Fine, I'll take the risk. If the videos don't sell I'll personally buy back the entire inventory." The series sold almost 5000 complete sets and made a good return for the business. According to A.J. Heightman, *JEMS* Editor-In-Chief, Page never did take a cut for himself.

In 1995 Page wrote the companion booklet to the videos, *Emergency! Companion,* which initially was free with video sales. The 32-page booklet featuring information about the cast and six early episodes now fetches high prices on Internet auction sites.

Ed Self

A writer and a producer for *Emergency!*, he also produced *The Rangers,* the pilot for the 1974 short-lived series *Sierra* with James G. Richardson (*Emergency!*'s Craig Brice), which featured a crossover episode with Johnny and Roy on a training exercise. Self later produced *Code R* for CBS in 1977, a combination fire, lifeguard, and police series based on Catalina Island.

Self tried his hand at another firefighting program, joining up with another *Emergency!* producer Gino Grimaldi, with *Vegas Firefighters*, the working title of a preview film for studio executives. This less-than-30-minute reality-based film featured the men and women of Las Vegas Fire & Rescue (LVFR) Station 4 on and off the job. Filmed in 2000, the project remains unsold. "To date (2007), nothing has happened with the project," said Self, "a pilot was never made. Gino and I spent a great deal of time at Station 4, and we made what amounted to a home movie, but it fell far short of a pilot. We just couldn't get a broadcaster interested." The technical consultant for LVFR was Deputy Chief Ken Riddle. Riddle worked on other non-fire TV programs when it involved fire or paramedic scenes. They include *VEGA$* starring Robert Urich, *Knight Rider* with David Hasslehoff, and others.

Christian I. Nyby II

A director of several episodes of *Emergency!*, Nyby II would also direct other related Robert A. Cinader projects, *The Rangers*, *Sierra*, and *Pine Canyon Is Burning*.

Rampart Hospital

In the *Quincy, M.E.* (1976–1983) episode "Cover Up" (5.15), which aired February 7, 1980, a paramedic is caring for a patient and says, "I think we should take him to Rampart" and calls the hospital, "Rampart Emergency, this is Squad 44". Also in this episode, Colby Chester (from the *Emergency!* World Premier, two episodes of *Emergency!*, and the series *Sierra*) appeared as a lawyer, and Michael Fox (*Emergency!* episode 3.9) portrays a Fire Captain. In the first episode of this series, Randy Mantooth's brother, Donald Mantooth (*Emergency!* episodes 3.17 and 4.9 and a *Sierra* episode), appeared on October 3, 1976.

Code F

In the County of Los Angeles a Code F is transmitted when a firefighter dies in the line of duty. Dispatch is notified in the same manner for any civilian death. Elsewhere throughout the United States the signal 5 – 5 – 5 – 5 may be transmitted. This is a signal, an alarm code that dates back to the beginning of the fire service. It was sent by the dispatchers through the old bell system to signal that a member had died in the line of duty and that stations should fly their flags at half-staff. It is still used in New York City, where it began in the 1860s, and other departments to alert the stations of a fallen comrade. The bell is rung in this manner each year at the International Association of Firefighters Fallen Firefighter Memorial event in Colorado Springs, Colorado.

The following people involved in *Emergency!* have passed on.

William Boyett
Captain at Station 39 and Battalion Chief McConnike in seven episodes
    and two movies
December 29, 2004

William Bryant
Various engine company Captains in multiple episodes
June 26, 2001

Robert A. Cinader
Writer and executive producer
November 16, 1982

Gary Crosby
Four *Emergency!* episodes; also appeared in *905-Wild*
August 24, 1995

Howard Curtis
Stuntman; also appeared in *Towering Inferno* and *Firehouse (1973 Movie)*
September 2, 1979

Paul Donnelly
Unit manager
October 7, 1990

Richard A. Friend
LACoFD liaison to *Emergency!*; LACoFD Public Information Officer
June 24, 2005

Kenneth Hahn
Los Angeles County Board of Supervisors, 1952–1992
October 12, 1997

Dick Hammer
LA County Fire Captain Dick Hammer, season 1, episodes 1–9
October 18, 1999

Sam Lanier
LA County civilian fire dispatcher
May 21, 1997

Julie London
Nurse Dixie McCall
October 18, 2000

Mickey Michaels
Set decorator
March 20, 1999

George Orrison
Stunt double for Kevin Tighe
March 1, 2001

James O. Page
LACoFD Battalion Chief, technical consultant, and writer
September 4, 2004

Albert Popwell
Animal control officer, episode 4.22 ("905-WILD")
April 9, 1999

James Gilbert "Jim" Richardson III
Paramedic Craig Brice and writer; also appeared in *Sierra, The Rangers, Weekend with a Bear*, and *Adam-12*
February 20, 1983

Nelson Riddle
Composer, *Emergency!* theme
October 6, 1985

John Smith (nee Robert Van Orden)
Captain Hammer, season 1, episodes 10 and 11
January 25, 1995

Kenneth Tobey
Various characters
December 22, 2002

Robert "Bobby" W. Troup, Jr.
Dr. Joe Early
February 7, 1999

Kelly Troup Romick (daughter of Bobby Troup and Julie London)
Debbi, episode 2.6
March 11, 2002

Jack Randolph Webb[3] (pen name, John Randolph)
Director, writer, and executive producer
December 23, 1982

---

[3] The pair of hands seen hammering the "Mark VII" logo at the end of every episode are Jack Webb's.

EMERGENCY! *Behind the Scene*

CHAPTER **22**

Comments from the Fans

Emergency! fans are everywhere. The following are just some of the many comments received by some fans of *Emergency!*—those who either chose their profession or changed it because of the impact that the show had on them. The show proved to many of these people that better emergency medical services (EMS) *had* to be provided, and they worked within their profession to make it happen.

At the *Emergency!* Convention held in Burbank, California, in 1998, firefighters, emergency medical technicians (EMTs), ambulance personnel, rescue squad personnel, and even nurses and doctors gave their reasons for choosing their profession; a TV program called *Emergency!*

"I grew up with this show and yes, I am a firefighter because of it, and I still love it."
—Phillip Stewart

"Thanks for allowing me to be a part of this great thing you are doing. When I started at my current job, we would often have to relieve the dispatchers in our stations for a few minutes or so. I was thrilled the first time I got to repeat our frequency designator after a transmission, which was KOL-808. Immediately the show's tones and theme song started playing in my mind. I remember watching Emergency!, thinking how cool it would be to do the kinds of things that they do. Repelling down an embankment to rescue a victim, masking up and going into a burning building, rescuing an injured worker from high atop a crane or scaffold, even just hanging around the hospital after a run, trying to make time with a pretty nurse. Every week John, Roy, Chet, Marco, Mike, and Captain Stanley were there to fulfill those dreams. I have been in the fire service almost 20 years now and still haven't done all those things, probably never will either. It's funny, though, how things stay with you. There are times when I get to do something on the job that reminds me of an episode that I saw as a kid, and after I have cleared the scene from whatever it was that we had been doing, I'll jokingly say without even thinking about it, 'KMG-365.' (After I have released the mic button of course)."
—Forester Sinclair, firefighter/EMT, Boeing Fire Department

"I would not be a firefighter/EMT if not for Emergency!. I found, after watching this particular show that I wanted to help people—real-time—not just doing other people's paperwork. I wanted to see their faces, talk to them, and lay a hand on theirs, hoping I could possibly make their situation easier. As an example, I remember a patient I had a few years ago. She broke water 3 months premature. She was scared, crying. She was at work. Her coworkers were present (which can be very humiliating and embarrassing). My crew was able to give her privacy, humor, comfort, and—by the time she was shipped off—she was smiling and laughing despite the situation. I think we made a difference. (Her husband called to thank us later.) It's not frequent, rare actually, but despite the mundane crap, picky stuff, swishy press, and budget cuts we deal with every day—it all comes down to the patient. I've been an EMT since '82. Wow. Way to go Emergency!"
—Michele

"The show is what inspired me and as you know a lot of people to become a firefighter. Since I was about 5 years old, I have known I wanted to be in this profession due to Emergency!. I have been a professional firefighter for 9 years, first in the Marine Corps and now in Fresno, California."
—Ryan Blankenship

"My earliest memories of the Fire Service would have to be when I was a toddler living in the Sunnyside section of Queens, New York. My mother would take me *to the park and I would regularly see FDNY Rescue Company 4 shooting up and down Queens Boulevard. I was enthralled with the sight of this truck, a 1971 Mack with a painting of a knight's helmet and a shield with the number 4 on the door, and the sound of its old mechanical siren as it sped off to another major fire. As I got a little older and my family relocated to another part of Queens, on Saturday afternoons at 5 P.M. EVERYTHING stopped. I would run inside from whatever I was doing and click on the old black-and-white TV to tune into WPIX TV-Channel 11. And there would be E! in syndication. I remember watching the show, saying to myself, I could do that. I would sit, eyes glued to the screen, listening for those tones and Sam Lanier's voice sending Station 51 and other stations to yet another calamity. From a plane crash to man down, nothing fazed this guy, wondering . . . could I do that too?*

I would play with my friends and we'd pretend to be talking to Rampart on the biophone . . . I kind of lost track with watching the show as I got older, as it was switched to time filler at 2 in the morning on WPIX, nestled in between the Honeymooners and TV Preachers. My family moved to a small community in Upstate New York, where I eventually became a volunteer firefighter/EMT.

My interest in E! was piqued a few years ago, while I worked as a fire alarm dispatcher for FDNY in Manhattan. A few of my colleagues cited E! as an influence on them and we would bring in videos to watch during the slower hours of our night tours. After having most of my senses overloaded by the terror attacks of September 11th, I clearly remember one of the only things that brought me a little bit of happiness was sitting at my desk in the dispatcher's office the night following the attack, watching a rerun on TV Land. [The show] was also an influence, slightly, on my brother, who is now an FDNY paramedic.

In medic jargon, someone who is a real hard charger is referred to as "Johnny-Roy" and usually greeted with the two thumbs up, mimicking Randy Mantooth's flipping the caps in the E! opening sequence.

[I've had the] opportunity to meet Randy and a couple of the producers of the show, Ed Self, and Gino Grimaldi. Hard to put into words the feelings to describe meeting one of your childhood heroes and thanking him for being such an influence. Strangely though, this meeting occurred a few months after the attacks of September 11th, it seemed like more people wanted to meet me because of my affiliation, and all I wanted to do was thank them for all the influences they had on me."

—James P. Raftery, "Jimmy Raf," Supervising Fire Alarm Dispatcher, FDNY Communications

Author's note: Jimmy is the recipient of FDNY's Chief O'Brien Award for his efforts on 9/11. It is the second highest award given out to a civilian employee of the Department.

"[Nurse] Dixie was the reason I went to nursing school, and [my daughter Aimee] says she is going to be one of the next generation of nurses. I bet these people had no idea that even 30 years later they were still going to be influencing people's lives."
—Kathy Tumbleson

"With respect to Jim Page—a visionary in EMS who influenced me toward getting to where I am—I can only hope to make a fraction of the impact on others lives that he did."
—Ken Phillips, Chief of Emergency Services, Grand Canyon National Park

"It is funny that after 30 years, nobody can seem to duplicate what Roy and Johnny did week in and week out. You'd think that there would be a firefighter reality show like Cops by now. I guess the original was done so well that nothing can stand up to it."
—John A. Weeks III, Newave Communications, Burnsville, MN

"No one will ever measure up to the cast of Emergency!. It's a classic. I don't think there will ever be a team of people who work together so well to make a show seem so real."
—Lisa Sutton Thomas, San Antonio, TX

"I don't know what I would have done without Emergency!. Seeing Captain Hank Stanley, Mike Stoker, Roy De Soto, John Gage, Chet Kelly, and Marco López save the day always put the spark back into my mind."
—Katie Allen

"Emergency! is one of those rare TV shows like Adam-12 and Dragnet that one could actually learn something while watching TV . . . .It certainly was one of those shows that actually did something big for North America."
—Paul Keenleyside, Canada

"That was a GREAT show that really put the EMS on the medical map. It changed a lot of things, and legitimized firefighters as real medical personnel."
—DeWitt Morgan, retired Fire Captain, LACoFD

"The 'seeds' of Emergency! were planted early for me [as a filmmaker]. I recall KTLA-TV/Channel 5 in Los Angeles ran Emergency! at noon and sometimes during the dinner hour. These were the days before first-run syndicated programming was readily available. I caught EVERY airing of that series and can boast I have seen all of the episodes multiple times. For its time, the series had great production value. There was excellent writing, and the cast was absolutely top-rate. Who could beat the adventures of Johnny and Roy? Who could beat the ever-ready Rampart staff of Kelly Brackett, Joe Early, and Nurse Dixie McCall?

One thing that sticks in my mind is the portrayal of African Americans. These days, we talk about having more positive images of blacks on TV. Jack Webb and R. A. Cinader did it 30 years ago with Ron Pinkard as Dr. Mike Morton, Vince Howard as, well, Vince Howard, and real-life dispatcher Sam Lanier. When I started screenwriting, my style was formulated from the Jack Webb model. I like to keep my characters 'on the real.'

I wrote/produced an indie [independent] film, The C-Shift, which looked at the 1992 L.A. riots from the eyes of a firefighter. Again, I did it with the Jack Webb model in mind. I sneaked in a few tributes to Jack and Emergency!. I told the actors to wear their helmets in the rescue while driving. Well, some real firefighters in L.A. City don't always do that, but that's what I wanted. Some shots at our fire station were shot based on Emergency! scenes. We shot a movie that had our own stamp on it, but it was a great thing to sneak those elements in. In fact, Jack Webb's name appears in the credits of the aforementioned film!

Two years later, I embarked on an all-new firefighter project, Engine Company X. This time, it was a documentary. I got the rare opportunity to spend a lot of time in the L.A. City and County fire stations. For me, it was like being in my own world of Emergency!. I spent two years building this history (of African-American firefighters), and I think it is something Jack would be proud of if he were here. Even with this project, keeping it 'on the real' was my personal directive. I even got a chance to sneak in a short 'bit' on Jack and Emergency!. Those two films are now part of a museum archive and have sold several copies across the United States and as far as England."
—Chin Thammasaengsri, independent screenwriter/filmmaker, Westlake Signal Group, Los Angeles, CA

"Since I was a basic EMT in 1972 and not a paramedic, there weren't many things I could do to emulate Johnny or Roy, medically. However, in the episode 'School Days' (2.14), the squad's crew assists in removing a dangerous snake from a man's chest. After sweeping off the man's chest, the paramedic trainee grabbed a CO_2 extinguisher and sprayed the snake to cool it sufficiently so that it could be removed safely. (In the episode, the snake turned out to be a phony rubber snake, but that is beside the point.)

The technique was also used with a cobra in 'Transition' (4.15) and with a real rattlesnake in a garage in 'On Camera' (5.12).

On my engine, we carried a small CO_2 extinguisher and worked in a rural area with several calls for snakes each summer, most of which were rattlesnakes. One day, an incident arose where we could try this technique out in a safe manner (obviously not on someone's chest), and it worked. The CO_2 did not freeze the snake, but it did restrict its movements so it could be removed safely."

—Richard Yokley, former EMT, Bonita-Sunnyside Fire Department, and co-author

"When I completed my tour of duty as a flight surgeon with the Navy in early 1971, I began working full time in the emergency department of Bay General Hospital in Chula Vista, California. In those days, moonlighting Navy physicians covered all the emergency departments in the evenings and on the weekends . . . . Patients were brought to the ER by old Cadillac ambulances or in station wagons by basic first-aid trained ambulance attendants. The San Diego Police Department, who ran the ambulance service at the time from Chevy vans, delivered patients within the boundaries of the city with a relayed phone message to us announcing the sex of the victim and the body part that was injured.

Pre-arrival notice went something like, 'We are en route with a male head!' or 'We are en route with a female leg.' We had private providers, fire service providers, and the police department responding to local hospitals. On one occasion, as the attendant was casually off-loading his very elderly patient, I looked into the back of the rig and asked, 'How long has your patient been dead?' Overall, it was apparent that we needed some better training in the field.

About this time, the American Academy of Orthopedic Surgeons had taken the lead in developing a training program for emergency medical technicians. Dr. Tom Elo, who was a staff physician at Naval Hospital San Diego emergency department took it upon himself to put together the first EMT training class in San Diego at one of the community colleges and asked a number of the community physicians to guest lecture. I was one of the physicians who assisted and immediately felt that we needed to bring that improved level of prehospital training to the South Bay.

Bay General Hospital was extremely interested in assisting and made space available in the hospital for classes and we set up an EMT program through Southwestern College for the fall semester of 1972. A number of firefighters, lifeguards, some police officers, and all of the ambulance attendants from the local private company attended. Over the years, it has been most interesting to see a number of those original EMT students become paramedics or fire chiefs!

The classes were a tremendous success . . . . Sergeant Frank Kral of the San Diego Police Department . . . [added] EMT training to the academy for the department. This was a great upgrade and began the course of steady improvement in pre-hospital care in San Diego. Paramedic services came to San Diego in the mid 1970s, and we convinced Bay General to become the first base station in the South Bay and employ the first set of medics in Chula Vista, they were called

'LifeSaver I.' The paramedics, based at the hospital, helped out in the ER when they were not out on calls."

—Dr. Mel Ochs, inventor, innovator, former Medical Director for San Diego County, and more importantly, co-author Richard Yokley's EMT instructor in 1972.

"Only nostalgic for but a moment, those family gatherings around the TV to view Johnny and Roy were more influential than ever credited to be. Within our household, it was a time to debate the poignant humor found in M*A*S*H, along with the frankness and reality of Emergency!. Ragingly popular then, the cast of characters was as much 'family' as the viewers watching. Driven by the nature of the profession, we were exposed to the camaraderie of the fire service, to the paramedics, the hospital staff, and police. In as much as 'reality television' has mesmerized today's audiences, Emergency! opened the door for an early peek inside our complex EMS world.

I can only imagine the tremendous educational component this show provided our nation, whether we knew it or not. Important issues now entwined with solid entertainment, imagine. Perhaps back then, the glamour of nurse Dixie, or the thrill of the paramedic role took life in many of our souls working in the field today. Certainly Emergency!'s success must have been linked to its human quality. Watching people, like you and me, faced with life's challenges, a blend of tragic and ridiculous. Reflecting back to Station 51, then fast forward to today, you may believe what you will, but we all know there are pooches still roaming in some stations today, cleverly conceived pranks run rampant everywhere, and when the alarm tones blare, adrenaline rushes, just as it did when we were 14.

My husband [Richard Forman, cameraman for COPS] told me . . . he wanted to be a fireman every time he watched Emergency! . . . how in this world he turned out to be a cameraman, I'll never figure!"

—Kelly Forman, RN, MICN, CEN, Flight Nurse LifeFlight San Diego, Mercy Air in San Diego

Authors' Notes

As with any television program, Emergency! had its detractors as well. For all the good Emergency! was able to accomplish across the country in getting communities to provide more advanced medical care, some felt that it did have a real downside. They say that the program created false expectations in many young people who were attracted into EMS for the wrong reasons—not to help people but to become heroes—and evolved into horrible caregivers. Some good medical providers quit because they could not deal with those who were in it for the glory and the power.

Many firefighters in the 1970s were not excited by the new EMS program because they felt they should concentrate on fighting fires, not providing first aid. (This theme was incorporated into episode 4.16, "The Smoke Eater.")

Others felt that the program demeaned ambulance companies, perpetuating the old "scoop and haul" syndrome. This may have more to do with the nature of how LA County built and handled its EMS system, because LA County paramedics do not have to ride with every patient transport. However, this method is popular among the paramedics because it allows them to "clear" much quicker.

Nonetheless, *Emergency!* did something no other television program before or after has been able to accomplish—through this new and innovative program called paramedics (whether through fire departments or private ambulance companies, volunteer or paid)—it saved lives!

EMERGENCY! *Behind the Scene*

APPENDIX **A**

The Wedworth-Townsend Act

Effective January 1975, and includes the original act and subsequent legislation.

HEALTH and SAFETY CODE

WEDWORTH–TOWNSEND ACT

MOBILE INTENSIVE CARE PARAMEDICS

1480. Pilot program

Any general acute care hospital operated by, or contracting with, a county may conduct a pilot program which provides services utilizing mobile intensive care paramedics for the delivery of emergency medical care to the sick and injured at the scene of an emergency, during transport to a general acute care hospital, while in the emergency department of the general acute care hospital until care responsibility is assumed by the regular staff of the general acute care hospital, and during training within the facilities of the sponsoring general acute care hospital.

1480.1 Pilot program

The training of mobile intensive care paramedics may only be conducted by a community college, college, university, or hospital that has a certificate of approval for its curriculum and training program from the county health officer of the county in which it is located.

1481. Definitions

As used in this article:
  (a) "Mobile intensive care paramedics" means personnel who have been trained in the provision of emergency cardiac and noncardiac care in a training program certified by the county health officer of the county giving certification or a certified training program in another county that has been evaluated and approved by the county health officer of the county giving certification, and who pass the performance and written examinations required for certification by the officer as qualified to render the services enumerated in this article in the county giving such certification.
  (b) "Mobile intensive care nurse" means a registered nurse who has been certified by a county health officer as qualified in the provision of emergency cardiac care and noncardiac care and the issuance of emergency instruction to mobile intensive care paramedics.
  (c) "Mobile intensive care units" means any emergency vehicles staffed by mobile intensive care paramedics or mobile intensive care nurses and equipped to provide remote intensive care or cardiac care to the sick or injured at the scene of medical emergencies or during transport to general acute care hospitals.
  (d) "Emergency department" means any department or separate area within a general acute care hospital, which is staffed and equipped to provide emergency medical care to the sick or injured.

1481.1 Minimum training; experience

The training program for mobile intensive care paramedics shall consist of a minimum of 200 hours of didactic training, a minimum of 100 hours of clinical experience, and a field internship of at least 200 hours.

However, all or any portion of the required training program for a mobile intensive care paramedic may be waived by the county health officer of the county giving certification if the applicant passes the performance and written examinations required for certification or the appropriate portion of the performance examination.

1481.2 Program evaluation report

Each county conducting a pilot program pursuant to this article shall submit an annual report to the Legislature and to the State Department of Health, not later than January 31 of each calendar year, evaluating any such pilot program conducted at any general acute care hospital operated by the county or under contract with the county. The report shall include an evaluation of the competency and effectiveness of the performance by the mobile intensive care paramedics in their duties in staffing rescue units and in the rendering of medical and nursing care pursuant to this article. The report may include recommendations relating to the extension or modification of the provisions of this article.

1481.3 Courses of instruction and training; certification; fees; reimbursement by federal funds

Any county conducting a pilot program under this article may provide courses of instruction and training leading to certification as a mobile intensive care paramedic. Where such instruction and training is provided to public employees other than employees of the county or employees of the fire protection district within the county, a fee may be charged sufficient to defray the cost of such instruction and training. Where such instruction and training is provided to any other persons such fee shall be charged. However, such fee may be reduced to the extent of any federal funds obtained by the county for the purpose of providing such instruction and training.

1482. Duties

Notwithstanding any other provision of law mobile intensive care paramedics may do any of the following:

(1) Render rescue, first aid and resuscitation services.
(2) Perform cardiopulmonary resuscitation and defibrillation.
(3) During training and while caring for patients in the sponsor general acute care hospital under the direct supervision of a physician or registered nurse, or while at the scene of a medical emergency where voice contact or a telemetered electrocardiogram is

monitored by a physician or a certified mobile intensive care nurse where authorized by a physician, and where direct communication is maintained, upon order of such physician or such nurse:

(a) Administer intravenous saline, glucose, or volume expanding agents or solutions.

(b) Perform gastric suction by intubation.

(c) Perform pulmonary ventilation by use of esophageal airway.

(d) Obtain blood for laboratory analysis.

(e) Apply rotating tourniquets.

(f) Administer parenterally, orally, or topically any of the following classes of drugs or solutions:

(i)   Antiarrhythmic agents.

(ii)   Vagolytic agents.

(iii) Chronotropic agents.

(iv)   Analgesic agents.

(v)   Alkalinizing agents.

(vi)   Vasopressor agents.

(vii) Narcotic antagonists.

(viii) Diuretics.

(ix)   Anticonvulsants.

(x)   Ophthalmic agents.

(xi)   Oxytocic agents.

(xii) Antihistaminics.

(xiii) Bronchodilators.

(xiv) Emetics.

(g) Assist in childbirth

1483. Liability for instructions given paramedics

No physician or nurse, who in good faith gives emergency instructions to a paramedic at the scene of an emergency, shall be liable for any civil damages as a result of issuing the instructions.

1484. Duration of article

(a) This article shall remain in effect only until July 1, 1976, and shall have no force or effect after that date.

(b) On or before July 1, 1975, the State Department of Health shall submit to the Legislature a comprehensive report on emergency medical services in California. Such report shall include a thorough review and evaluation of the mobile intensive care paramedic pilot program authorized by this article and shall make specific recommendations on the following:

(1) Development of statewide coordination of emergency medical service systems, including appropriate communications systems and equipment;

(2) Development of manpower certification standards for all types of emergency medical service personnel to include specifically the training and scope of practice requirements for the categories of ambulance personnel (E.M.T. I) and paramedics (E.M.T. II);

(3) Standards for local paramedic programs including location, qualifications for appropriate teaching institutions, performance standards, and the curriculum necessary for state accreditation of the local program; and

(4) Standards for the staffing and equipping of hospital emergency rooms.

(c) In developing such report, the department shall solicit the advice and recommendations of the Advisory Committee on Emergency Medical Services.

1484.1 Duration of article

During the clinical internship portion of the training program specified in Section 1481.1, mobile intensive care paramedic interns shall be supervised continuously by a physician or registered nurse.

During the field internship portion of the training program specified in Section 1481.1, mobile intensive care paramedic trainees may perform all the services enumerated in this article, provided that they are supervised and accompanied by a certified mobile intensive care paramedic, a physician, or a mobile intensive care nurse.

1484.2 Duration of article

The county health officer shall establish criteria necessary to maintain certification as a mobile intensive care paramedic or a mobile intensive care nurse including, but not limited to:

(a) A formal program of continuing education.

(b) Continuous service as a mobile intensive care paramedic or a certified mobile intensive care nurse.

(C) Retesting at two-year intervals, which shall include a performance examination and may include written examinations and oral examinations.

1484.3 Duration of article

No agency, public or private, shall advertise or disseminate information to the public that the agency provides paramedic rescue or paramedic ambulance service unless that agency does, in fact, provide mobile intensive care units on a continuous 24-hours-per-day basis. If advertising or information regarding the agency's paramedic rescue or paramedic ambulance service appears on any vehicle it may only appear on those mobile intensive-care-unit vehicles utilized solely to provide service on a continuous 24-hours-per-day basis.

1484.4 Duration of article

It shall be a misdemeanor for ambulance personnel to impersonate or refer to themselves as paramedics unless the person has been certified as a mobile intensive care paramedic and currently maintains that certification.

1485. Short title

This article shall be known and may be cited as the Wedworth-Townsend Paramedic Act. It is the intent of this article to respond to the critical shortage of professionally trained medical and nursing personnel for the fast, efficient medical care of the sick or injured at the scene of a medical emergency, during transport to a general acute care hospital, and in the emergency department of the general acute care hospital until care responsibility is assumed by the regular staff of the general acute care hospital. Improved emergency medical service is required to reduce the mortality and morbidity rates during the initial treatment phases of the onset of an acute illness or following an accident. Within the goals of this act is the provision of the best and most efficient and economical delivery of emergency medical care.

APPENDIX **B**

Robert A. Cinader and the Trauma Center Concept

The following is recounted by Tom Hibbard, Deputy First Supervisorial District for LA County Supervisor Pete Schabarum, from March 1973 to February 1991. Frank "Pete" Schabarum (R) was a three-term State Assemblyman before becoming Supervisor for the First District from 1972 to 1991. Schabarum's uncle, P. K. Schabarum, worked for the City of Los Angeles as an architect. It was he who designed LA City Fire Station 27, which opened in 1930 at 1355 N. Cahuenga Boulevard in North Hollywood. The station is now a Fire Museum.

Los Angeles County First District Supervisor Pete Schabarum asked me in 1973 to join his staff to deal with issues related to the county's Department of Health Services. The paramedic program was in its infancy, and the county had contracts with some 100 or more hospital emergency rooms to provide care for the medically indigent.

I was introduced to Bob Cinader, who was doing his *Emergency!* television program. He was intensely interested in the county's emergency medical services (EMS) system, and it didn't take long to realize that his knowledge of EMS issues was excellent. Bob would call the office several times a week to discuss what he saw as flaws in the system, mainly related to the paramedic program. I asked Schabarum to appoint him to what was initially called the Paramedic Commission to make use of his knowledge of EMS.

During this time, I had the county health department draft what is known as a Special Motion calling for a feasibility study regarding developing not just a single facility but a network of trauma centers within the county to handle trauma patients. Schabarum opposed it for about 3 years. I even took my case to Supervisor Kenneth Hahn. He at that time also did not understand the concept. I told Kenny that Pete was not interested in bringing in the motion to do a feasibility study and that I would give it to him to bring in should he be interested in doing so; Kenny declined.

I finally made my case with Supervisor Schabarum, which caused him to agree to bring the motion in and at least have the feasibility of the concept looked at. I needed three votes among the five members of the Board of Supervisors to approve the study, and this is where Bob Cinader came in. Once he endorsed the concept, he went about getting support for it. In fact, I credit Bob with making it possible to get the votes needed to go ahead with trauma centers. He had a wide circle of people he talked to, and he literally jawboned the concept into acceptance.

Today, people have forgotten—and would no doubt be astounded—but hospitals and emergency rooms were initially adamantly opposed to the concept of trauma centers. They formed a well-organized effort to kill the feasibility study. They got the medical profession, city councils, fire departments, etc., to oppose the idea. The world was told what a bad idea trauma centers were.

Bob Cinader was a diplomat on a mission. I don't really know how he did it, who all he talked to, but I have no doubt it was Bob Cinader who caused opposition to slowly turn to support. I credit him for his work not only in the paramedic program but the development of the trauma centers as being the individual who did more to improve EMS for people across our nation than any other person. He accomplished this not only by his television show but by his personal contact with decision-makers.

It took several years once it was decided to go ahead with trauma centers before the first center (LAC/USC Medical Center) came on line. In the meantime, Bob came to suffer with esophageal cancer while he was working on the *Knight Rider* television show. Despite his illness and work, he championed the trauma center concept. He died before the first trauma center was opened in the county, but it was already a foregone conclusion that trauma centers would become a reality.

After Bob's death I asked Supervisor Pete Schabarum to have the name of the fire station in Carson, which was the site used in the opening of the *Emergency!* television show, named the Robert A. Cinader Memorial Fire Station. This was done. I'm not sure but what this is the only fire station in the county named after an individual—an honor Bob rightly deserved.

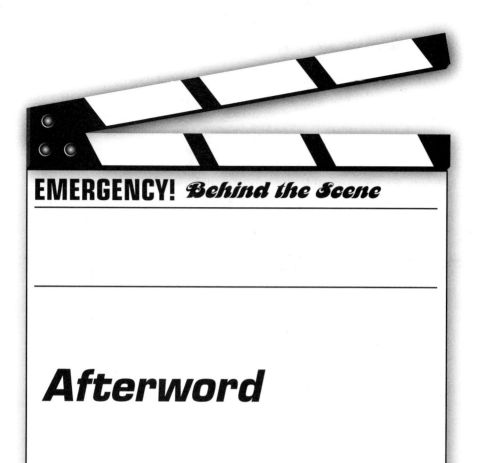

EMERGENCY! *Behind the Scene*

Afterword

"This book captures the essence of an important chapter in television history. Particularly, the coverage of the origins of the Emergency! series is significant beyond entertainment. When the World Premiere of Emergency! was first broadcast in 1972, there were only twelve paramedic units in all of North America. Ten years later, more than half of all Americans were within 10 minutes of a paramedic rescue or ambulance unit. That simply would not have happened without the influence of Emergency!. Without this book, this historical fact might have been lost to succeeding generations."

—James O. Page
Los Angeles County Fire Department Battalion Chief (retired 1973),
founder *JEMS* magazine, and
Technical Consultant and writer to *Emergency!*

These words were written by Jim Page about *Emergency! Behind the Scene*. When work on this book began, Jim said he would be proud to write the Introduction. Sadly, he passed away before this could be realized. Jim contributed greatly to this book and looked forward to its release.

As a firefighter, chief officer, magazine editor, author, lecturer, consultant, and lawyer, Jim's contributions to the health and well-being of our society are immeasurable. He most certainly will be missed, not only as an expert, but also as a wonderful person. His death was a sad day for emergency medical service, fire service, and for all of those who had the opportunity to know him and learn from him.

Jim once gave me a copy of his book, *The Paramedics,* and wrote on the cover: "With appreciation for your dedication to the history of modern EMS and to your important contributions to the preservation of that history." It is my fondest wish that this book he was so looking forward to meets with his approval in that regard.

Our heartfelt sympathies go out to his family, friends, acquaintances, and to all the lives he has touched. Jim leaves his mother, sister, wife, two sons (one of whom is a firefighter), two daughters, six grandchildren, and a legacy not to be forgotten.

—Richard Yokley

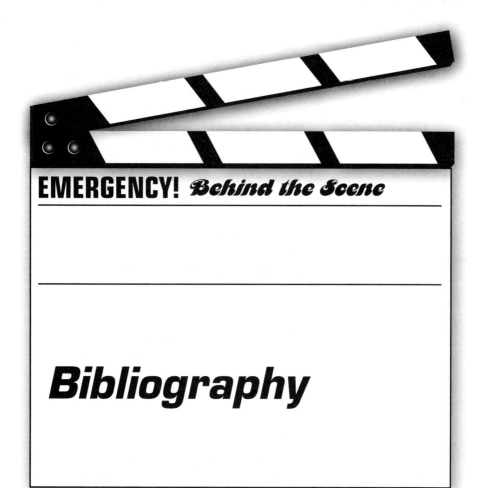

EMERGENCY! *Behind the Scene*

Bibliography

Books, Journals, Magazines, and Papers

Brooks, Tim, and Earle Marsh. *The Complete Directory to Prime Time Network TV Shows, 1946—Present.* 3rd ed. and 6th ed. New York: Ballantine Publishing, 1985 and 1995.

Burzichelli, John J., and Richard J. Gergel. *Ward LaFrance Fire Trucks, 1918–1978,* photo archive. Hudson, WI: Iconographix Publishing, 2000.

Calderone, John A. *"Emergency!," Fire Apparatus Journal,* November/December 1999.

Coleman, Ronny J., and Raymond M. Russell. *Fire Truck Toys for Men and Boys,* Vol. 2. San Clemente, CA: Phoenix Press, 1985.

Drucker, Malka, and Elizabeth James. *Series TV—How a Television Show Is Made.* New York: Clarion Books, 1983.

Emergency! '98 Convention Program, produced by Erika Bartlett, 1998.

Farabee, Charles R. "Butch," Jr. *Death Daring and Disaster, Search and Rescue in the National Parks.* Lanham, MD: Taylor Trade Publishing, 2005.

Since 1965 Farabee worked in ten different U.S. National Parks and served a 4-year stint as the U.S. National Park Service's emergency services coordinator. He retired in 1999 as assistant superintendent of Montana's Glacier National Park.

Fireman, Judy, ed. *TV Book: The Ultimate Television Book.* New York: Workman Publishing Co., 1977.

Freeman, Lisa. *TV80.* New York: Scholastic Book Services, 1979.

Force, Edward. *Miniature Emergency Vehicles.* Atglen, PA: Schiffer Publishing Ltd., 1985.

Friend, Dick. "The Los Angeles County Fire Department." Unpublished document, 1999 (revised 2002).

Friend, Dick. "On the Road to DC—Project 51." Unpublished document, 2000 (revised 2003).

Friend, Dick. "*Emergency!*, This Is a Story about a TV Show." Unpublished document, 2003.

Herz, Peggy. *TV Album.* New York: Scholastic Book Services, 1978

Herz, Peggy. *TV Time '74.* New York: Scholastic Book Services, 1974.

Herz, Peggy. *TV's Top Ten Shows, and Their Stars.* New York: Scholastic Book Services, 1976.

Liversidge, Jim. University of Florida, Belknap Collection for the Performing Arts, George A. Smathers Libraries, Department of Special and Area Studies Collections.

Los Angeles County Fire Department, *1939 Annual Report.*

Los Angeles County Fire Department, 1975 Yearbook, published by the Los Angeles County Firemen's Benefit & Welfare Association, Inc., Los Angeles, CA, 1975.

Marill, Alvin H. *Movies Made for TV—1964–1984.* New York: Baseline Books, 1984.

Martindale, David. *Television Detective Shows of the 1970s.* Jefferson, NC: McFarland & Co., 1991.

Page, James O. *The Paramedics.* Morristown, NJ: Backdraft Publications, 1979.

Page, Jim. *The Emergency! Companion.* Carlsbad, CA: Jems Communications, 1995.

Page, James O. *Effective Company Command.* Alhambra, CA: Borden Publishing, 1973.

Paramedics International 1, no. 2, Spring 1976.

Perry, Jeb H. *Universal Television: The Studio and Its Programs, 1950–1980.* Metuchen, NJ: Scarecrow Press, 1983.

Podrazik, Walter, and Harry Castleman. *Harry & Wally's Favorite TV Shows.* Englewood Cliffs, NJ: Prentice Hall, 1989.

Solomon, Louis. *The TV Doctors.* New York: Scholastic Book Services, January 1, 1974.

Spring, Laurence. *The Dennis Ace Fire Engine.* Dennis Pamphlet Series No. 2. Surrey, UK: Surrey Record Office, 1995.

Stewart, Ronald. *A Paramedic Handbook of Pharmacology* (1975). For use by the Mobile Intensive Care Unit Paramedics within the County of Los Angeles.

Straight Streams, a magazine of the Los Angeles County Fire Department, August 1971.

Strauss. Michael Thomas. *Hot Wheels Price Guide,* 5th ed. Dayton, OH: Tomart Press, 2002.

Turow, Joseph. *Playing Doctor: Television, Storytelling, and Medical Power.* New York: Oxford University Press, 1989.

van Heerden, Bill. *Film and Television In-Jokes.* Jefferson, NC: McFarland & Company, 1998.

Woodard, Clarence C. "The General: Apparatus from the Motor City," *Enjine!-Enjine!* 2 (Summer 1978); reprinted, 1994.

Woolery, George W. *Children's Television: The First Thirty-Five Years 1946–1981.* Metuchen, NJ: Scarecrow Press, 1983–1985.

Yokley, Richard. *TV Firefighters.* Chula Vista, CA: Black Forest Press, 2003.

Entertainment Industry Publications

The Internet Movie Database (IMDB)

Entertainment industry publications from around the world, such as *TV Guide* (American and Canadian), *Entertainment Weekly,* Britain's *TV Week,* Australia's *TV Week,* America's *TV Week,* Mexico's *Tele*Guia,* Argentina's *TV Guia,* and other regional weekly TV magazines as noted throughout the book.

Websites

The official website of the Los Angeles County Fire Department, *www.lacofd.org/.*

The County of Los Angeles Fire Museum Association website, *www.LACountyFireMuseum.com.*

Erika and Rozane's *Emergency!* website, *www.emergencyfans.com/.*

Nexxie's *Emergency!* website, *http://www.nexxie.0catch.com*

Paul's Emergency Equipment Manifest website, *http://modena.intergate.ca/personal/p18s/E!Manifest.htm*

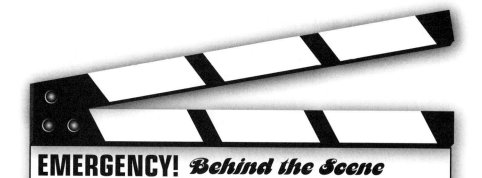

EMERGENCY! *Behind the Scene*

Glossary of Terms

Medical Terms as Used on Emergency!

Advanced life support (ALS)
Medical care provided by paramedics trained to assess a patient's condition, administer drugs, defibrillate, and provide advanced airway management prior to transportation to the hospital.

Basic life support (BLS)
Level of care provided to patients requiring transportation to the hospital. BLS does not include extensive medical supervision or treatment.

Blood pressure
The pressure of the blood in the arteries that rises and falls as the muscles of the body cope with exercise, stress, sleep, etc. There are two types of

pressure that are measured: (1) systolic pressure, created by the contraction of the heart muscle pushing blood into the vessels, and (2) diastolic pressure, when the heart is at rest between beats. A reading of 120/80 is said to be the normal range.

Carotid pulse
Pulse obtained from the carotid artery in the neck.

Codes
Not all of these radio codes were used on *Emergency!* but this is a complete list.

Code A   Request arson/fire investigator
Code C   Child abuse
Code D   Request for a "cause investigator" for an undetermined fire cause
Code E   Escaped inmate (fire crew)
Code F   Transmitted when a firefighter has died in the line of duty in the County of Los Angeles; similarly used when there is a civilian death
Code I   Injured firefighter
Code L   Request law enforcement (no longer used)
Code N   Notify news agencies of a newsworthy event: fire, rescue, etc.
Code R   LA County speak for the more commonly used "Code 3" or "Priority 1," that is, "red lights and siren"
Code T   Terrorism notification

CPR (cardiopulmonary resuscitation)
The emergency substitution of heart and lung action to restore life to someone who appears dead. The two main components of CPR are chest compression to make the heart pump and mouth-to-mouth ventilation to breathe for the victim.

Diaphoretic
Sweaty

D5W
A solution of 5 percent glucose in distilled water within an IV bag; a TKO (to keep open) IV utilized in the field as a vehicle for administering medications intravenously.

EKG
Electrocardiogram. Used to monitor the patient's heart rhythm.

FACEP
As in Dr. Early, MD, FACEP; Fellow of the American College of Emergency Physicians

Fibrillation
A rapid and irregular contraction of the heart muscle causing an irregular heartbeat.

Hare traction splint
A splint used on femur (thigh bone) fractures. It applies a constant pull along the length of the leg to help stabilize the fractured bone and reduce muscle spasms.

The Johnny Gage thump
See Precordial thump. Patients on *Emergency!* were usually subjected to a blow to the chest from a height of approximately 3 feet (91 centimeters); arm's length over the head (as if swinging a hammer).

Lactated Ringer's
See Ringer's lactate.

Leads
Lead placement on the patient's chest for transmitting cardiac information to the hospital via the BioPhone.

Lead 1   In recording lead 1 on an electrocardiogram, the negative terminal of the electrocardiograph is connected to the right arm and the positive terminal to the left arm.

Lead 2   In recording limb lead 2, the negative terminal of the electrocardiograph is connected to the right arm and the positive terminal to the left leg.

Lead 3   In recording limb lead 3, the negative terminal of the electrocardiograph is connected to the left arm and the positive terminal to the left leg.

MAST pants
Medical anti-shock trousers. Also called PASG (pneumatic anti-shock garment) pants. It is a pant-like device used to control bleeding from areas that the garment covers. It is also used to force blood from the lower extremities

to the upper torso as needed. It controls external bleeding from the lower extremities by direct pressure, similarly to the air splint. It is also useful in providing indirect pressure to help control internal bleeding in the pelvic and abdominal cavities.

The Precordial thump

A precordial thump is a thump administered to the front of the chest, over the sternum, in cardiac resuscitation of *witnessed* ventricular fibrillation.

The American Heart Association (AHA) recommends the precordial thump as the initial maneuver in treatment of ventricular tachycardia (VT) and monitored ventricular fibrillation (VF). The precordial thump is still included in the advanced cardiac life support (ACLS) paramedic-training program, and it is used in the approach to the pulseless, nonbreathing patient. San Diego County also has a protocol for "thump pacing," which is used for symptomatic bradycardia prior to medication administration.

Technique:

1. Confirm pulselessness.
2. Expose chest and visualize center of chest.
3. Strike the middle of the sternum with a sharp, quick blow, using a clenched fist. Strike the chest with fleshy part of the fist (hypothenar eminence). The blow should be from a height of 8 to 12 inches (20 to 30 centimeters) maximum.

Note: The force of the blow should not break ribs.

Ringer's lactate (or Lactated Ringer's)

An electrolyte solution for management of shock and dehydration. Ringer's is used similarly to normal saline solution to help correct fluid imbalances and fight hypovolemic (blood loss) shock. Especially used for surgical or traumatic blood loss, burns, or fluids lost such as vomitus or diarrhea. Dr. Ringer created the solution, thus it is known as "Ringer's." Not given in cases of cardiac failure.

STAT

A common medical abbreviation that is used to imply "urgent" or "rush." It is derived from a Latin word *statim,* which means immediately.

Syncope episode

A loss of consciousness due to inadequate blood flow to the brain. It is basically light-headedness or dizziness, commonly referred to as fainting.

TKO (to keep open) or **KVO** (keep vein open)
Maintaining just enough of a drip rate to keep the IV from clotting.

Firefighter Terms

Attic ladder
A ladder, usually 8 to 10 feet long, that can be folded so that the two beams touch each other. Also called a *scuttle hull* or *pencil ladder* in some parts of the country.

Backdraft
A backdraft occurs when an oxygen-starved fire suddenly receives oxygen. The sudden rush of oxygen causes all of the superheated gases to ignite at the same time, which causes an explosion. While the risk of such an occurrence is low, a backdraft is almost always fatal to anyone caught in it.

Booster tank
The tank on a pumper that supplies booster lines and hand lines at a fire until a connection with a water source can be made. The booster tank on most pumpers is between 500 and 1000 gallons.

Call firefighter
The Los Angeles County Fire Department, as of this writing, employs approximately 100 call firefighters. These personnel staff eleven engine companies assigned to areas that include Catalina Island, Malibu, and the Antelope Valley. Call firefighters, when alerted by a paging system, respond to all types of emergencies. There are three levels of staffing: "first responder" engines are staffed by paid firefighters, respond to all emergency incidents within their jurisdictional areas, and are supported by full-time companies; "supplemental" call firefighters staff a second engine company from a station that is also staffed by a full-time company; and "augmentation" call firefighters are assigned to an existing career company and respond directly to the scene to augment that company's staffing. (As referenced in Chapter 8 with the still in-service 1972/1973 Ward LaFrance engines.)

Deck gun
A large and usually fixed water nozzle attached to an engine. Deck guns deliver larger amounts of water than hand-held hose.

Engine
An engine carries small ground ladders, 1000 feet of supply line to connect it with a hydrant, hand lines to fight the fire with, and a tank holding

between 500 and 1000 gallons of water. Often called a *pumper* or a *triple* (triple combination—pump, hose, water tank).

Engine company
An engine company is a combination of a fire engine and the manpower used to staff it. A standard engine company will include an officer (Captain or Lieutenant), driver (Engineer), and one to two Firefighters.

Forcible entry
An act of gaining access to a structure through means other than an open window or door. Frequently, firefighters must force open doors that are locked or remove security doors or window bars to enter the structure to search for victims and/or extinguish a fire. A variety of hand, power, and hydraulic tools can be used for forcible entry.

Forward lay
A forward lay is when fire hose is laid from the hydrant to the fire. Usually with a 2.5-inch or 4-inch hose coming off the back of the engine.

Hand line
A hand line is a small-diameter hose usually used inside a burning structure to directly apply water onto the fire. Hand lines are usually 1.5 or 1.75 inches in diameter. Lines 2.5 inches in diameter are used for heavy fire conditions.

Hose
Hose is used to deliver water onto a fire and to provide water from hydrants to firefighting apparatus. The types of hose used include hand lines, booster lines, and large-diameter hose.

Hydrant
An above-ground steel or bronze metal casting connected to a water supply system and equipped with one or more valved outlets to which a pumper or hose line can be connected. Typically on street corners, painted yellow. May be either wet or dry, depending on local and weather conditions.

Jaws
A term applied to a rescue tool that can cut, push, or pull material (most often automobiles). "Jaws of Life" is a trademarked name of Hurst. Holmatro and Amkus are also major manufacturers of Jaws.

Kelly schedule

Denotes a scheduled amount of time off from work; had its beginnings in Chicago. In 1933 the son of a Chicago fireman, Edward J. Kelly, was elected mayor. Kelly began his term by partially restoring firemen's salaries, and in 1934 Mayor Edward Kelly was named an Honorary Fire Chief. In 1936 Kelly would continue his work toward improving fireman conditions, and he instituted a day off for every 7 days on duty for Chicago firemen, beginning a new terminology that they used for additional days off, a "Kelly day." Prior to this, firemen received only 1 day off per month. This term has stuck and spread across the country, and it is still used today to denote the firefighter schedule of work/days off.

There are different variations to the firefighter schedule all across the country, but roughly all amounting to three complete crews (shifts) of firefighters working an average 56-hour workweek. Typically starting their shift at 7 or 8 A.M. and being relieved by the next crew at the same time the next day. LA County, as well as most of all the West Coast departments, works a 24-hour shift. The current LA County work schedule can be found at: http://www.lacofd.org/ShiftCalendar.htm.

Ladder company (truck company)

A ladder company is a combination of a fire truck with an aerial ladder (75 to 125 feet extended). It will have an assortment of ground ladders and forcible entry tools and the manpower used to staff it. Required to carry a minimum of 115 feet of ground ladders broken down to at least one attic ladder, two extension ladders, and two roof-style straight ladders. Ladder companies are responsible for ventilation, forcible entry duties, securing utilities, and rescue. A standard ladder company will include an officer (Captain or Lieutenant), driver/operator (Engineer), and two or more firefighters. May or may not have a pump.

Overhaul

Commonly viewed as "cleaning up" after a fire; the process of putting a structure in the safest condition following a fire. Additionally, it is during the overhaul phase of an incident that firefighters verify that the fire has not extended into unknown areas and that hidden "hot spots" are extinguished.

Quint

A pump with a capacity of at least 1000 gallons per minute, with a booster tank that holds 300 gallons or more of water. Has at least 800 feet of 2.5-inch or larger supply line (usually 4-inch) and at least 400 feet of attack line. Ground ladders total 85 feet and include one attic ladder, one straight ladder, and one extension ladder. And an aerial or platform with a permanently pre-piped waterway.

Red line
Red line is a hose that is usually 1-inch in diameter, rubber jacketed and actually red. This type of hose is used on small fires using the water carried in an engine's booster tank and is stored on reels on top of the engine (sometimes located in a rear compartment). Same as *booster line* and *hard line.*

SCBA
Self-Contained Breathing Apparatus; contains compressed air, not oxygen. Early models contained about 2200 pounds per square inch (psi) of oxygen in heavy steel tanks, and lasted about 15 minutes even though rated at 30 minutes; they could be easily sucked down in about 10 minutes or less in tense situations. The complete set could weigh up to 45 pounds. Current breathing apparatus (BA) sets now made of lighter-weight aluminum have up to 5000-psi bottles that weigh only about 13 pounds, with some configured to last up to an hour; combined with a backpack and harness assembly, the system weighs approximately 5 to 10 pounds. These are not to be confused with SCUBA tanks that are strictly for use under water, although current SCBA sets have been used in shallow bodies of water such as pools during a rescue.

Ventilation
Ventilation is the systematic removal of smoke from a building. Ventilation is accomplished with one of two methods: positive or negative pressure ventilation. Positive pressure ventilation increases the atmospheric pressure by forcing air inside the structure until it is greater than the pressure outside the building. With negative pressure ventilation, the pressure inside the building is reduced by exhausting the air until it has less pressure than outside the building. This is accomplished by the use of high-volume portable fans (carried on the trucks) placed near the front (or rear) door of the structure.

Movie and TV Terms

Arc light
A high-intensity light used to supply very bright illumination—provided by an electric flow (or "arc") crossing the gap between two electrodes. Used primarily for studio lighting, to create artificial daylight from the outside of interior sets, or to enhance or simulate sunlight for exterior scenes.

Associate producer
Normally a producer's second-in-command; often shares both creative and business responsibilities with the producer. Is sometimes the actual producer of a film with the credited producer functioning only as a figurehead.

Best boy
In film-set jargon, an assistant or apprentice, such as the assistant to the gaffer or the key grip.

Bobbed
In TV-ese, this term refers to the unceremonious deleting of regular or recurring program characters, without explanation or future mention. This term was allegedly created as a result of a character on *ER* named Bogdanalivetsky Romansky (played by Malgoscha Gebel), nicknamed Bob, who disappeared from the cast minus explanation. *Emergency!* fans will note this event occurred several years earlier with the departure of the first two Captains at Station 51, who left without explanation (in the show) in the first season. Ironically, the first two Captains on *Third Watch* unceremoniously disappeared during the first season as well.

Body makeup artist
According to Hollywood union regulations, the ordinary makeup artist is allowed to apply cosmetics only from the top of the head to the apex of the breastbone and from the tips of the fingers to the elbows. All other areas of the body are the province of the body makeup artist.

Dailies
Similar to rushes where the director, producers, and other members of the crew can see the footage filmed that day. It shows whether a scene needs to be reshot and gives the editor an idea of how the scene will work in the film as a whole.

Director
Generally considered the most important person on a set. The director usually, but not always, has the clearest vision of the final product, is in charge of the actors and technicians, and often has a say in both the pre- and post-production aspects of filmmaking.

Editor
In motion picture production, the person responsible for editing a film. Working behind the scenes, away from the glare of publicity and the glamorous surroundings of the film set, the film editor is an unsung member of

a motion picture's creative team. Yet the success or failure of a production may hinge on the quality of this person's work. Sharp film editing can make a mediocre production look good and a good production look even better. Conversely, sloppy editing can undo a solid script and even negate fine efforts by the director, the actors, and technical crews.

Fade (fade in, fade out)
An optical effect that causes a scene to emerge gradually on the screen from complete blackness (fade in) or that causes a bright image to dim gradually into blackness (fade out). The fade is a transitional device usually signifying a distinct break in a film's continuity and indicating a change in time, location, or subject matter. Most films begin with a fade-in and end with a fade-out. The use of a fade-in/fade-out between sequences within a film is similar to the function of the beginning or end of a chapter in a book or an act in a play. In television, it is used when going to the commercial break. The length of the fade should be in keeping with the film's tempo and mood. Technically, a fade-in is achieved by a gradual increase of exposure for each frame until the image reaches full brightness; a fade-out is obtained by a gradual decrease of exposure for each frame with the last frame completely black. Normally, the optical printer makes fades, but some cameras can also satisfactorily achieve them. Amateurs often use a fading solution to obtain fades chemically. The gradual increase or decrease in the level of sound in a film is similarly known as a fade-in or fade-out. Thus, typically, a motion picture script would start with the instruction "fade in" on the picture side and "fade in music" (or sound effects) on the sound side.

Gaffer
The chief electrician on a film unit; responsible for the lighting of a set under instructions from the director of photography. Under his or her supervision, the electrical crew positions the appropriate lamps before and during a shooting session.

Grip
A general-purpose handyperson, the TV or movie set's counterpart of the theater's stagehand. His or her duties include laying dolly tracks, moving flats, setting up parallels, building platforms, placing reflectors and gobos, doing light carpentry, and generally performing tasks that require brawn.

Key Grip
The head grip on a TV or film set, in charge of a group, usually numbering from five to fifteen.

ND (nondescript)

Seen on the shooting schedules and script cast pages for a non-speaking role or a prominent background character is the term "ND firefighter" or similar. These "no-name" people are called *supernumeraries*—a long word for a background character who has no lines, as one who appears in a crowd scene or assists a "regular." These people did not get end credit mention on *Emergency!*. It would not be until the mid 1980s that longer end credits would begin to be seen on television programs and the term "ND firefighter...actor name," for example, would appear.

Post-production

The period after principal photography when the film undergoes editing, sound dubbing, and optical effects. The post-production time period is often equal to that of the initial shoot. *See also* pre-production.

Pre-production

The period before photography begins when final script changes are made, the cast and crew are hired, locations are scouted, and other preliminary work is finished. *See also* post-production.

Producer

The person exercising overall control over the production of a motion picture and holding ultimate responsibility for its success or failure. Ideally, a producer should be a combination of shrewd businessperson, tough taskmaster, prudent cost accountant, flexible diplomat, and creative visionary. But producers vary widely in personality, in the extent of their authority, and in the degree of their involvement in the various phases of production. Typically, however, their job begins long before the start of production and does not end until long after the film is "in the can." Their involvement begins where all films begin, with an idea or the acquisition of a promising property.

Whether he or she has chosen the idea or the property personally or was assigned one by a studio's executive producer, his or her responsibility is the same: to guide the development of the property into a successful motion picture or TV series.

Meanwhile, the producer proceeds with the selection of a director. Again, the director may be assigned to the project by studio management. The uppermost factor in the producer's mind is the limitations of the budget, whether these are set by the studio or by him- or herself if he or she is an independent producer. The goal is to achieve maximum quality at a minimum price tag.

Once the actual shooting begins, the producer removes him- or herself from the set to allow the director freedom of action. But he or she must not let control leave his or her grasp. The producer keeps abreast of the daily progress in production and ascertains that the director and the crew are functioning smoothly in adherence to the timetable and within the boundaries of the budget. He or she must be available at all times as a troubleshooter, in case of personality or labor conflicts on the set, or if some unforeseeable technical problems arise during shooting. Once shooting is completed, the producer becomes involved in the post-production phase of filmmaking. His or her functions would normally include supervision of the editing, scoring, sound effects, dubbing, mixing, opticals, titles, and all other steps that must be taken before a film or series is ready for release.

Ritter fans
Also called "E-fans," these are electric wind machine fans that are 7-foot-diameter units with eight propped blades. Some of the effects created are blowing smoke, snow, dust, turbulence, rain, rippled water, and tumbleweed, as well as exhausting sets and waving flag effects. Some units are gas powered and also come in various sizes. Ritter fans can weigh between 1750 and 2000 pounds.

Script
A general term for a written work, detailing story, setting, and dialogue. A script may take the form of a screenplay, a shooting script, a lined script, continuity script, or a spec script. A spec script is often sold for a particular price, which is increased to a second price if the script is produced as a movie or TV program.

Script supervisor
A person who tracks which parts have been filmed and how the filmed scenes deviated from the script; he or she also makes continuity notes, creating a lined script. The script supervisor sits there with the script, marking each camera angle that is shot and printed. He or she times the length of each shot and keeps track of props and wardrobe. If an actor is holding a drink in his or her right hand at the end of the shot, the script supervisor makes sure it is in the right hand when filming resumes. On that note, how often have you been able to spot a glass of wine or iced tea go from full to half full and back to full again during different camera angles of the same scene?!

Sequence
A number of scenes linked together by time, location, or narrative continuity to form a unified episode in a motion picture. It is often likened

to a chapter in a book, the scene being the equivalent of a paragraph and the shot the equivalent of a sentence. Traditionally, but not necessarily, a sequence begins with a fade-in and ends with a fade-out or some other optical transitional device. *See also* fade.

Set decorator
A person who has total charge of decorating the set with all furnishings, draperies, interior plants, and anything seen on indoor or outdoor sets.

Shooting schedule
Because scenes are filmed out of sequence and out of a continuous line of progression, daily schedules must be planned. The shooting schedule contains the locations, times, equipment, and personnel required for a day's shoot. The schedule itself may be compiled for a single day but is usually planned ahead for a number of days if not for the entire episode.

The shooting schedule for the *Emergency!* World Premier was twenty-six pages long while the 60-minute episodes ran from nine to eleven pages.

Shooting schedules, along with cast schedules or call sheets, are often attached to the scripts given to the cast and crew.

Shooting schedules were extensively used for this book for identifying many of the shooting locations, along with the assistance of the technical advisors, some of the cast and crew, and other sources.

Soundbite
Not always heard but used for background fill; for example, the public address announcements at Rampart or the radio chatter overheard on the squads radio that has nothing to do with the incident that the squad is responding too, such as "Squad 209 10-7 at St. Francis" or other similar chatter.

Stand-in
A substitute for a motion picture star during the tedious process of preparing scenes, setting up the camera, taking light-meter readings, adjusting lights, etc. The men or women in question are chosen for their physical resemblance to a particular star, in size, coloring, and facial features. The stand-in may occasionally be used to substitute for the star in long shots or crowd scenes that require no acting. Note that in some of the stock footage used in *Emergency!* of the Crown leaving the station, Mike Stoker is definitely the driver, but the two "firemen" in the seats behind are not López or Donnelly.

When a stand-in is used as a substitute for the star in potentially hazardous situations or in stunts requiring specialized physical agility, he or she is better known as a "double." *See also* stunt person.

Standing sets
Soundstage sets used every week that don't change. What is in place for filming, like the fire station or Rampart's emergency room interiors. These sets have moveable walls for camera placement.

Stock footage
Scenes used repeatedly, thus saving money, such as the clips of the squad and engine leaving the station.

Stunt person
A highly trained person who performs potentially dangerous scenes in a film. A stunt performer specifically takes the part of another actor for a stunt. Stunt doubles rarely (if ever) speak and are typically chosen to resemble the actors that they are replacing as much as possible. While the director is in control of most aspects of a film, the stunt coordinator or head stunt person has the final say on all stunts. Strict union regulations state that the stunt coordinator and the actual stunt people involved must sign off on any stunt before it is attempted. There is a current trend for younger actors to perform their own stunts. In these cases, stunt persons must work with the star and certify his or her readiness.

Swing sets
A collection of walls/flats that are frequently reused and redressed to be different sets such as apartments or office areas.

Technical advisor
The technical advisors (TAs) have a dual role: they help the production company provide the viewer with a sense of realism and ensure that the agency is being portrayed in the most positive light (although this is not always possible). In many cases, the technical advisor is a retired member of a department, a firefighter, police officer, or physician, who has many years of experience and knowledge about the job. The TA will be a source of valuable information, as well as a resource for props, personnel, and technical jargon. TAs review the scripts and offer creative changes and enhancements.

In this case, *Emergency!*'s TAs were all Los Angeles County Fire Department firefighter/paramedics, except where otherwise noted.

Unit manager
The person in charge of logistics ranging from hiring of caterers to feed everybody while on location to working out the myriad of details of the shooting schedule to making sure the project stays within budget.

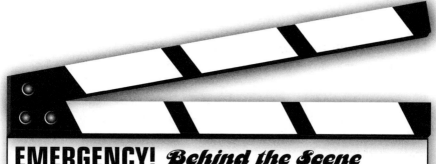

EMERGENCY! *Behind the Scene*

About the Authors

Richard Yokley

Born and raised in San Diego, California, Richard Yokley joined the ranks of the Bonita-Sunnyside Fire Department (near San Diego) in 1972. He became an Emergency Medical Technician (EMT) that first year and soon became the department's historian. Progressing through the ranks, he became the department's Public Information Officer and fire marshal and then rose to the rank of Operations Chief. Richard retired in December 1999 after almost 28 years of service.

As a firefighter/EMT, Richard worked alongside one of the first paramedic ambulances in San Diego County (which began service in March 1977), *LifeSaver 1*, operating out of Bay General Hospital in Chula Vista (now Scripps Memorial Hospital). During his off time he also worked for Pacific Ambulance (mid 1970s), for Hartson's Ambulance service as an

EMT-D/C (1978–1980), and in Bay General Memorial Hospital's emergency department as an emergency room technician (1980–1983).

Richard is the author of *The History of Fire Protection in Sweetwater Valley* (an unpublished document), a 50-year history of the Bonita-Sunnyside Fire Department, and *TV Firefighters,* published in 2003. He has written many articles for newspapers and contributed to trade journals such as *JEMS, Firehouse, California Fire Service* (CSFA), *London Firefighter,* and *Fire International.* He received *Firehouse* magazine's Heroism & Community Service Award in 1987. Along with several other community awards, he was also awarded his fire department's only Exemplary Service Award.

Richard studied in England at the Fire Service College at Moreton-in-Marsh and went through training at the London Fire Brigade Training Academy at Southwark, where he also was able to spend some time on the fireboat London Phoenix. In 2004 he was awarded the Friends of the Society certificate from Britain's Royal Life Saving Society.

He also spent some time with fire departments in Helsinki, Finland; St. Petersburg, Russia (as Leningrad in the Soviet Union at the time of visit); Dublin and Waterford, Ireland; Edinburgh, Scotland; Paris, France; and Vienna, Austria.

Richard is a California state-certified fire officer, fire instructor, and fire investigator. Richard has an AS degree in fire science with a minor in radio and television broadcasting.

Of the many offices held and committees served on over the years, Richard considers his appointment to the Emergency Medical Care Committee for the County of San Diego among the most rewarding. Representing 1st District Supervisor Greg Cox, Richard served from 2001 through 2004.

In 2004, after spending 7 years at SeaWorld San Diego (where he received the SeaWorld Excellence Award in 2000) in the medical services and aviculture departments, he and his wife moved to Tucson, Arizona, in retirement. He now volunteers at the Arizona-Sonora Desert Museum in the mammalogy and ornithology department as a keeper's assistant. Richard continues his research for a second edition of *TV Firefighters* and hopefully will publish it in a few years.

Rozane Sutherland

Rozane Sutherland wanted to be a Forest Ranger when she was a teenager. While a senior in high school in Washington state, she enrolled in the environmental conservation aide class. The teacher got the "assignments" from the rangers for that day or week. The students did everything from putting gravel on trails, to clearing paths after a storm, to taking out an old dock on Lake Crescent that was part of the Olympic National Park. Whatever the rangers needed/wanted them to do for them, the students did. They carried all their own equipment, which included chainsaws, axes, and shovels.

After graduation, Rozane moved to Texas, where she met her future husband Kent, who was in the Air Force, while he was on Christmas leave visiting his family. They met on a blind date. "There is love at first sight!" says Rozane. They have been married for over 27 years and have three boys. They live on 50 acres with all the two- and four-legged critters they have adopted (or that adopted them) over the years!

Erika Bartlett and Rozane started the *Emergency!* website in 1997. They met online in early 1997 while looking for someone to trade episodes with. Erika mentioned she was going to start a website on the show, and Rozane offered to help. They both had wondered what had become of the cast and crew, and so they went to work on finding all of them. Mike Norell was the first, and Rozane said, "If he was not as sweet and gracious as he was to me when I called him...I probably would not have had the courage to keep looking for the others! So, everyone has Mike Norell to thank for all those interviews on the site."

Rozane started working on the *Emergency!* Convention as co-chair in May 1998. She stated that it was well worth all the work to see all the faces of the fans as they saw their heroes together again for the first time in more than 20 years.

Ode to *Emergency!*

By Marina Baker

As a thirty-something beneficiary of something called syndication,
I happily tune in these days to my local cable station.

To visit with some friends I met a long time ago.

At a time when the grown-up world was still very far away,
And I lived my life in a two-story house in a city north of L.A.

As a child I watched it every week, and one certain episode stands out for me,
It was filmed in a town not far from my own, and I was excited to see…
Ferries taking familiar routes, the Kingdome—which will soon be torn down—
And so many other familiar places around the Puget Sound.

Today my life has changed, and TV is no longer a daily affair.
I see the same shows differently; observations I'd like to share.

The contest and quiz shows—opportunities to shine.
All the things we could do (and would do) if we just had the time.

The death of a friend, a mealtime faux pas—
An act of heroics it seems nobody saw.

Convinced that an idea we have is certain to be great;
Then finding out that it's come just a little too late.
These are just some of the things my older eyes now see—
On those oh so rare occasions when they can rest in front of a TV.

These days, when I go shopping, I can take heart,
In knowing that I am not the only one who's ever kicked her cart!

I am still wondering why we never saw Joanne;
Or if it's really possible to start each sentence with, "Man!"

When reference is made to Johnny's glory days in track;
I can't help but smile because this always takes me back…
To a time when I ran the exact same race, and my aspirations were very high.
Yet I am pretty sure that this was not because I wished to impress some guy.

I can now understand Roy's mother in law troubles, and the Cap's fear of arthritis
because I wasn't the one good enough for her son and cope daily with bursitis.

I'm humbled and truly inspired by the guy's dedication,
When they're driving to a parade and even while on vacation!

When there's laundry, and dishes, and kids, and groceries…well, believe me,
    I'm NO SLOUCH…
But I have wished on those days, that I, like Henry, could have spent them on
    the couch.

As a stressed out adult in this technical world, it's strangely comforting to see;
That the person who's just saved somebody's life can also blow up a TV!

Every now and then I'm joined by my twelve-year-old son;
Who *really* likes the explosions but just mostly makes fun
Of the clothes and hairstyles because, as he fervently believes,
I'm only watching because I've been stricken with "Old Person's Disease"!

Any attempts to explain the significance of some particular scene
Are most often met with the "Yeah right!" expression of the 1990s teen.

But as for me I remain impressed by each rescue that takes place, and *all* those
    happy endings make me glad,
because the younger fan did not know, that "real" paramedics would one day
    save my dad.

A prime slice from the seventies; a blast from the past;
A poignant reminder that youthful days did not last.

For all these reasons, I still watch *Emergency*!; yet also 'cause I've come to know
That more than twenty years later I can still relate to my all time favorite show!

Thanks for the Memories!

Reprinted with permission, written for the Emergency! *convention in 1998.*